Pitt Ford's Problem-Based Learning in Endodontology

T0338032

Pitt Ford's Problem-Based Learning in Endodontology

Second Edition

Edited by

Elizabeth Shin Perry DMD FICD
Division of Postgraduate Endodontics
Department of Restorative Dentistry and Biomaterial Sciences
Harvard School of Dental Medicine
Boston, MA, USA

Shanon Patel BDS MSc MClinDent MRD PhD FDS FHEA
Postgraduate Endodontic Unit
King's College London Dental Institute
London, UK

Shalini Kanagasingam BDS MClinDent MFDS MRestDent
FHEA
School of Medicine and Dentistry
University of Central Lancashire
Preston, UK

Samantha Hamer BDS MFDS MSc MClinDent MEndo
Postgraduate Endodontic Unit
King's College London Dental Institute
London, UK

WILEY Blackwell

The right of Elizabeth Shin Perry, Shanon Patel, Shalini Kanagasingam, and Samantha Hamer to be identified as the authors of the editorial material in this work has been asserted in accordance with law.

Registered Office(s)
John Wiley & Sons, Inc., 111 River Street, Hoboken, NJ 07030, USA
John Wiley & Sons Ltd, The Atrium, Southern Gate, Chichester, West Sussex, PO19 8SQ, UK

For details of our global editorial offices, customer services, and more information about Wiley products visit us at www.wiley.com.

Wiley also publishes its books in a variety of electronic formats and by print-on-demand. Some content that appears in standard print versions of this book may not be available in other formats.

Library of Congress Cataloging-in-Publication Data

Names: Perry, Elizabeth Shin, editor. | Patel, Shanon, editor. |
    Kanagasingam, Shalini, editor. | Hamer, Samantha, editor.
Title: Pitt Ford's problem-based learning in endodontology / edited by
    Elizabeth Shin Perry, Shanon Patel, Shalini Kanagasingam, Samantha
    Hamer.
Other titles: Problem-based learning in endodontology
Description: Second edition. | Hoboken, NJ : Wiley, 2025. | Includes
    bibliographical references and index.
Identifiers: LCCN 2023017104 (print) | LCCN 2023017105 (ebook) | ISBN
    9781119565970 (paperback) | ISBN 9781119566014 (adobe pdf) | ISBN
    9781119565963 (epub)
Subjects: MESH: Dental Pulp Diseases–diagnosis | Dental Pulp
    Diseases–therapy | Endodontics | Problems and Exercises | Case Reports
Classification: LCC RK351 (print) | LCC RK351 (ebook) | NLM WU 18.2 |
    DDC 617.6/342–dc23/eng/20230901
LC record available at https://lccn.loc.gov/2023017104
LC ebook record available at https://lccn.loc.gov/2023017105

Cover Design: Wiley
Cover Image: Courtesy of Elizabeth Perry

Set in 11/13pt STIXTwoText by Straive, Pondicherry, India

Printed and bound in Great Britain by Bell & Bain Ltd, Glasgow

B001024 300924

The publishers thank the contributors and acknowledge that the images used in this textbook are owned by the individual contributors except where indicated.

Contents

Contributors

Abdulaziz A. Bakhsh
BDS MClinDent MEndo PhD
Department of Restorative Dentistry, Endodontic Division
Faculty of Dental Medicine
Umm Al-Qura University
Makkah, Saudi Arabia

Benoit Ballester
DDS MSc
Department of Endodontics and Restorative Dentistry
Aix-Marseille Université
Marseille, France

and

Practice Limited to Restorative Dentistry
Assistance Publique des Hôpitaux de Marseille
Marseille, France

Bhavin Bhuva
BDS MFDS RCS MClinDent, MRD FHEA
Postgraduate Endodontic Unit
Faculty of Dentistry, Oral & Craniofacial Sciences
King's College London, UK

and

Practice Limited to Endodontics, UK

Rahul Bose
BDS MFDS MClinDent MEndo
Postgraduate Endodontic Unit
King's College London Dental Institute
London, UK

and

Practice Limited to Endodontics, UK

Frédéric Bukiet
DDS MSc PhD HDR
Department of Endodontics and Restorative Dentistry
Aix-Marseille Université
Marseille, France

and

Practice Limited to Endodontics
Assistance Publique des Hôpitaux de Marseille
Marseille, France

Dermot Canavan
BDentSc MGDS MS
Dublin Dental School & Hospital
Trinity College Dublin
Dublin, Ireland

and

Practice Limited to Orofacial Pain Management
Dublin, Ireland

Nadia Chugal
DDS MS MPH
Division of Regenerative and Reconstructive Sciences
Section of Endodontics
UCLA School of Dentistry
Los Angeles, CA, USA

and

Practice Limited to Endodontics
Los Angeles, CA, USA

Nestor Cohenca
DDS FIADT
Department of Pediatric Dentistry
University of Washington and Seattle Children's Hospital
Seattle, WA, USA

and

Practice Limited to Endodontics
Kirkland, WA, USA

Raul Costa
LMD Lisbon
Practice limited to Restorative Dentistry
London, UK

Matthew C. Davis
DDS
Practice Limited to Endodontics
Winnetka, IL, USA

Luis Ferrandez
BDS MSc
Practice Limited to Endodontics
Poole, UK

David Figdor
BDSc LDS MDSc FRACDS Dip Endo FPFA PhD FASM FADI FICD
Department of Microbiology
Biomedical Discovery Institute
Monash University
Melbourne, Australia

and

Specialist Endodontic Practice
Melbourne, Australia

Massimo Giovarruscio
Dip Dent MSc
Practice Limited to Endodontics
Bristol, UK

Thomas Giraud
DDS MSc PhD
Department of Biomaterials
Aix-Marseille Université
Marseille, France

and

Practice Limited to Endodontics
Marseille, France

Maud Guivarc'h
DDS MSc PhD
Department of Endodontics and Restorative Dentistry
Aix-Marseille Université
Marseille, France

and

Practice Limited to Endodontics
Marseille, France

Samantha Hamer
BDS MFDS MSc MClinDent MEndo
Postgraduate Endodontic Unit
King's College London
London, UK

and

Practice Limited to Endodontics
London, UK

Simon Harvey
BDS MFDS MA
The Eastman Dental Hospital
London, UK

and

Queen Victoria Hospital
East Grinstead, West Sussex, UK

Jianing He
DMD PhD
Department of Endodontics
Texas A&M University College of Dentistry
Dallas, TX, USA

and

Practice Limited to Endodontics
Flower Mound, TX, USA

Ali Hilmi
BDS BSc MJDF RCS MClinDent MEndo
Practice Limited to Endodontics
London, UK

Shalini Kanagasingam
BDS MClinDent MFDS MRestDent FHEA
School of Medicine and Dentistry
University of Central Lancashire
Preston, UK

and

Practice Limited to Endodontics
Preston, UK

Maria Lessani
BDS MFDS MClinDent MRD
Unit of Endodontology,
Eastman Dental Institute, UCL, London, UK

and

Practice Limited to Endodontics
London, UK

Francesco Mannocci
DDS MD PhD
Postgraduate Endodontic Unit
Dental Institute, King's College London
London, UK

Philip Mitchell
BDS MSc MRD
Postgraduate Endodontic Unit
Dental Institute, King's College London
London, UK

Garry L. Myers
DDS FICD FACD
Department of Oral Diagnostic Sciences and Endodontics
Virginia Commonwealth University
Richmond, VA, USA

Kreena Patel
BDS(Hons) MJDF MClinDent MEndo
Practice Limited to Endodontics
London & Reading, UK

Neha Patel
BDS MJDF MClinDent MEndo FHEA
Postgraduate Endodontic Unit
King's College London Dental Institute
London, UK

and

Practice Limited to Endodontics
London, UK

Shanon Patel
BDS MSc MClinDent MRD PhD FDS FHEA
Postgraduate Endodontic Unit
King's College London Dental Institute
London, UK

and

Practice Limited to Endodontics
London, UK

Elizabeth Shin Perry
DMD FICD
Division of Postgraduate Endodontics
Department of Restorative Dentistry and Biomaterial Sciences
Harvard School of Dental Medicine
Boston, MA, USA

and

Practice Limited to Endodontics
Westfield, MA, USA

Tiago Pimentel
LMD MSc MClinDent MEndo RCSEdin
Postgraduate Endodontic Unit
King's College London
London, UK

and

Practice Limited to Endodontics
London, UK

Taranpreet Puri
BDS (Hons) MFGDP MFDS RCS PG Cert MClinDent MEndo RCSEng MEndo RCSEd
Practice Limited to Endodontics
London, UK

John Rhodes
BDS FDS MSc MFGDP MRD RCS
Practice Limited to Endodontics
Dorset, UK

Isabela N. Rôças
DDS MSc PhD
Laboratory of Molecular Microbiology
Postgraduate Program in Endodontics
Grande Rio University
Rio de Janeiro, Brazil

Suhaila S. Shariff
DMD MPH
Practice Limited to Endodontics
Illinois, USA

José F. Siqueira Jr
DDS MSc PhD
Postgraduate Endodontics Unit
Grande Rio University
Rio de Janeiro, RJ
Brazil

Nargis Sonde
BDS MFDS MSc Periodontology
School of Medicine & Dentistry
University of Central Lancashire
Preston, UK

Peng-Hui Teng
DDS MFDS MClinDent MEndo
Postgraduate Endodontic Unit
King's College London Dental Institute
London, UK

Shatha Zahran
BDS MSD FRCDC ABE PhD
Department of Endodontics
King Abdulaziz University
Jeddah, Saudi Arabia

First Foreword

Over the last 50 years of endodontics, we have witnessed immense technical and biological advances that have helped to underpin our understanding of pulpal and apical disease and the appropriate therapies to manage these conditions. Notably, many of these advancements have not been fully translated into practice with shortcomings in educational dissemination and limitations to conventional teaching methodology highlighted. *Pitt Ford's Problem Solving in Endodontology*, now in its second edition, uniquely addresses this in that it challenges the reader to be the problem solver, asking pertinent questions based around every day clinical vignettes. This form of case-based learning increases the relevance for the reader and also challenges them to consider how best to manage these scenarios with a research-led mindset. A particularly welcome facet of the book is that it does not aim to provide all the answers, but rather stimulates the reader to further develop their knowledge.

The book covers a wide range of topics from the biological rationale for endodontic treatment, diagnosis, and treatment planning, through vital pulp treatment, root canal treatment, regenerative endodontics, and endodontic microsurgery, while also covering critical areas that are often ignored such as pain of non-odontogenic origin, dental trauma, and medico-legal aspects. The topics have been brought together in such a way that the overall scope of this text is much greater than the simple summation of the individual components. It will appeal to postgraduates, residents in training, researchers, and practicing clinicians, and I am sure it will help to inspire many people in the clinical endodontic area. It is led by a talented and experienced editorial group that has recruited an exceptional range of talented and prominent endodontists working and researching globally. I am grateful to the editors and authors for providing us with this valuable insight and know that the text will become essential reading for those working in the area.

Of particular pride to me to see that the book carries the name and legacy of Tom Pitt Ford, a personal mentor and pioneer in the field and development of the science endodontology. I know he would have been immensely proud of the new edition of this important text.

Henry (Hal) Duncan BDS, FDS RCS, FFD RCSI,
MClin Dent, MRD RCS, PhD
Professor in Endodontology, Dublin Dental University Hospital,
Trinity College Dublin, Ireland
President of the European Society of Endodontology

Second Foreword

In clinical dentistry, problem solving and critical thinking are crucial in the accurate diagnosis and delivery of clinical care for patients. In this second edition of *Pitt Ford's Problem Solving in Endodontology*, the editors have produced an outstanding pragmatic guide to endodontic therapy. Since the first edition, the field of endodontics has undergone impressive developments in the evolution of more conservative minimally invasive therapies that incorporate innovations in biomedical imaging, microscopy, and risk factor discovery to benefit patients. This edition beautifully holds up the legacy of Professor Tom Pitt Ford. The book brings together real-life clinical scenarios to enhance the education of dental and postgraduate students alike on key principles involved in patient management, especially in situations of traumatic injury to the dentition and/or alveolus for the promotion of tooth support, function, aesthetics, and long-term survival.

The book is subdivided into nine valuable sections that comprehensively address areas such as aetiology, diagnosis, and treatment planning. Pertinent new chapters have been added on vital pulp therapy and regenerative endodontics and reflect the rapidly evolving area of tissue engineering and regenerative medicine, leading much of dentistry to improve clinical outcomes for enhanced delivery of the minimally invasive treatments that patients have come to expect. Chapters on management of both failure and/or complications during endodontic therapy are also very relevant, as we know that it is desirable to retain teeth for as long as practically possible. Advancements in endodontic microsurgery and the many challenges in managing exquisite restorative work to preserve teeth that require either initial endodontic treatment or retreatment have also been updated.

Additional considerations for patient management such as the (potential) association between apical periodontitis and systemic disease, medicolegal issues, and determining prognosis of teeth that may eventually support clinical decision making in patient risk stratification have been added in this second addition.

In summary, I am excited for readers to delve into this second edition of *Pitt Ford's Problem Solving in Endodontology* to partake in this assembly of pertinent clinical scenarios. This text will advance students' understanding in order to better deliver clinical care to preserve the dentition by enhancing long-term endodontic outcomes. Please enjoy!

William V. Giannobile, DDS, MS, DMedSc
Dean, Harvard University School of Dental Medicine
Boston, MA, USA

Preface

The success and positive feedback of the first edition of Pitt Ford's Problem-Based Learning in Endodontics led to the commissioning of this second edition. As with the first edition, the aim of this novel textbook is to enable readers to become adept problem solvers in real-life clinical scenarios, mirroring their experiences in patient care. This case-based approach fosters problem-solving skills and cultivates critical thinking.

This book does not replace traditional Endodontology textbooks but is intended as a supplementary resource to help readers consolidate their knowledge. Each chapter maintains an accessible question-and-answer format, covering the core topics of endodontics. This approach encourages inquisitive readers to delve deeper into specific subjects and cultivates a self-learning approach throughout their careers.

This textbook is designed to benefit undergraduate dental students in their final years looking to enhance their clinical skills, as well as postgraduates preparing for Royal College Diplomas or advanced graduate programs in North America. It is also a valuable resource for specialists in training in non-endodontic disciplines who seek to understand the relevance of endodontics. Additionally, it serves as a contemporary reference for experienced endodontic specialists looking to update their core clinical knowledge. In recognition of its global scope, this book has been crafted to serve the needs of endodontists worldwide, embracing the universal tooth numbering system to ensure a consistent and comprehensive approach.

From the outset, we were committed to upholding the first edition's focus on the biological rationale behind Endodontology, rather than merely providing a step-by-step guide. Each chapter and clinical case is intentionally structured to encourage readers to systematically and logically assess patients' presenting complaints and clinical information. This edition has been thoroughly revised and incorporates the latest advances in our specialty where appropriate.

As with the first edition, the contributors and editors represent a spectrum of expertise, encompassing a range of backgrounds in academia, clinical practice, and professional development. The result is a publication that is richly diverse in its content and perspectives.

The original concept for this book originated from the late Professor Tom Pitt Ford, a true pioneer and well-respected clinical academic. We hope you enjoy reading this new edition of Pitt Ford's Problem-Based Learning in Endodontology and that it contributes to the elevation of excellence in our specialty worldwide.

Elizabeth Shin Perry
Shanon Patel
Shalini Kanagasingam
Samantha Hamer
2025

Acknowledgements

We extend our heartfelt gratitude to our families, whose unwavering support and understanding have been instrumental in our journey to bring the second edition of "Pitt Ford's Problem-Based Learning in Endodontology" to fruition. Your patience and encouragement have been our pillars of strength.

We would also like to extend our thanks the dental teams we collaborate with daily in our specialist practices and within the universities where we are affiliated, as their dedication has been invaluable in shaping this work.

Furthermore, we wish to express our deep appreciation to the contributors who generously shared their knowledge, insights, and expertise to make this publication a comprehensive and valuable resource for the field of Endodontology.

This publication stands as a testament to the collective effort of many, and we are truly grateful for the support and collaboration of all those who have played a role in its creation.

Elizabeth Shin Perry

Shanon Patel

Shalini Kanagasingam

Samantha Hamer

Aetiology, Diagnosis, Treatment Planning

1.1 *Microbiology of Primary Apical Periodontitis*

José F. Siqueira Jr and Isabela N. Rôças

Objectives

Apical periodontitis is an inflammatory disease that affects the tissues surrounding the apical portion of the dental root and is primarily caused by bacteria infecting the root canal system. At the end of this case the reader should be able to recognise the infectious origin of apical periodontitis as well as understand some basic aspects of the microbiology of endodontic infections.

Introduction

A 34-year-old female was seeking replacement of defective and aesthetically unpleasant composite restorations in the maxillary incisors. The teeth had been restored more than five years previously. No significant symptoms were reported at the time of consultation.

Chief Complaint

The patient complained of the aesthetic appearance of the coronal restorations in all the maxillary incisors. She recalled having the restorations about five years ago due to decay in the teeth. Except for a mild sensitivity to sweet food in the UL2 a few years ago, all the maxillary incisors had been asymptomatic.

Medical History

Unremarkable.

Pitt Ford's Problem-Based Learning in Endodontology, Second Edition. Edited by Elizabeth Shin Perry, Shanon Patel, Shalini Kanagasingam, and Samantha Hamer.
© 2025 John Wiley & Sons Ltd. Published 2025 by John Wiley & Sons Ltd.

Dental History

Last visit to a dental office for a check-up appointment was two years previously. At that time, no apical periodontitis lesion was evident in the maxillary anterior region.

Clinical Examination

Extraoral examination was unremarkable. The patient had a moderately restored dentition, and her oral hygiene status was satisfactory. Composite restorations in all maxillary incisors were defective and discoloured.

All anterior teeth responded normally to thermal and electric sensitivity testing, except for the UL2, which was non-responsive. No swelling or sinus tract was evident on the mucosa over the apices of the anterior teeth. The UL2 was discoloured with an existing restoration with marginal deficiencies.

Radiographic Examination

Periapical radiograph revealed (Figure 1.1.1):

- Normal bone levels.
- The UL2 with an existing restoration with secondary caries in proximity to the pulp chamber.
- A radiolucency involving the apical region of the UL2.

Diagnosis and Treatment Planning

What was the diagnosis?

The diagnosis was asymptomatic apical periodontitis associated with pulp necrosis. The pulp became necrotic as a consequence of frank exposure to the bacterial biofilm associated with the recurrent/secondary caries.

What treatment should be carried out in this case?

Diet advice and caries removal with replacement of discoloured and deficient coronal restorations in the maxillary incisor teeth and endodontic treatment on the UL2.

What are the goals of antimicrobial endodontic treatment?

The ultimate goal of the endodontic treatment is to maintain or restore the health of the periradicular tissues. The treatment of teeth with irreversibly inflamed pulps is essentially a prophylactic approach, since the radicular vital pulp is usually free of infection and the rationale is to treat so as to prevent further pulp necrosis and infection, with consequent emergence of apical periodontitis. On the other hand, in cases like the one reported here, an intraradicular infection is already established and, consequently, endodontic procedures should focus not only on prevention of introduction of new bacteria in the canal, but also on elimination of those occurring therein.

Entrenched in the root canal system, bacteria are beyond the reach of the host defences and systemically administered antibiotics. Therefore, endodontic infections can only be treated by means of professional intervention using antibacterial procedures based on mechanical, chemical, and ecological effects.

Treatment procedures should ideally render the root canal system free of bacteria. Nevertheless, given the complex anatomy of the system, it is widely recognised that, with available instruments, irrigating substances and preparation techniques, fulfilling this goal is virtually impossible for most cases. Therefore, the reachable goal is to reduce bacterial populations to levels below those necessary to induce or sustain disease. The clinician should adopt an evidence-based antibacterial protocol that predictably disinfects the root canal and allows this goal to be accomplished.

Discussion

How does caries cause pulp necrosis and subsequent apical periodontitis?

Bacteria involved with caries are organised in authentic biofilms that advance towards the pulp as the tooth structure is destroyed in the process. Diffusion of bacterial products through dentinal tubules induces pulp inflammation long before this tissue is exposed. After exposure, the pulp surface is colonised and covered by bacteria composing the caries biofilm and the subjacent tissue becomes severely inflamed (Figure 1.1.2). Some tissue invasion by bacteria may occur. As a response to direct bacterial challenge, the pulp tissue invariably undergoes necrosis and then loses the ability to contain bacterial invasion. Eventually, invading bacteria colonise the necrotic tissue. These events of bacterial aggression, pulp inflammation, pulp necrosis and pulp infection occur in the tissue compartments, which coalesce and move towards the apical part of the canal until virtually the entire root canal is necrotic and infected.

Bacteria colonising the necrotic apical root canal induce damage to the periradicular tissues and give rise to inflammatory changes therein (Figure 1.1.3). Bacteria exert their pathogenicity by wreaking havoc on the host tissues through direct and/or indirect mechanisms. Bacterial virulence factors that cause direct tissue-harmful effects include those that are toxic to host cells and/or disrupt the intercellular matrix of the connective tissue. Furthermore, bacterial structural components stimulate the development of host immune reactions capable not only of defending the host against infection, but also of causing severe tissue destruction. Pus formation in acute apical abscess and bone resorption associated with asymptomatic apical periodontitis are clear examples of tissue-destructive effects indirectly caused by bacteria; that is, they are promoted by the host itself in defence against bacterial infection.

In addition to caries lesions, are there other avenues for endodontic infection?

Under normal conditions, the pulp–dentine complex is isolated and protected from the oral microbiota by overlying enamel and cementum, the same way the connective tissues elsewhere in the body are segregated from the microbiota residing in body cavities and surfaces by the epithelium of mucosa or skin. Once the integrity of these natural layers is breached (e.g. as a result of caries, trauma-induced fractures and cracks, restorative procedures, scaling and root planing, attrition or abrasion) or naturally absent (e.g. because of gaps in the cemental coating at the cervical root surface), the pulp–dentine complex is exposed to the oral environment. This complex is then challenged by bacteria present in carious lesions, in saliva bathing the exposed dentinal area and/or in the dental biofilm formed on the exposed surface. The subgingival biofilm associated with periodontal pockets may also represent a source of bacteria to reach the pulp via dentinal tubules at the cervical region of the tooth, or through lateral and apical foramina.

Whatever the route of bacterial access to the root canal, necrosis of pulp tissue is a prerequisite for the establishment of primary endodontic infections. As long as the pulp is vital, it can protect itself against bacterial invasion and colonisation by mounting an immune defence response. However, if the pulp becomes necrotic as a result of caries, trauma, operative procedures or periodontal disease, the necrotic tissue can be very easily invaded and colonised (infection). This is because host defences do not function in the necrotic pulp tissue.

Microorganisms can also have access to the root canal any time after professional endodontic intervention (secondary infection), either by a breach in the aseptic chain during treatment, by coronal leakage through temporary/definitive restorations or by tooth/restoration fracture.

Why do some traumatised teeth develop apical periodontitis even when the unrestored tooth crown looks intact?

Bacteria have been isolated from the root canal of traumatised teeth whose pulps became necrotic and apical periodontitis developed, even in circumstances where the tooth crown was apparently intact. How did those bacteria invade the pulp space? In the past, it was believed that such bacteria originated from the gingival sulcus or periodontal pockets and reached the necrotic canal via severed blood vessels of the periodontium, a phenomenon called anachoresis. This theory was never supported by scientific evidence. Actually, trauma can induce exposure of dentine by fracturing the crown or inducing the formation of enamel cracks, which can be macroscopic or microscopic. A large number of dentinal tubules can be exposed to the oral environment by a single crack. These cracks can be colonised and clogged with oral bacterial biofilm, serving as potential portals of bacterial entry to the pulp. If the pulp remains vital after trauma, bacterial penetration into tubules is counteracted by the dentinal fluid and tubular contents. On the other hand, if the pulp becomes necrotic as a consequence of trauma, it loses the ability to protect itself against bacterial invasion and the dentinal tubules become true avenues through which bacteria can reach the pulp.

Which microorganisms are commonly found in primary endodontic infections?

Although fungi, archaea and herpesviruses have been found in association with apical periodontitis, bacteria are the major microorganisms implicated in the pathogenesis of the different forms of this disease. Therefore, one can state that apical periodontitis is a disease primarily caused by bacterial infection.

Primary endodontic infections are dominated by anaerobic bacteria organised in a mixed community (Table 1.1.1). Overall, a mean number of 10–30 different species can be found per canal. As for population density, each canal can harbour from 10^3 to 10^8 bacterial cells in asymptomatic apical periodontitis cases and from 10^4 to 10^9 in acute forms of the disease (symptomatic apical periodontitis and acute apical abscess). The larger the size of the apical periodontitis lesion, the more diverse and populous the root canal microbiota. The named bacterial species frequently detected in primary infections of teeth with either symptomatic (acute) or asymptomatic (chronic) apical periodontitis are depicted in Table 1.1.1.

Table 1.1.1 Features of the endodontic microbiota in primary apical periodontitis.

Features	Primary infections	
	Asymptomatic apical periodontitis	**Acute apical abscess**
Community	Mixed	Mixed
Mean number of species/case	10–30	10–30
Mean number of cells/case	$10^3–10^8$	$10^4–10^9$
Most prevalent groups	Gram-negative/Gram-positive anaerobes	Gram-negative anaerobes
Most frequent taxa	Gram-negative *Fusobacterium nucleatum* *Porphyromonas* spp. *Dialister* spp. *Treponema* spp. *Tannerela forsythia* *Synergistetes* phylum *Prevotella* spp. *Campylobacter* spp. Gram-positive *Filifactor alocis* *Pseudoramibacter alactolyticus* *Olsenella* spp. *Parvimonas micra* *Peptostreptococcus* spp. *Streptococcus* spp.	Gram-negative *Fusobacterium nucleatum* *Porphyromonas* spp. *Dialister* spp. *Treponema* spp. *Tannerela forsythia* *Synergistetes* phylum *Prevotella* spp. Gram-positive *Olsenella* spp. *Parvimonas micra* *Streptococcus* spp.

*Is there a difference between the endodontic microbiota
in symptomatic (acute apical abscess) and asymptomatic apical
periodontitis cases?*

Diversity of bacterial communities is comparatively higher in symptomatic cases than in canals of teeth with asymptomatic apical periodontitis. Differences are essentially represented by different dominant species in the communities associated with symptomatic and asymptomatic disease and larger number of species in symptomatic cases. However, there is no clear evidence supporting the specific involvement of a single species with any particular sign or symptom of apical periodontitis. Some Gram-negative anaerobic bacteria have been claimed to be the main culprits for symptomatic disease, but the same species also have been encountered in asymptomatic cases. Other factors, in addition to the presence of pathogenic species, are thought to influence the emergence of symptoms (Table 1.1.2).

Table 1.1.2 Factors influencing the development of symptomatic apical periodontitis.

Factors influencing the emergence of symptoms

- Differences in virulence ability among strains of the same species
- Additive or synergistic effects among species in mixed communities
- Total number of bacterial cells (total bacterial load)
- Number of cells of certain pathogenic species (specific bacterial load)
- Environment-regulated expression of virulence factors
- Host resistance (can be modulated by systemic diseases, concomitant virus infection, environmental factors and genetic patterns)

*How do bacteria flourish in the necrotic root canal? Is there
selective pressure dictating the composition of the infecting
microbiota?*

A root canal with necrotic pulp provides a space for bacterial colonisation and affords bacteria a moist, warm, nutritious, and anaerobic environment. This environment is by and large protected from the host defences because of lack of active blood circulation in the necrotic tissue. The main sources of nutrients for bacteria in the necrotic root canal are shown in Table 1.1.3. Although a large number of bacterial species (100–200) can be found in

Table 1.1.3 Main sources of nutrients for bacteria colonising the root canal system.

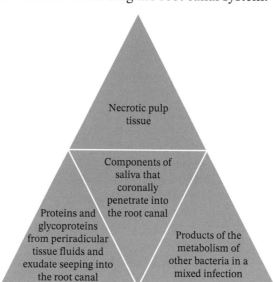

the oral cavity of a particular individual, only a limited assortment of these species (about 10–30) is selected out for growth and survival within the root canal. The major ecological determinants that influence the composition of the root canal microbiota include oxygen tension, type and amount of available nutrients and bacterial interactions.

The ecology of the endodontic microbiota is influenced by different physico-chemical conditions and type of nutrient availability in the different regions of the root canal. Gradients of oxygen tension and available nutrients are established along the extent of the root canal in such a way that the apical region contains the lowest oxygen tension and the highest concentration of proteins, while in the most coronal region the oxygen tension and amount of available carbohydrates may be higher. These gradients allow the dominance of certain groups of bacteria in different regions of the canal according to their relationship to oxygen and metabolic demands. Hence, asaccharolytic and/or proteolytic anaerobic species are expected to dominate at the apical region and saccharolytic anaerobic or facultative species dominate at the most coronal parts of the canal.

What is the pattern of bacterial colonisation in the necrotic root canal system?

In advanced stages of the endodontic infectious process, bacterial organisations resembling biofilms can be observed adhered to the dentinal root canal walls (Figure 1.1.4). For this reason, apical periodontitis has been included in the group of biofilm-induced oral diseases along with caries and marginal periodontitis. In addition to forming biofilms adhered on the canal walls, bacteria can also be observed as planktonic cells suspended in fluid or enmeshed in the necrotic tissue present in the main canal lumen (Figure 1.1.5). Lateral canals and isthmuses connecting main canals may also be clogged with bacteria, primarily organised in biofilms. Bacterial cells originating from biofilms adhered to the root canal walls are often seen penetrating the subjacent dentinal tubules. Dentinal tubule infection can occur in about 70–80% of the teeth with apical periodontitis lesions. Shallow penetration is more common, but bacterial cells can be observed reaching approximately 300 µm in some teeth (Figures 1.1.6 and 1.1.7).

While bacteria present as planktonic cells floating in the main root canal may be easily accessed and eliminated by instruments and substances used during endodontic treatment, bacterial biofilms attached to the canal walls or located in isthmuses, lateral canals and dentinal tubules are definitely more difficult to reach and may require special therapeutic strategies to disrupt and eliminate them.

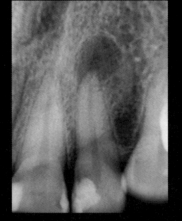

Figure 1.1.1 Periapical radiograph of tooth UL2, showing an apical radiolucency. The root canal is necrotic and infected, and an inflammatory response associated with bone resorption has developed at the periradicular tissues (apical periodontitis) in an attempt to prevent spread of the infection to the bone and other body sites.

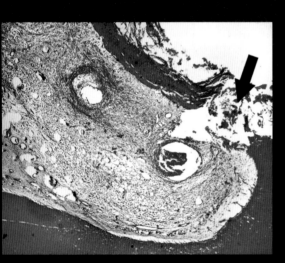

Figure 1.1.2 Histological section of a tooth with caries exposure (arrow). The pulp was vital, but severely inflamed at the area of exposure.

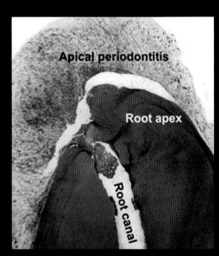

Figure 1.1.3 Histological section of a tooth with necrotic pulp and apical periodontitis.

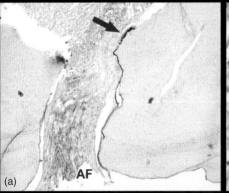
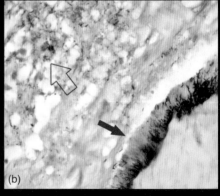

Figure 1.1.4 (a) Histological section of the very apical part of the root canal of a tooth evincing apical periodontitis. A bacterial biofilm (red arrow) is seen adhered to the canal wall very close to the apical foramen (AF). (b) Higher magnification of the biofilm shown in (a). Planktonic bacterial cells are also seen in the main canal (empty arrow).

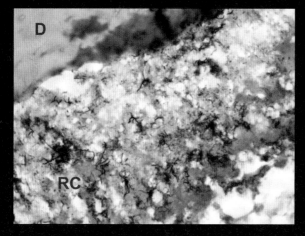

Figure 1.1.5 Histological section showing the main root canal of a tooth with apical periodontitis. Bacteria are seen intermixed with necrotic tissue. D, dentine; RC, root canal.

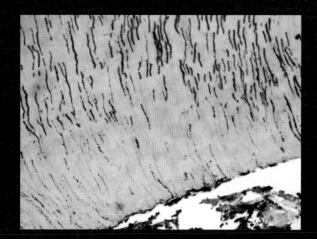

Figure 1.1.6 Histological section of a tooth with apical periodontitis showing bacteria adhered to the canal walls and invading dentinal tubules to a deep extent.

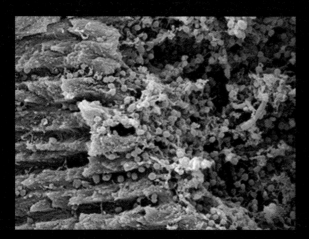

Figure 1.1.7 Scanning electron micrograph showing bacterial cells from the main root canal invading dentinal tubules. Source: Reproduced with permission from S. Patel, et al. © 2005, Oxford University Press.

Further Reading

Fouad, A.F. (2017). Endodontic microbiology and pathobiology: current state of knowledge. *Dental Clinics of North America* 61: 1–15.

Kakehashi, S., Stanley, H.R., and Fitzgerald, R.J. (1965). The effects of surgical exposures of dental pulps in germ-free and conventional laboratory rats. *Oral Surgery, Oral Medicine Oral Pathology* 20: 340–349.

Love, R.M. (2004). Invasion of dentinal tubules by root canal bacteria. *Endodontic Topics* 9: 52–65.

Möller, A.J.R., Fabricius, L., Dahlén, G. et al. (1981). Influence on periapical tissues of indigenous oral bacteria and necrotic pulp tissue in monkeys. *Scandinavian Journal of Dental Research* 89: 475–484.

Ordinola-Zapata, R., Costalonga, M, Dietz M., Lima, B.P., and Staley, C. (2023). The root canal microbiome diversity and function. A whole-metagenome shotgun analysis. *International Endodontic Journal* doi: 10.1111/iej.13911.

Ricucci, D. and Siqueira, J.F. Jr. (2010). Biofilms and apical periodontitis: study of prevalence and association with clinical and histopathologic findings. *Journal of Endodontics* 36: 1277–1288.

Siqueira, J.F. Jr. and Rôças, I.N. (2022). Present status and future directions: microbiology of endodontic infections. *International Endodontic Journal* 55 (Suppl 3): 512–530.

Vianna, M.E., Conrads, G., Gomes, B.P.F.A., and Horz, H.P. (2006). Identification and quantification of archaea involved in primary endodontic infections. *Journal of Clinical Microbiology* 44: 1274–1282.

1.2 Reversible Pulpitis

Tiago Pimentel and Raul Costa

Objectives

At the end of this case, the reader should be able to appreciate the characteristic symptoms and signs of reversibly inflamed pulps and how to manage them.

Introduction

A 67-year-old patient presented with sensitivity to cold and sweets on her lower left first premolar (LL4).

Chief Complaint

Sensitivity to cold and sweet drinks lasting for a few seconds, localised to the lower left quadrant. The pain had been present intermittently over the last few months, becoming progressively worse recently. There was no episode of nocturnal or spontaneous pain, and none of the teeth were tender on biting.

Medical History

Unremarkable.

Dental History

The patient had fair oral hygiene and was a regular attendee at her dentist. Periodontal probing depths in all four quadrants were 2–3 mm.

Clinical Examination

Extraoral examination was unremarkable. The patient had a moderately restored dentition, generalised tooth wear and large posterior edentulous areas.

Pitt Ford's Problem-Based Learning in Endodontology, Second Edition. Edited by Elizabeth Shin Perry, Shanon Patel, Shalini Kanagasingam, and Samantha Hamer.
© 2025 John Wiley & Sons Ltd. Published 2025 by John Wiley & Sons Ltd.

LL4 was carious, but was not tender to percussion or buccal palpation. The cavity was tender to probe.

The cold sensibility test (Endo-Frost) revealed heightened sensitivity lasting for 5–7 seconds compared to the lower left canine (LL3) and the contralateral premolar (LR4). The symptoms did not linger.

What did the periapical radiograph show about the LL4?

The periapical radiograph showed:

- Approximately 15% interproximal bone loss on the mesial aspect of the LL4 and 30% on the distal.
- LL2 and LL3 show tooth surface loss with intact and uniform periodontal ligament.
- LL4 extensive distal root caries in proximity to the pulp (Figure 1.2.1a) with intact and uniform periodontal ligament.
- LL5 has been replaced with an implant-supported crown.

The LL5 implant-supported crown was removed to allow direct assessment of the cavity on the distal aspect of the LL4 (Figure 1.2.1b).

Diagnosis and Treatment Planning

What was the diagnosis?

The diagnosis for the LL4 was reversible pulpitis associated with a carious cavity.

What are the treatment options?

- Direct restoration with or without pulp capping
- Non-surgical root canal treatment
- Extraction
- No treatment

The fact that the tooth sensitivity to stimuli was limited to a few seconds, spontaneous pain was absent and there was no tenderness to percussion indicated that the pulp was reversibly inflamed. Endodontic treatment was therefore not indicated. In the presence of contradictory or non-specific signs and/or symptoms, cone beam computed tomography may be indicated to investigate the periapical status of the tooth. Previous studies have demonstrated that periapical lesions were present in teeth with reversible pulpitis, leading to high failure rates of vital pulp therapy when compared with teeth with no preoperative lesions. In this case, it was decided to perform a direct restoration of the tooth. If the pulp was exposed during caries excavation, a pulp capping or pulpotomy procedure would be considered.

Treatment

The tooth was anaesthetized and isolated with dental dam. The caries was removed using a round bur in a slow handpiece from the periphery. The infected dentine was then removed carefully from the pulpal aspect of the cavity using the same bur and hand excavators (Figure 1.2.2a). The demineralized infected dentine was completely removed, exposing the dark caries-affected dentine. As the bonding strength is lower and less predictable in affected dentine, a peripheral zone of sound intact dentine was prepared during excavation to obtain a more reliable bonding.

Polytetrafluoroethylene (PTFE) was used to improve isolation and retraction of the soft tissues/dental dam, helping the correct visualisation of the margins of the cavity to be restored (Figure 1.2.2b).

The cavity was restored with a direct composite resin restoration (Figure 1.2.3a–c).

Care was taken in this case to check and adjust the contact point, to prevent food trapping between the restored tooth and crown of the implant (Figure 1.2.4a, b). The need for review appointments was stressed to the patient, who was instructed to be attentive to signs of potential aggravation of the pulpal status, such as spontaneous and/or lingering pain, increased sensitivity to thermal stimuli (particularly heat) and tenderness on biting.

Discussion

The prognosis for this tooth is good. The treatment aimed to preserve the pulp vitality by removing bacteria of the contaminated carious lesion and at the same time provide a tight seal to arrest caries progression and preserve tooth function (Table 1.2.1). Improvement of the interproximal contour and contact point between the restored tooth and the implant-retained crown is also crucial for the longevity of the restoration, as it prevents food trapping and allows for more effective interdental cleaning.

Table 1.2.1 Benefits of maintaining pulp vitality.

- Preservation of dental structure
- Retention of the pulp's protective mechanisms
- May help prolong the survival of teeth
- Maintenance of proprioception
- Less time-consuming and technically demanding than non-surgical root canal treatment
- Improves the cost-effectiveness of treatment
- Reduces the chances of biological complications (such as apical periodontitis)

The minimally invasive approach means that the tooth does need to be restored with a cuspal coverage restoration, which would have been indicated if root canal treatment had been carried out.

The ability to remove the crown of the implant during the restoration of the lower left first premolar allowed perfect direct visualisation of the lesion.

In this case, a selective caries removal technique was utilised, all peripheral caries was removed to hard dentine and caries affected dentine (firm, dark coloured dentine) was left on the pulpal aspect of the cavity only. This technique minimises the risk of pulp exposure and has been supported by the European Association of Endodontists. An alternative approach is complete caries removal, which is considered essential to eliminate infected tissue. Histology has shown chronic inflammatory cell infiltrates and subclinical pulp inflammation where caries has remained. This approach is supported by the American Association of Endodontists. Both techniques agree that complete caries removal at the periphery is essential for improved adhesion of bonding resins, to create the most important cavity seal. It is also best, where possible, to manage the treatment under dental dam and with magnification.

The materials employed to restore the tooth may be important, because it is very difficult to determine the thickness of the remaining dentine over the pulp. Calcium silicate cements may be used as a base over which a permanent direct plastic is placed.

When discussing treatment options, it is essential that patients are made aware that should their symptoms persist or deteriorate, endodontic treatment would be indicated.

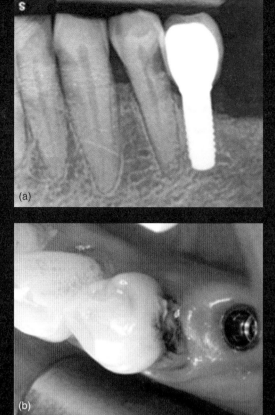

Figure 1.2.1 (a) Periapical radiograph of the LL4 demonstrating the extension and proximity to the pulp of the distal interproximal carious lesion. There appeared to be reactionary dentine in close relation to the carious lesion. No noticeable changes in the periapical tissues could be appreciated. (b) After removal of the implant-supported crown, the size of the carious lesion was assessed. The deep cavity was darkened and covered with soft plaque. It was also possible to visualise the undermined enamel in relation to the lesion.

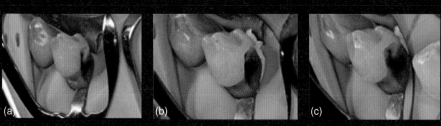

Figure 1.2.2 (a) Dental dam isolation and excavation of the peripheral area; (b) retraction of the dental dam/soft tissues with PTFE; (c) detail of the cavity after caries excavation, etching, rinsing and drying. Note the affected dentine and the peripheral area of sound dentine.

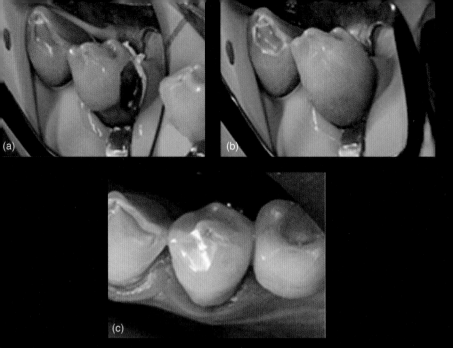

Figure 1.2.3 (a) After bonding application; (b) after restoration with composite resin; (c) view after completion and with implant crown in situ, showing an adequate contact point.

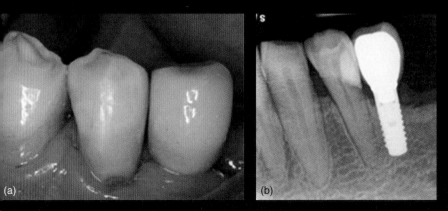

Figure 1.2.4 (a) Buccal view of the restored tooth. The interproximal contour and contact point were optimised to prevent food trapping and allow the facilitated

Further Reading

Alleman, D.S. and Magne, P. (2012). A systematic approach to deep caries removal end points: the peripheral seal concept in adhesive dentistry. *Quintessence International* 43 (3): 197–208.

American Association of Endodontists (2021). Position statement on vital pulp therapy. Chicago, IL: AAE. `https://www.aae.org/wp-content/uploads/2021/05/VitalPulpTherapyPositionStatement_v2.pdf`.

Dummer, P.M., Hicks, R., and Huws, D. (1980). Clinical signs and symptoms in pulp disease. *International Endodontic Journal* 13: 27–35.

Duncan, H., Galler, K., Tomson, P. et al. (2019). European Society of Endodontology position statement: management of deep caries and the exposed pulp. *International Endodontic Journal* 52 (7): 923–934.

Mainkar, A. and Kim, S.G. (2018). Diagnostic accuracy of 5 dental pulp tests: a systematic review and meta-analysis. *Journal of Endodontics* 44: 694–702.

Maltz, M., Koppe, B., Jardim, J.J. et al. (2017). Partial caries removal in deep caries lesions: a 5-year multicenter randomized controlled trial. *Clinical Oral Investigations* 22: 1337–1343.

Ricucci, D., Loghin, S., and Siqueira, J. Jr. (2014). Correlation between clinical and histologic pulp diagnoses. *Journal of Endodontics* 40: 1932–1939.

Schwendicke, F., Frencken, J.E., Bjørndal, L. et al. (2016). Managing carious lesions: consensus recommendations on carious tissue removal. *Advances in Dental Research* 28: 58–67.

1.3 *Symptomatic Irreversible Pulpitis*

Shatha Zahran

Objectives

At the end of this case the reader should be able to understand and differentiate the characteristic signs and symptoms of irreversibly inflamed pulps.

Introduction

A 33-year-old male presented to his dentist with severe sensitivity on his upper right first molar (UR6).

Chief Complaint

The patient complained of severe pain to cold and sometimes spontaneous pain that lasted for minutes. He was avoiding eating on the right side of his mouth due to this sensitivity.

Medical History

Unremarkable.

Dental History

The patient was a regular attender at his dentist. He had several restorations in the past and the UR6 was restored with an amalgam restoration more than six years ago.

Clinical Examination

Extraoral examination was unremarkable. Intraoral examination revealed no swelling or tenderness in the buccal sulcus associated with UR6. The oral hygiene was fair. The probing around the UR6 was 1–3 mm. The UR6 was

Pitt Ford's Problem-Based Learning in Endodontology, Second Edition. Edited by Elizabeth Shin Perry, Shanon Patel, Shalini Kanagasingam, and Samantha Hamer.
© 2025 John Wiley & Sons Ltd. Published 2025 by John Wiley & Sons Ltd.

tender to percussion. Cold sensibility testing (Endo-Frost) elicited a severe pain response that lingered for over 30 seconds. Teeth UR5 and UR7 were both responsive to Endo-Frost, with the sensation fully resolving on removal of the stimulus within a few seconds.

Radiographic Examination

- Alveolar bone levels were within normal limits.
- UR4, UR5, and UR8 amalgam restorations with intact and uniform periodontal ligament (PDL).
- UR7 occlusal amalgam restoration, intact and uniform PDL.
- UR6 amalgam restoration with distal overhang and proximity to the pulp chamber with distal pulp horn and root canal sclerosis, with no visible root canal in the mesio-buccal or palatal roots, with a visible canal in the disto-buccal root. There is loss of lamina dura on the palatal root apex with no apical radiolucency. The root apices overlie the maxillary sinus (Figure 1.3.1).

Diagnosis and Treatment Planning

What is the diagnosis for the UR6?

The diagnosis for the UR6 was symptomatic irreversible pulpitis.

What are the treatment options for tooth UR6?

- Root canal treatment
- Pulpotomy
- Extraction
- No treatment

After discussion with the patient, informed consent was gained for root canal treatment.

Treatment

Root canal treatment was carried out in a single visit under local anaesthetic and dental dam. The working length was measured using an electronic apex locator. Canals were apically prepared with no. 15 K hand file followed by rotary instrumentation in a crown-down technique. Patency was maintained with a no. 10 K file in all canals. Irrigation was carried out with sodium hypochlorite and ethylenediaminetetraacetic acid (EDTA) utilising passive ultrasonic activation.

The root canal system was obturated with gutta percha (GP) and root canal sealer using a warm vertical condensation technique (Figures 1.3.2 and 1.3.3). A composite resin was placed in the access cavity and the tooth was restored with a ceramic onlay. The one-year follow-up periapical radiograph revealed normal PDL and lamina dura, intact coronal filling and normal pocket depths (Figure 1.3.4). The tooth was not tender to percussion or palpation and was normally functioning.

Discussion

How can one differentiate between reversible and irreversible pulpitis?

See Table 1.3.1 for details.

Table 1.3.1 Comparing the symptoms of reversible and irreversible pulpitis.

	Reversible pulpitis	Irreversible pulpitis
Nature of the pain	Discomfort is experienced when a stimulus such as cold or sweet is applied and it goes away 5–10 seconds following removal of the stimulus. Pain is not spontaneous	Exaggerated pain on thermal stimulus, lingering pain (often 30 seconds or longer after stimulus removal), spontaneity (unprovoked pain) and referred pain. Sometimes the pain may be accentuated by postural changes such as lying down or bending over. Over-the-counter analgesics are typically ineffective
Aetiologies	Typical aetiologies may include exposed dentine (dentinal sensitivity), caries or deep restorations	Common aetiologies may include deep caries, extensive restorations or fractures exposing the pulpal tissues
Cold sensibility test	Sharp pain that disappears immediately after removal of the cold test stimulus	Sharp, severe pain that lingers on removal of the cold test stimulus
Percussion	Not tender to percussion	May or may not be tender to percussion
Radiographically	No significant radiographic changes in the periapical region	No significant radiographic changes in the periapical region. Some cases might exhibit widening of the periodontal ligament

What can help with diagnosis?

Diagnosis of irreversible pulpitis can be challenging, with difficulty local-ising the source of the pain. This may be because one neuron innervates multiple teeth or due to the lower density of proprioceptors in the pulp, so that the inflammatory mediators need to have reached the more highly innervated PDL for the patient to be able to localise the pain.

Pulp sensibility tests can aid in diagnosis via using a thermal or electrical stimulus to indirectly determine the pulp status by assessing the condition of the nerves; they do not assess the blood flow in the pulp. The cold tests that have been used are Endo-Frost, ethyl chloride and carbon dioxide snow, with Endo-Frost being favoured due to its ease of use and −50 °C temperature. The warm tests that can be used are a warmed GP stick (using a lubricant to ensure it does not stick to the tooth surface), frictional heat generated from a rubber cup, or isolating the tooth with dental dam and applying warm water to the tooth. For some patients the tooth is sensitive to heat and the symptoms resolve with the application of a cold stimulus, so relieving the patient's symp-toms with the application of a cold stimulus could aid in the identification of the symptomatic tooth. A positive reading by an electric pulp test (EPT) only indicates that there are some viable nerve fibres capable of response. The numerical reading obtained is compared with a control tooth and it is most accurate when no response is obtained, suggesting a possible necrotic pulp.

Pulpal sensibility testing with Endo-Frost and EPT is an accurate and reliable method, with cold test results showing accuracy of 0.904, while the EPT results showed accuracy of 0.75. However, all sensibility tests are highly subjective and must be used in conjunction with other signs and symptoms to aid in diagnosis, as false positives and false negatives are possible (Table 1.3.2).

Table 1.3.2 Causes of inaccurate pulp sensibility test results.

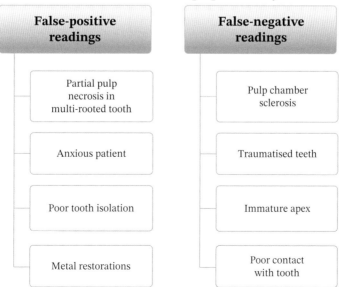

Do the clinical findings correspond to the histological status of the pulp?

Irreversible pulpitis is a clinical diagnosis based on subjective and objective findings. Historical studies had reported a poor correlation between the patients' symptoms/diagnostic test findings and the histological status of the pulp. A more recent study in 2014 of 95 teeth showed good agreement between the clinical findings and histological findings, with 96.6% agreement for the diagnosis of reversible pulpitis and 84.4% for irreversible pulpitis.

Why is pulpitis so painful?

An increase in inflammatory mediators within the inflamed pulp tissue repeatedly stimulates the nociceptors, causing sensitisation. The peripheral sensitisation results in a lower excitation threshold, so that even usually non-painful stimuli cause pain (allodynia), the response to the pain is heightened and prolonged (hyperalgesia) and a pain response can occur spontaneously. Within the pulp the main nociceptive primary afferent nerve fibres are A (90% are A-delta) and C fibres. The A-delta fibres are myelinated, with a fast conduction and lower stimulation threshold. They are located in the periphery of the pulp and respond to hydrodynamic stimuli, producing an initial sharp shooting pain. C fibres are unmyelinated, with low conduction and a higher excitation threshold, and are located in the central region of the pulp, a location that may explain the diffusely located pain felt by patients as nerve fibres may innervate multiple teeth. The pain is described as a diffuse, burning, throbbing pain that comes on several seconds after a warm drink and lingers following removal of the stimuli. C fibres have been shown to be able to function in a hypoxic environment, which would be present in the reduced blood flow of a necrotic pulp. This could be why some patients feel pain on instrumentation on a seemingly necrotic tooth.

Why can it be difficult to anaesthetise teeth with irreversible pulpitis?

Anaesthetising teeth with irreversible pulpitis can be problematic, and unsuccessful anaesthesia is distressing for both patient and clinician. Mandibular molars are the most difficult to anaesthetise, then mandibular premolars, maxillary molars, maxillary premolars and lower anterior teeth, and there is the highest success in maxillary anterior teeth. Theories behind why anaesthesia is more difficult to achieve include:

- Localised elevations in tissue pressure and inflammatory mediators in acute inflammation that results in hyperalgesia.
- The lower pH in inflamed tissues reducing anaesthetic penetration.
- Inflamed tissues have decreased excitability thresholds or altered sodium channels, which both affect the success of local anaesthetic agents.

- Anxious patients (pre-existing apprehension lowers pain threshold).
- Patients with moderate to severe pain or spontaneous pain have less successful IANB than patients who only have pain on stimulation.

What can be done to improve anaesthesia?

- Ask the patient about previous difficulties with anaesthesia, consider anxiety levels and assess patients presenting with pain – forewarned is forearmed.
- Give pre-operative non-steroidal anti-inflammatory drugs one hour prior to treatment.
- For mandibular teeth:
  - IANB with supplemental:
    - Articaine infiltrations
    - Lignocaine or mepivacaine intraosseous injections
    - Lignocaine intraligamental injections
    - Gow-Gates technique.
- For maxillary teeth:
  - Buccal/labial and palatal infiltrations
  - Supplemental intraosseous or intraligamental injections.
- Intrapulpal injections – which have the downsides of being painful for the patient and that you need to have accessed the pulp chamber.
- Conscious sedation.

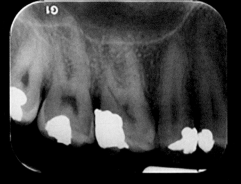

Figure 1.3.1 Pre-operative periapical radiograph of the upper right sextant.

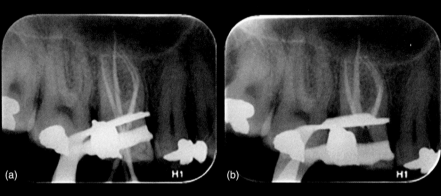

Figure 1.3.2 (a) Master cone radiograph and (b) obturation radiograph.

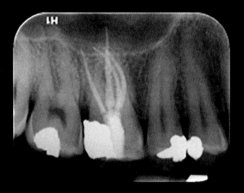

Figure 1.3.3 Post-operative radiograph.

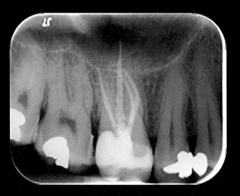

Figure 1.3.4 One-year follow-up.

Further Reading

Jespersen, J.J., Hellstein, J., Williamson, A. et al. (2014). Evaluation of dental pulp sensibility tests in a clinical setting. *Journal of Endodontics* 40 (3): 351–354.

Keiser, K. and Hargreaves, K.M. (2002). Building effective strategies for the management of endodontic pain. *Endodontic Topics* 3 (1): 93–105.

Ricucci, D., Loghin, S., and Siqueira, J.F. (2014). Correlation between clinical and histologic pulp diagnoses. *Journal of Endodontics* 40 (12): 1932–1939.

Seltzer, S., Bender, I.B., and Ziontz, M. (1963). The dynamics of pulp inflammation: correlations between diagnostic data and the actual histologic findings in the pulp. *Oral Surgery, Oral Medicine, Oral Pathology* 16: 969–977.

1.4 Treatment Planning
Samantha Hamer

Objectives

At the end of this case, the reader should understand the importance of treatment planning in endodontic cases and be aware of the key clinical features and differing treatment protocols that will affect the complexity of the treatment.

Introduction

A female, 63 years old, presented to her dentist regarding the lower right second molar (LR7). The tooth was restored with a crown about 20 years ago.

Chief Complaint

Tooth was tender on biting.

Medical History

The patient was a non-smoker and had well-controlled hypertension.

Dental History

Regular dental attendance since joining the practice eight years ago. When she was a child some molar teeth were extracted, and she wore a removable brace for the upper teeth.

Clinical Examination

Extraoral examination was unremarkable. Intraoral examination revealed a moderately restored dentition with good oral hygiene. The LR6 and LL6 had been extracted and there was some space closure.

Pitt Ford's Problem-Based Learning in Endodontology, Second Edition. Edited by Elizabeth Shin Perry, Shanon Patel, Shalini Kanagasingam, and Samantha Hamer.

The LR7 was firm, with tenderness to palpation and percussion. The LR7 had periodontal probing of less than 2 mm, with no bleeding on probing. It was restored with a metal–ceramic full-coverage crown and was unresponsive to sensibility tests.

What did the radiograph reveal?

- 15% bone loss LR5.
- Mesial angulation of LR7 and LR8 and distal angulation of LR5, following loss of LR6.
- LR7 metal–ceramic crown with negative distal margin.
- LR7 existing root canal filling, sparsely condensed, short of the radiographic apex. The canal beyond the root filling was visible on the mesial root but not on the distal root.
- Apical radiolucency associated with the mesial and distal root apices (Figure 1.4.1).

Diagnosis and Treatment Planning

The diagnosis for the LR7 was symptomatic apical periodontitis associated with an existing root canal treatment.

What are the treatment options for this patient?

- Non-surgical root canal retreatment
- Surgical endodontic treatment
- Extraction
- No treatment

Is there a systematic way to plan the treatment of endodontic cases?

Treatment planning requires the clinician to consider many inter-related factors. Planning for endodontic treatment is not only about the complexity of the root canal system, but must also take into account the periodontal condition, the integrity of the remaining tooth structure, the patient's medical history, dental conditions and patient expectations and wishes. This can be challenging and employing a methodical treatment planning tool can assist in making logical and coherent treatment planning decisions.

The Dental Practicality Index (DPI) aims to break down treatment planning into four categories (Table 1.4.1):

- Tooth structural integrity:
  - How much sound tooth structure remains?
  - Is it restorable?
- Endodontic considerations:
  - Are the canals easily identifiable on the radiograph?

Table 1.4.1 The Dental Practicality Index.

Weighting	Tooth integrity	Endodontic	Periodontal	Extra considerations
0 No treatment required	Unrestored	Vital pulp	Probing <3.5 mm	Local: Adjacent teeth are healthy
	Existing restoration OK	Existing root canal treatment OK	Periodontal disease treated	General: History of intravenous bisphosphonates, head and neck radiotherapy
1 Simple treatment required	Simple direct or indirect restoration	Simple root canal treatment	Probing 3.5–5.5 mm	Local: Whether this tooth will be a bridge abutment
	Suitable for general dental practitioner	Canal(s) visible, straight	Root surface debridement suitable for hygienist or general dental practitioner	General: Planned radiotherapy of head and neck region Immunocompromised patient
2 Complex treatment required	Minimal sound tooth	Complex root canal system	Probing >5.5 mm	Local: Prosthodontic treatment planned of multiple teeth
	Subgingival margins	Sclerosed canal(s)	Short root	General:High caries rate Poor oral hygiene, active perio
	Post-core	Acute curvatures	Crown lengthening	Parafunctional habits/ tooth surface loss
		Fractured instrument Perforation	Grade 2 mobility Grade 2–3 furcation involvement	Limited mouth opening/severe gags Anxious, requiring sedation
6 Impractical to treat	Inadequate structure for ferrule	Untreatable root canal system	Untreatable periodontal disease	Local: Keeping the tooth would complicate a simple plan, e.g. one remaining over-erupted tooth affecting denture construction
				General: Potentially life-threatening medical conditions where the objective of dental treatment is pain relief only

- Are the canals sclerosed or curved, or are there fractured instruments, perforations or resorption?
- Are there signs of a crack?
- Periodontal condition:
  - Can the patient maintain good oral hygiene?
  - Is there gingival inflammation?
  - Is there an isolated deep probing depth? (indicates a crack)
  - Will crown lengthening be required?
- Extra considerations/context:
  - Medical history, bisphosphonates, radiotherapy
  - Is the patient anxious and will sedation be required?
  - Can the patient lay flat for long treatment?
  - Is there limited mouth opening?
  - Will the tooth be used as a bridge abutment?
  - Would retaining this tooth compromise other restorative treatment?

Each category is given a score, 0, 1, 2 or 6 to indicate the complexity of the treatment. The sum of the category scores indicates the complexity of the treatment (Table 1.4.2).

Table 1.4.2 Explanation of Dental Practicality Index (DPI) scoring, indicating the complexity of the proposed treatment.

DPI score	
Maximum Score 0 in all categories	No treatment
Maximum Score 1 in any category	Simple, predictable treatment
Maximum Score 2 in any category	Complex treatment (possibly requiring advanced training or referral)
Score 6 in any category or total score > 6	Impractical to definitively treat (does not mean the tooth should not be restored or requires immediate extraction, but accentuates the need for a discussion with the patient about the poor long-term prognosis)

It is important that the patient is fully aware of the potential complications associated with the proposed treatment to be able to give informed consent. Every patient is unique: some patients are willing to go ahead with a complicated treatment, even with the knowledge that it may not be successful, but others would not.

Properly assessing the case and its potential complications will help you know whether the treatment is within your capabilities to treat or whether it should be referred; it will also help you to better inform your patients. Dento-legally this will be of benefit to you and the patient.

Assessing this case using the dental practicality index

The LR7 is restored with a metal ceramic crown. The existing root canal filling is sparsely condensed and short of the radiographic apex. The canal beyond the root filling is not visible in the distal root and is visible in the mesial canal. The canals are straight. There is a periapical radiolucency associated with the mesial and distal root. The patient has pain on biting and is keen to save the tooth.

- *Tooth integrity*: What core material is under the crown and how much tooth remains? Will the core fracture if the crown is removed? With only 1 mm of tooth above the level of the adjacent alveolar bone, can a ferrule for the new crown be achieved? Will the mesial angulation of the LR8 make it difficult to achieve a good margin on the distal of the LR7? If the access was made through the crown, how much tooth would be left to retain the crown? This case presents many potential complications, with a best-case scenario of DPI = 2 (challenging but restorable). It is possible that once the crown is removed or accessed, the tooth could be found to be unrestorable (DPI = 6). It is always better to have a discussion of all possibilities before starting treatment, rather than trying to explain afterwards.
- *Endodontic*: There is a sparsely condensed existing root canal filling material short of the radiographic apex. The tooth has a mesial angulation, which will affect access to the mesial canals. The canals look straight on the radiograph and the canal is visible beyond the root filling on the mesial root, but not visible on the distal root. Ask yourself whether you can remove the existing root canal filling, find the other canal in the mesial root and get to the radiographic apex. Why did the previous dentist have difficulties? DPI = 2.
- *Periodontal*: Good bone levels, clinically good oral hygiene. DPI = 0.
- *Extra considerations*: Non-smoker, unremarkable medical history. No dental anxiety, good mouth opening and able to lie in the dental chair. Most importantly the patient fully understands the risks associated with the treatment, as the tooth could be found to be unrestorable and require extraction. DPI = 0.
- *Summary*: This is a challenging case that could present multiple complications. If the tooth is restorable it would be DPI = 2, indicating that additional training may be required to successfully manage this case.

What are the advantages and disadvantages of each treatment option?

Non-surgical root canal retreatment

Non-surgical root canal retreatment treats the most common cause of root canal failure, which is intraradicular infection. Removing the existing crown facilitates a full assessment of the remaining tooth structure for restorability, cracks and planning for the new core. The access to the root canals is improved with better illumination and orientation. The clinician will need to fabricate a well-fitting temporary crown that maintains the marginal seal, good gingival health and aesthetics throughout treatment. It is important to have a discussion with the patient about the benefits of removing the crown, which can be difficult if the existing crown is quite new or if the crown is part of a bridge, as this will significantly increase the cost and the amount of treatment required.

If the root canal treatment is performed by accessing through the existing crown, this will increase the complexity of the treatment for the clinician. It will not be possible to fully assess the restorability of the tooth. The crown may be masking the fact that the original tooth was rotated, making location of the canals more difficult and making the risk of becoming disorientated higher, leading to a greater risk of perforation. Placing the dental dam clamp and accessing through a crown may fracture the porcelain and the access preparation may weaken the remaining core, resulting in core fracture.

Surgical endodontic treatment

The 2016 update of the Cochrane review of endodontic procedures for retreatment of periapical lesions examined the evidence comparing surgical and non-surgical retreatment of apical periodontitis. The quality of the evidence was poor and did not show any difference in the healing at one year between the two groups, and further research was advised. Non-surgical root canal treatment is generally the preferred option, as it is less invasive and treats the most common cause of apical periodontitis, which is bacteria within the root canal system. However, in a situation where the existing root canal filling and coronal seal are good, ask yourself what you will improve by performing non-surgical retreatment. In another situation, for example a tooth with a crown and long post, would it be possible to remove the post–crown without further damage to the tooth? Surgical treatment is performed when the risks of non-surgical treatment outweigh the benefits.

Extraction

There is a degree of subjectivity when deciding on where to draw the line between restorable and unrestorable, and a patient may decide to have a tooth extracted, even though it is technically possible to perform endodontic treatment. Patients base their decision on their own perception of the options available and what is best for them. Situations that are unrestorable include:

- Extensive caries or fracture extending beyond the cemento-enamel junction.
- Advanced periodontal disease.
- Irretrievable instrument, perforation or infection, where non-surgical treatment is not viable and surgical endodontic treatment is not practical due to the proximity to the inferior alveolar nerve or sinus.

If heroic attempts to save a tooth are unlikely to be successful, then extraction and replacement with an implant are an option. However, remember that not all teeth need to be replaced following extraction and implants are not without complications and compromises.

No treatment

The incidence of exacerbation of chronic apical periodontitis becoming symptomatic is less than 5% a year and less than 6% after 20 years.

It is not fully understood why some chronic apical periodontitis evolves into an acute apical abscess. It may be due to an increase in the number of bacteria present, the virulence of the bacteria present or host-related factors. Conditions such as diabetes, herpesvirus infection, stress and autoimmune conditions may act as disease modifiers and can influence the severity of apical periodontitis. Most apical abscesses localise intraorally and respond to local intervention; however, there is the risk that an apical abscess can spread regionally to fascial spaces or haematogenously, causing a potentially life-threatening systemic infection.

What factors can affect the complexity of endodontic treatment?

Patient

- *Patient disposition*: Anxious patients feel more pain.
- *Restriction in mouth opening*: It is usually possible to instrument most teeth, if it is possible to place two fingers between the maxillary and mandibular incisor tips.
- *Gag reflex.*
- *Trauma history*: Traumatised teeth may have arrested root development, with thin walls and an open apex, or there may be canal obliteration or resorption or cracks.

Intraoral examination

- *Ability to position radiograph*: Presence of tori, height of palatal vault.

- *Presence of a sinus*: The presence of a pre-operative sinus tract has been associated with a reduced prognosis. Trace the sinus tract with a gutta percha point when taking a radiograph to identify the source of the sinus; it is not always the tooth adjacent to the sinus opening.
- *Probing depth*: An isolated narrow, deep probing depth can indicate the presence of a vertical root fracture or sinus tract lying within the periodontal ligament.
- *Tooth*:
  - Position, rotation and angulation can affect access and risk disorientation, and increase the risk of perforation and difficulty visualising pulpal anatomy.
  - Accessing through a crown is more challenging due to risk of porcelain fracture, core fracture, difficult illumination and loss of anatomical map.
  - Can dental dam be placed? If dental dam cannot be placed, the root canal treatment should not be done.

Radiograph

- *Bone levels*: Vertical alveolar bone loss can be a sign of a vertical crack/ fracture in the tooth (Figure 1.4.2a and b).
- *Tooth angulation*: Moderate angulation is 10–30° and severe is >30°, which makes it difficult to achieve straight-line access for instrumentation.
- *Pulp chamber*: Look at the depth of the pulp chamber and measure it against your bur, so you know how far down you are expecting to reach the chamber. If the pulp chamber is reduced in height, there will not be the classic drop feeling into the chamber, so be careful not to perforate. Look for pulp stones and how the canals exit the chamber.
- *Canals*:
  - Length >25 mm is more difficult.
  - Open apex makes obturation difficult, with high risk of extrusion.
  - If the canals are not visible on the radiograph and are sclerosed, preparation will be challenging. Canals that are visible and then disappear midway can be a sign of a dividing canal.
  - A moderate curvature is 10–30° and a severe curvature is >30°; the risk of causing a ledge in the preparation is high.
  - Resorption requires cone-beam computed tomography for full analysis and treatment planning to assess size and location.
- *Previous root treatment*:
  - Teeth with perforations have a reduced success rate.
  - Anatomical changes or ledges will make instrumenting the canal difficult as the file catches in the ledge.
  - Can fractured instruments be removed or bypassed?
  - Missed canals.

- *Apical periodontitis*: Teeth with pre-operative apical periodontitis have a reduced healing rate compared to teeth with no pre-operative apical periodontitis. The size of the lesion has also been shown to be a prognostic indicator.

Single or multiple visits for endodontic treatment

The 2016 Cochrane review of 25 randomised control trials found no difference between root canal treatments performed in a single visit or over multiple visits, although the quality of the evidence was poor. The frequency of short- and long-term complications was similar in both groups and neither regime can prevent all complications. However, there was a higher frequency of post-operative pain requiring analgesia in the first week after treatment for single-visit root canal treatment.

Discussion

Treatment planning is fundamental to treatment success. Identify the signs that will make treatment more complicated, have a good knowledge of the potential risks and benefits of each treatment option, understand the limitations of your own clinical skills, and communicate well with the patient to help them choose the best treatment option for their own unique circumstances. This is in line with shared decision making and should be integral to the informed consent process.

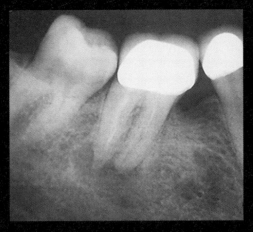

Figure 1.4.1 Periapical radiograph of the LR7, showing negative crown margin, sparsely condensed root canal filling with apical radiolucency.

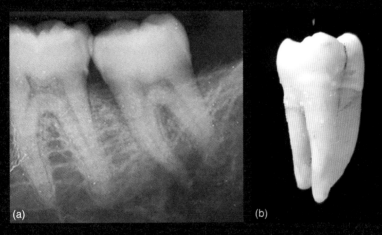

(a)   (b)

Figure 1.4.2a and b Periapical radiograph and photograph of the LL7 with intact clinical crown. Note the mesial vertical bone loss with apical radiolucency and the corresponding crack with radicular extension on the mesial root.

Further Reading

AAE Endodontic Case Difficulty Assessment Form and Guidelines. Chicago, IL: AAE. https://www.aae.org/specialty/wp-content/uploads/sites/2/2022/01/CaseDifficultyAssessmentFormFINAL2022.pdf.

AAE Treatment Standards. (2020) Chicago, IL: https://www.aae.org/specialty/wp-content/uploads/sites/2/2018/04/TreatmentStandards_Whitepaper.pdf.

Dawood, A. and Patel, S. (2017). The dental practicality index – assessing the restorability of teeth. *British Dental Journal* 222: 755–758.

Del Fabbro, M., Corbella, S., Sequeira-Byron, P. et al. (2016). Endodontic procedures for retreatment of periapical lesions *Cochrane Database of Systematic Reviews* 10(10): CD005511.

Eriksen, H.M. (2008). Epidemiology of apical periodontitis. In: *Essential Endodontology*, 2e (ed. D. Ørstavik and T. Pitt Ford), 262–274. Oxford: Blackwell Science.

Manfredi, M., Figini, L., Gagliani, M., and Lodi, G. (2016). Single versus multiple visits for endodontic treatment of permanent teeth (review). *Cochrane Database of Systematic Reviews* 12 (12): CD005296.

Nair, P.N.R. (2006). On the causes of persistent apical periodontitis: a review. *International Endodontic Journal* 39: 249–281.

Ng, Y.L., Mann, V., and Gulabivala, K. (2011). A prospective study of the factors affecting outcomes of non-surgical root canal treatment: Part 1: Periapical health. *International Endodontic Journal* 44: 583–609.

Siqueira, J.F. and Rôças, I.N. (2013). Microbiology and treatment of acute apical abscesses. *Clinical Microbiology Review* 26: 255–273.

Torabinejad, M., Cymerman, J.J., Frankson, M. et al. (1994). Effectiveness of various medications on postoperative pain following complete instrumentation. *Journal of Endodontics* 20: 345–354.

Yu, V.S., Messer, H.H., Yee, R., and Shen, L. (2012). Incidence and impact of painful exacerbations in a cohort with post-treatment persistent endodontic lesions. *Journal of Endodontics* 38 (1): 41–46.

1.5 Maxillary Sinusitis of Endodontic Origin

Maria Lessani and Shalini Kanagasingam

Objectives

Periapical infections involving the maxillary sinus are frequently undetected by both dental and medical professionals, due to the varied clinical and radiographic presentation. At the end of this case, the reader should be able to accurately diagnose and gain an understanding of the management of maxillary sinusitis of endodontic origin (MSEO), including the indications for referral to the Ear, Nose and Throat (ENT) specialist.

Introduction

The patient was a female aged 58 with history of sinusitis on and off for many years. She had seen ENT specialists on a few occasions and had been prescribed various antibiotics, steroids, and sinus washes, which did not completely resolve her symptoms. The patient reported that over the years she had learnt to live with one side of her nose feeling more or less blocked and heavy. She had not been seen by ENT for the past three years.

Chief Complaint

The patient reported a heavy feeling from the right sinus region and no symptoms from the teeth. There was no discomfort on biting and no sensitivity to hot or cold drinks.

Medical History

Unremarkable.

Pitt Ford's Problem-Based Learning in Endodontology, Second Edition. Edited by Elizabeth Shin Perry, Shanon Patel, Shalini Kanagasingam, and Samantha Hamer.
© 2025 John Wiley & Sons Ltd. Published 2025 by John Wiley & Sons Ltd.

Dental History

The patient was a regular attender at her dentist and hygienist. The UR7 had been previously root canal treated over 20 years ago.

Clinical Examination

Extraoral examination revealed slight tenderness to palpation around the upper border of the masseter muscle on the right side and was otherwise unremarkable. Intraoral examination revealed a moderately restored dentition. Oral hygiene was good and generalised periodontal bone loss of about 30% was noted.

The UR7 was restored with a gold onlay and the UR6 had a disto-occlusal composite restoration. The margins were sound and there was generalised recession noted around these teeth. The teeth were not tender to percussion or palpation.

Can we pulp test teeth with existing crowns?

Cold tests using certain refrigerant sprays (at temperatures as low as −50 °C) can penetrate through the restorations and elicit a response from a vital tooth. Hence, in this case Endo-Ice was utilised, which provoked a positive response from the UR6 and no response from the UR7.

What did the radiograph reveal about the upper left molar region?

The periapical radiograph (Figure 1.5.1a) revealed:

- 30% horizontal bone loss.
- UR7 had an occlusal restoration that extended into its pulp chamber. UR7 has been inadequately filled with single cone gutta-percha cones in the mesio-buccal and disto-buccal canals with multiple voids noted. The palatal canal does not appear to have been obturated. External inflammatory apical resorption was seen on the disto-buccal, mesio-buccal and palatal roots. The presence of periapical lesions could not be ascertained.
- UR6 had a disto-occlusal restoration with intact margins and intact and uniform periodontal ligament space.
- The presence of the low-lying maxillary sinus floor was noted.

Diagnosis and Treatment Planning

What was the diagnosis?

The provisional diagnosis was previously root treated with asymptomatic apical periodontitis associated with the UR7. The presence of periapical lesions could not be ascertained from the periapical radiograph. A discussion was carried out with the patient and a small field-of-view (40×40 mm) cone beam computed tomography (CBCT) was carried out in order to accurately visualise the apices of the maxillary posterior teeth and their relationship to the maxillary sinus.

What did the CBCT scan reveal?

The CBCT scan was reported on by a radiologist, who identified dehiscence of the floor of the maxillary sinus and the presence of sclerosing osteitis associated with the root apices of the UR7. Periapical lesions were associated with the mesio-buccal, disto-buccal, and palatal root apices. External inflammatory root resorption was noted on all three root apices. The partially visualised maxillary sinus was fully opacified and the patient was advised that an ENT opinion may be sought after endodontic intervention. There was an untreated mesio-buccal canal. (Figure 1.5.1b–d).

What were the potential treatment options for this patient?

- No treatment
- Root canal retreatment (non-surgical)
- Surgical retreatment
- Extraction

The CBCT report was discussed with the patient and she was made aware of the need for the ENT referral on completion of dental treatment.

Treatment

The patient opted to save the tooth. Root canal retreatment was carried out under local anaesthetic with dental dam isolation. The UR7 was accessed and gutta percha was removed using Hedstrom files. The root canal systems were prepared using stainless steel hand instruments and reciprocating nickel titanium instruments. Irrigation was carried out with sodium hypochlorite (NaOCl) and ethylenediaminetetraacetic acid (EDTA) solutions. The working length was measured on the pre-operative radiograph and CBCT, confirmed with a working length radiograph and an electronic apex locator. The root canals were dried with sterile paper points and dressed with calcium hydroxide (CH) for four weeks. The palatal canal had a large calcification projecting into it, which was removed using ultrasonics. Once removed it revealed a large canal diameter. The MB2 canal was identified and treated.

The patient returned for a review appointment after two weeks. She was still asymptomatic; however, she reported a slight improvement in her sinus symptoms. At the following treatment appointment, the teeth were once again isolated with dental dam, disinfected, irrigated with EDTA solution to remove the CH, and irrigated further using NaOCl solution. The canals were obturated with gutta-percha and calcium silicate sealer. The palatal canal was obturated based on the apex locator reading. The access cavity was restored with a composite core (Figure 1.5.2a).

A review CBCT scan was taken after six months, which revealed resolution of the periapical lesions. There was a significant reduction of the thickness of mucosal lining of the maxillary sinus on the right side, which appeared clear (radiolucent) compared to the pre-operative scan (Figure 1.5.2a–d).

How common is maxillary sinusitis of endodontic origin?

Contemporary literature reports a high prevalence of MSEO, as more than 40% of chronic rhinosinusitis cases have been reported to have a dental cause. Maxillary posterior dental infections are frequently associated with sinus mucosal inflammation. Therefore, dentists should be aware of the findings that may raise suspicion of MSEO and sinonasal symptoms (Table 1.5.1).

Is it always an endodontic problem or can both tooth and sinus problems occur simultaneously?

It is difficult to determine if the dental aetiology led to the sinus problem. When there is a fully opacified maxillary sinus or an unusual appearance of

Table 1.5.1 Commonly encountered findings that are most likely associated with maxillary sinusitis of endodontic origin (MSEO) compared to sinogenic-specific findings.

MSEO findings	Sinogenic-specific findings
• Repeated episodes of unilateral maxillary sinus infections including purulent sinusitis (especially associated with patent ostium)	• Unilateral nasal congestion or obstruction
• Previously unsuccessful sinus surgery	• Presence of nasal discharge (runny nose)
• No improvement after antibiotics	• Retrorhinorrhea (post-nasal drip)
• Recent dental procedure (assess for teeth with pulpal necrosis, evaluate the quality of previous endodontic treatment and the quality of the restoration)	• Concomitant or recent upper respiratory tract infection
• Symptomatic or asymptomatic apical periodontitis of posterior maxillary teeth with root apices near or in direct contact with antral mucosa	• Worsening pain on vertical change in head position
	• Facial pain
	• Foul odour
	• Observation of pus in the middle meatus (Ear, Nose and Throat observation)

Note: Patients may experience overlapping of symptoms.

a lesion in the sinus, the radiologist would advise an ENT opinion. In cases where the dental aetiology is obvious, once this has been managed (via endodontic treatment or extraction) the sinus problems are expected to resolve. Some cases may not completely heal after endodontic treatment, and this may be a situation where there is concurrent sinusitis and endodontic disease. This may necessitate further adjunctive surgical sinus procedures. Antibiotic therapy has been reported to be ineffective and unwarranted in the treatment of MSEO. Appropriate antibiotics are limited to cases of spreading infection and systemic involvement.

What are the advantages of referring to an ENT consultant?

It is essential for dentists and ENT consultants to collaborate in the diagnosis of MSEO, including differentiating this from sinogenic sinusitis or rhinosinusitis. ENT consultants would gain a full history of nasal and sinus symptoms and commonly examine the patient by using a surface local anaesthetic agent and dilating the nostrils to place a flexible or a rigid endoscope to examine the nasal cavity and maxillary sinus. They may then consider further investigation with computed tomography (CT) scans and magnetic resonance imaging (MRI). It is always helpful to provide them with the dental CBCT scan and a radiologist's report. A referral to ENT should be considered if a dentist suspects a non-odontogenic lesion, impending sinus complications (e.g. fistula, fungal balls), recalcitrant sinus disease post endodontic treatment or the presence of a foreign body (e.g. extruded dental materials) in the maxillary sinus and malignant lesions.

What did the ENT consultant say?

When the patient attended the ENT review about three months after root canal retreatment, her sinusitis symptoms had continued to improve. On examination, the ENT surgeon advised that no intervention was necessary at this time, as the patient had experienced significant improvement since the root canal retreatment was carried out (about nine months earlier). The patient was advised that it would be worth continuing to review the healing post endodontic treatment (with her endodontist) as well as resolution of the sinusitis symptoms over the next few months.

The discussion with the patient included potential indications for surgical intervention to remove diseased sinus tissue and establish drainage should her sinusitis symptoms persist or worsen over time. The goal for ENT treatment is to re-establish sinus aeration and drainage. However, it was acknowledged that medical and surgical therapies of the osteomeatal complex will not resolve MSEO without dental intervention, as seen in this case since the aetiology was linked to endodontic disease.

Discussion

In cases of MSEO, necrotic and infected posterior maxillary teeth have peri-apical lesions that extend into the sinus space. The expansion and discharge into the maxillary sinus result in no obvious swelling or draining intraoral sinus tract, as would be typically seen in mandibular teeth.

It is imperative to identify the different symptoms and their origins. The clinician needs to ask the questions that target signs and symptoms of sinusitis as well as endodontic disease. The dental history as well as medical history should also identify previous episodes of sinusitis and the dentist should consider referral to the ENT team, especially if there is a strong history of unilateral maxillary sinusitis.

Conventional periapical radiographs are unreliable in detecting periapical lesions as well as mucosal soft tissue changes or air–fluid levels in the maxillary sinus. Limited field-of-view CBCT scans are integral to being able to fully appreciate the anatomy of posterior maxillary teeth and the sinus floor. Having said this, it is important to note that dentists with access to CBCT will inadvertently obtain images of the paranasal sinuses. They are then responsible for accurately reporting on abnormalities or pathological findings, with appropriate onward referral where relevant. It would be prudent to request a report from a radiologist to ensure that the entire image dataset has been comprehensively analysed.

Management of MSEO will focus on resolving the periapical periodontitis in the first instance and may include treatment options such as non-surgical root canal therapy, periradicular surgery when indicated, intentional replantation or extraction of the infected tooth.

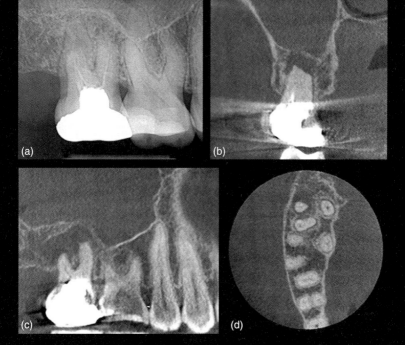

Figure 1.5.1 (a) The pre-operative periapical radiograph revealed inadequately filled root canals of the UR7. (b–d) The cone beam computed tomography images showed the apical periodontitis lesion associated with the mesio-buccal, disto-buccal and palatal root apices of the UR7 perforating the antral cortical floor and opacification of the maxillary sinus.

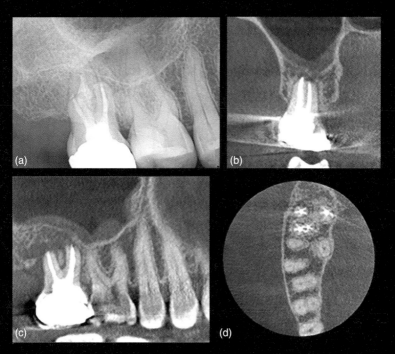

Figure 1.5.2 (a) Periapical radiograph following endodontic treatment of the UR7. The palatal root filling was obturated based on the apex locator reading. (b–d) Six-month review cone beam computed tomography images showed all four canals fully obturated and resolution of the mucosal oedema. The maxillary sinus appeared to be clear.

Further Reading

Bell, G., Joshi, B., and Macleod, R. (2011). Maxillary sinus disease: diagnosis and treatment. *British Dental Journal* 210: 113–118.

Longhini, A.B. and Ferguson, B.J. (2011). Clinical aspects of odontogenic maxillary sinusitis: a case series. *International Forum Allergy Rhinology* 1: 409–415.

Miller, S.O., Johnson, J.D., Allemang, J.D., and Strother, J.M. (2004). Cold testing through full-coverage restorations. *Journal of Endodontics* 30 (10): 695–700.

Patel, S., Brown, J., Semper, M. et al. (2019). European Society of Endodontology position statement: use of cone beam computed tomography in endodontics: European Society of Endodontology (ESE) developed by. *International Endodontic Journal* 52 (12): 1675–1678.

Segura-Egea, J.J., Gould, K., Şen, B.H. et al. (2018). European Society of Endodontology position statement: the use of antibiotics in endodontics. *International Endodontic Journal* 51 (1): 20–25.

Tataryn, R.W., Lewis, M.J., Horalek, M.L. et al. (2018). Maxillary sinusitis of endodontic origin. American Association of Endodontists position statement. Chicago, IL: AAE. https://www.aae.org/specialty/wp-content/uploads/sites/2/2018/04/AAE_PositionStatement_MaxillarySinusitis.pdf.

1.6 Cracked Tooth with Radicular Extension

Suhaila S. Shariff and Matthew C. Davis

Objectives

At the end of this case, the reader should be able to diagnose and prognose cracked teeth with cracks that extend onto the root surface. The reader should also understand treatment and post-treatment protocols that are likely to impact the treatment outcome.

Introduction

A 57-year-old male presented to the endodontist with pain on mastication and constant throbbing in the lower left quadrant.

Chief Complaint

The patient complained of moderate pain on biting and an ache that had progressively worsened over the past week. He had been unable to sleep for the past two nights.

Medical History

The patient had a history of mild hypertension that was controlled with diet and exercise. He had been taking 400 mg ibuprofen every six hours as needed for pain. His medical history was otherwise unremarkable.

Dental History

The patient was a routine attender to his dentist and hygienist. His most recent visit was three months ago, at which time he had lingering sensitivity to cold and spontaneous aching in the lower left quadrant. His dentist performed a pulpotomy on the lower left second molar (LL7) and referred him to an endodontist. The patient's pain resolved with the pulpotomy, so he did not see the endodontist until his pain returned.

Pitt Ford's Problem-Based Learning in Endodontology, Second Edition. Edited by Elizabeth Shin Perry, Shanon Patel, Shalini Kanagasingam, and Samantha Hamer.

Clinical Examination

The lower left second premolar and first molar (LL5 and LL6) were both responsive within normal limits to pulp sensibility testing and percussion and were ruled out as the cause of his symptoms. The LL7 was not responsive to pulp sensibility testing (cold and electric pulp testing) and was moderately tender to percussion. There was no swelling or sinus tract. Transillumination revealed a crack on the distal marginal ridge that extended subgingivally. There was a 5 mm probing depth on the direct distal of LL7 along the crack line.

Radiographic Examination

The radiograph of LL7 showed evidence of prior access with an occlusal restoration and a periapical radiolucency (see later Figure 1.6.5a).

Diagnosis

Endodontic diagnosis of LL7: Cracked tooth; previously initiated endodontic therapy with symptomatic apical periodontitis.

What are longitudinal tooth fractures?

Longitudinal tooth fractures are fractures that occur along the long axis of a tooth over time. They include craze lines, fractured cusps, cracked teeth, split teeth and vertical root fractures. It is imperative that the proper diagnosis is made regarding the type of longitudinal tooth fracture, since the recommended endodontic and restorative treatments vary significantly (Table 1.6.1).

What is a cracked tooth?

A cracked tooth is a restored or unrestored tooth with an incomplete longitudinal tooth fracture initiated at the occlusal surface that extends apically and potentially subgingivally over time. The crack is typically directed mesio-distally, but it can also be present in the bucco-lingual direction. The most commonly cracked teeth are mandibular molars, maxillary molars and maxillary premolars. Transillumination, dyes and increased magnification can improve the visualisation of cracks in a clinical setting (Figure 1.6.1).

What is a cracked tooth with radicular extension?

A cracked tooth with radicular extension is a subset of cracked teeth where an occlusal crack has extended apically from the crown onto the root surface and potentially into the periodontium (Figure 1.6.2). These teeth have traditionally been deemed unrestorable and have been extracted with little to no

Table 1.6.1 Longitudinal tooth fracture types and their respective characteristics and treatment plans.

Type of longitudinal tooth fracture	Characteristics	Endodontic treatment plan	Restorative treatment plan
Craze line	Confined to enamel only Transillumination: light transmits through a craze line	Not necessary	Not necessary unless a cosmetic issue
Cuspal fracture (complete and incomplete)	Initiates in the crown of the tooth, extends obliquely undermining cusp(s), involves enamel and dentine, and may or may not involve the pulp Incomplete cuspal fracture: a crack that undermine cusp(s) Complete cuspal fracture refers to those cases where the cusp is lost Transillumination: light will stop at the fracture for incomplete cuspal fracture	No endodontic treatment: ● If diagnosis is normal pulp or reversible pulpitis ● If no pulp exposure with complete cuspal fracture Root canal treatment: ● If diagnosis is irreversible pulpitis or pulpal necrosis ● If a post is necessary for complete cuspal fracture ● If the pulp is exposed in cases of complete cuspal fractures	No crown: ● If pulp is normal, the tooth is asymptomatic and minimal tooth structure is lost Crown as soon as possible: ● For all other pulpal diagnoses ● Consider crown lengthening for complete cuspal fractures encroaching on the periodontium Check and adjust occlusion, consider nightguard
Cracked tooth	Initiates in the crown of the tooth, extends apically along the long axis of the tooth, involves enamel and dentine, may or may not involve the pulp, and is confined to coronal tooth structure Transillumination: light will stop at the fracture	No endodontic treatment: ● If diagnosis is normal pulp or reversible pulpitis Root canal treatment: ● If diagnosis is irreversible pulpitis or pulpal necrosis	No crown: ● An option if pulp is normal and the tooth is asymptomatic Crown as soon as possible: ● If diagnosis is reversible pulpitis ● If root canal treatment is performed Check and adjust occlusion, consider nightguard

(Continued)

Table 1.6.1 (Continued)

Type of longitudinal tooth fracture	Characteristics	Endodontic treatment plan	Restorative treatment plan
Cracked tooth with radicular extension	A cracked tooth with further apical extension of a crack involves enamel, dentine, pulp, root structure, and potentially affects the periodontium Transillumination: light will stop at the fracture	Same as cracked tooth (above) Microscopic visualisation of the internal crack with intraradicular barrier placement	Same as cracked tooth (above)
Split tooth	Complete crack with separate, mobile segments; extends deep into root structures with potentially significant destruction to the periodontium	Most will require extraction	Extraction, then implant, bridge,or removable partial denture may be considered
Vertical root fracture	Initiates in the root and propagates apically and coronally Typically seen in root canal treated roots in the bucco-lingual dimension Transillumination: light will stop at the fracture	Most will require extraction; however, root amputation, hemisection and root resection are options in select cases	If extraction, then implant, bridge or removable partial denture may be considered

supporting evidence. However, recent studies have suggested that teeth with radicular cracks, the extent of which can be visualised into the root canal internally or with narrow, isolated vertical areas of bone loss externally, can potentially be retained for prolonged periods with successful outcomes.

Due to increased crack depth, the majority of cracked teeth with radicular extension will likely have irreversible pulpal disease, with a higher percentage of *pulp necrosis* over *irreversible pulpitis*. Since a wide variety of symptoms and presentations are possible, accurate pulp and periapical testing is paramount.

Due to bacterial ingress into tooth fractures, deeper cracks also affect the periodontium resulting in narrow areas of bone loss adjacent to the fracture. This can result in an isolated periodontal pocket, which due to its position and size, often eludes clinical probing.

What are the radiographic characteristics of cracked teeth with radicular extension?

Since cracks are typically oriented mesio-distally and run parallel to the plane of the radiograph, visualisation with traditional radiography is usually limited. We must instead rely on bone loss patterns suggestive of deeper cracks; that is, the bone loss that occurs along the root surface adjacent to a crack (Figure 1.6.3). However, these bony changes can often be difficult to observe with two-dimensional (2D) radiographs and superimposition of structures.

Unfortunately, as with radiographs, cracks are rarely visible even on high-resolution cone beam computed tomography (CBCT) images, since the cracks are usually narrower than the voxel size. Once again, in the cracked tooth with radicular extension, we must rely on bone loss patterns to indicate the potential presence and depth of a crack. A typical indication of a crack with radicular extension on CBCT is a narrow, isolated area of low density along the root surface in the three-dimensional (3D), axial, and sagittal sections (Figure 1.6.4). Unlike traditional radiography, the thin slices allowed by CBCT remove the problem of superimposed structures, making the angular defect more visible and making CBCT more reliable for detecting these bony changes. Periapical pathosis may or may not be present depending on the extent of endodontic disease progression.

Treatment

What are the treatment options?

- No treatment
- Root canal therapy followed by cuspal coverage crown
- Extraction

Treatment plan

The treatment plan included root canal treatment of the LL7 followed by a crown restoration.

The LL7 was anaesthetised and isolated under the dental dam. The existing temporary filling was removed and the initial access modified to deroof the chamber. A crack was visualised extending apically along the distal wall of the chamber into the area of the distal canal. Canal debridement was performed so that the extent of the crack, which extended 2 mm beyond the level of the canal orifice, could be visualised microscopically. After obturation with gutta percha and sealer, coronal gutta percha was removed and a resin-modified glass-ionomer was placed apical to the extent of the crack internally in the distal canal and as an orifice barrier in the mesial canals. A cotton pellet and glass-ionomer temporary were then placed to seal the access cavity. The tooth was adjusted out of occlusion. The patient was instructed not to chew on the treated tooth and to have a crown placed by his dentist as soon as possible. The patient was recalled periodically (Figure 1.6.5).

What are the treatment modifiers specific to cracked teeth with radicular extensions?

- Under the microscope, the endodontist should internally assess the extent of the crack into the canal space and place an intraradicular barrier (e.g. composite or glass-ionomer) into the canal orifice, ideally below the level of the visualised crack (Figure 1.6.6).
- After treatment, the tooth should be adjusted out of occlusion and the patient must be advised not to chew on that side of the mouth.
- A crown should be placed on the tooth as soon as possible, and care should be taken to ensure the tooth is not in hyperocclusion.
- The occlusion should be reevaluated periodically.

Discussion

Deeply cracked teeth pose challenges to the clinician in terms of diagnosis and treatment planning. The decision on whether to intervene endodontically is predicated on accurate clinical and radiographic assessment. A cracked tooth with a diagnosis of *reversible pulpitis* would be treatment planned for a crown without root canal treatment. A diagnosis of *irreversible pulpitis* or *pulp necrosis* would require endodontic intervention before crown placement as long as the tooth is restorable. A crack in a tooth with a depth that causes extensive damage to the periodontium or a split tooth with mobile segments carries a poor prognosis and will likely require extraction.

Cracked teeth with radicular extension are unique in that following root canal treatment, the crown will not entirely cover the crack. This radicular extension below the crown margin will continue to harbour bacterial biofilms that will likely create an asymptomatic, isolated periodontal defect (pocket). However, if managed appropriately with certain treatment and post-treatment modifiers as mentioned earlier, these deeper cracked teeth can survive, heal and remain asymptomatic for many years despite the presence of this persistent pocketing. Recent evidence indicates little to no change in this periodontal pocketing over time in most cases (Figure 1.6.7), but further studies are needed to verify this observation.

Endodontically treated posterior teeth have much higher success and survival if crowned expeditiously. This is especially true for cracked teeth. A full-coverage crown will limit propagation of cracks and progression of disease over time. Proper patient education on the importance of a crown and avoidance of chewing on the affected tooth in the interim are critical.

Following endodontic treatment, the tooth should be adjusted completely out of contact with the opposing teeth. After crown cementation, the occlusion should be carefully assessed immediately, at six weeks, at six months and at one year post-operatively to ensure no heavy contacts or excursive interferences. A night guard should be considered if parafunctional stresses are evident or suspected.

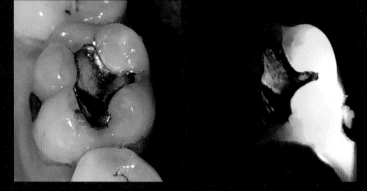

Figure 1.6.1 Example of transillumination of a lower right first molar reveals a distal marginal ridge crack.

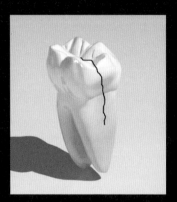

Figure 1.6.2 Illustration of a cracked tooth with radicular extension.

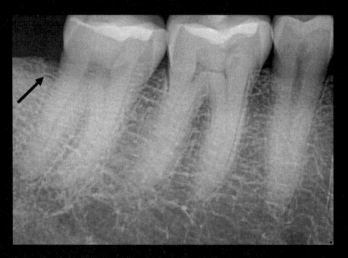

Figure 1.6.3 Radiographic angular bone loss (arrow) suggestive of cracked tooth with radicular extension.

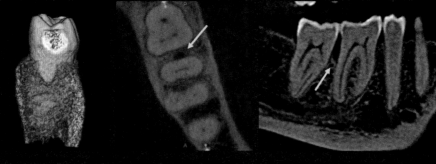

Figure 1.6.4 Cone beam computed tomography three-dimensional, axial and sagittal views of a cracked lower right first molar demonstrating the narrow area of low density in the periodontium (arrows), highly suggestive for a cracked tooth with radicular extension.

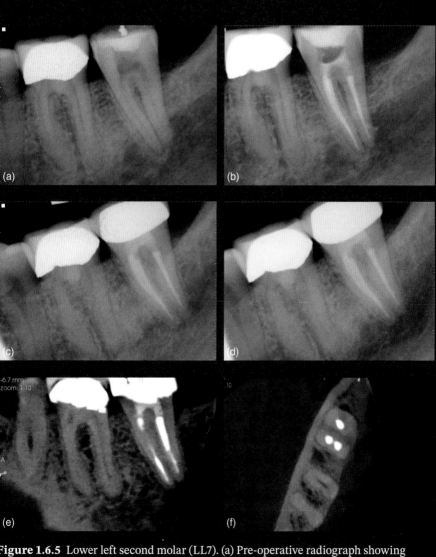

Figure 1.6.5 Lower left second molar (LL7). (a) Pre-operative radiograph showing periapical periodontitis. (b) Immediate post-operative radiograph. (c, d) Two- and eight-year follow-up radiographs, respectively, showing resolution of the apical lesion. (e, f) Eight-year sagittal and axial sections of cone beam computed tomography scan showing isolated distal periodontal defect.

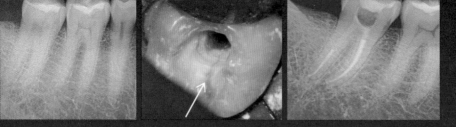

Figure 1.6.6 Angular bone loss on the radiograph suggesting a crack on the distal. Visualisation of the crack under the microscope with placement of a resin-modified glass ionomer intracanal barrier.

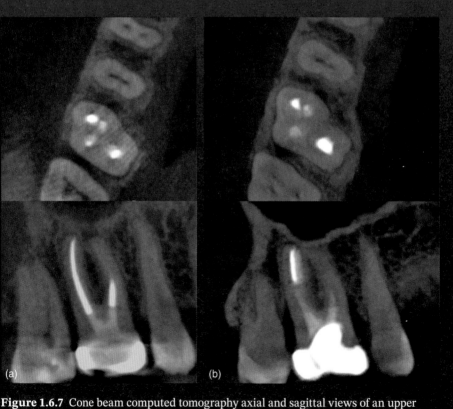

Figure 1.6.7 Cone beam computed tomography axial and sagittal views of an upper right first molar (UR6) exhibiting cracks with radicular extension at both the mesial and distal surfaces. (a) Three-year follow-up images and (b) seven-year follow-up images showing minimal to no change in the appearance of the isolated, narrow periodontal defects over four years.

Further Reading

Chen, Y., Hsu, T., Liu, H., and Chogle, S. (2021). Factors related to the outcomes of cracked teeth after endodontic treatment. *Journal of Endodontics* 47 (2): 215–220.

Davis, M.C. and Shariff, S.S. (2019). Success and survival of endodontically treated cracked teeth with radicular extensions: a 2- to 4-year prospective cohort. *Journal of Endodontics* 45 (7): 848–855.

Krell, K.V. and Rivera, E.M. (2007). A six year evaluation of cracked teeth diagnosed with reversible pulpitis: treatment and prognosis. *Journal of Endodontics* 33 (12): 1405–1407.

Rivera, E.M. and Walton, R.E. (2007). Longitudinal tooth fractures: findings that contribute to complex endodontic diagnoses. *Endodontic Topics* 13 (1): 82–111.

1.7 *Vertical Root Fracture*

Shanon Patel and Peng-Hui Teng

Objective

At the end of this case, the reader should be familiar with the diagnosis of vertical root fracture (VRF). The reader should also know the aetiology and treatment options available for VRF.

Introduction

A 62-year-old man presented to his general dental practitioner with intermittent dull ache associated with his previously root-treated lower right first molar (LR6). He was then referred to an endodontic specialist for further management of the LR6.

Chief Complaint

The patient complained of occasional episodes of dull pain on the LR6 for the last few weeks. The patient had the LR6 root canal treated and restored with a metal ceramic crown over 15 years ago by an endodontist and had been asymptomatic until now.

The patient was managing his symptoms with over-the-counter analgesics. However, the patient still experienced mild discomfort on biting on the tooth.

Medical History

Unremarkable.

Dental History

The patient was a regular dental attender for routine check-ups with his general dentist and twice-a-year maintenance appointments with his dental hygienist.

Pitt Ford's Problem-Based Learning in Endodontology, Second Edition. Edited by Elizabeth Shin Perry, Shanon Patel, Shalini Kanagasingam, and Samantha Hamer. © 2025 John Wiley & Sons Ltd. Published 2025 by John Wiley & Sons Ltd.

Clinical and Radiographic Examination

Extraoral examination was unremarkable. Intraoral examination revealed a moderately restored and well-maintained dentition with good levels of oral hygiene.

The LR6 was restored with a well-adapted metal ceramic crown. The LR6 was tender to percussion but not tender on palpation. The periodontal probing depths and mobility of the LR6 were within normal range. No swelling or sinus tract was associated with the LR6. There were no signs of endodontic or periodontal disease associated with the adjacent teeth or opposing teeth. Occlusal assessment revealed there was group function in lateral excursions.

A periapical radiograph (PR; Figure 1.7.1) was taken to investigate the LR6. What did the radiograph reveal about the LR6?

- Normal horizontal bone levels.
- Crown with well-adapted margins.
- Existing root canal filling had several voids at the canal entrance level.
- The mesial root fillings were approximately 2–3 mm short from the radiographic apex while the distal root fillings appeared to be well condensed and to length.
- A periapical radiolucency was associated with the mesial and distal roots of the LR6.

A small field-of-view cone beam computed tomography (CBCT) scan was taken to explore other causes, such as untreated root canal(s). The sagittal CBCT (Figure 1.7.2a) revealed similar findings to the PR with a well-defined periapical radiolucency on the LR6. However, in the coronal and axial slices (Figure 1.7.2b–d), periradicular radiolucencies were detected on the buccal aspect of the mesial root and lingual aspect of the distal root. These periradicular radiolucencies were separate to and not continuous with the periapical radiolucency.

What are the limitations of periapical radiographs?

PRs compress three-dimensional structures into two-dimensional images. While the radiographic changes on mesial and distal surfaces can be appreciated on PRs, the radiographic changes on the buccal or lingual surfaces will be either missed or underestimated, especially in the multi-rooted teeth where the buccal and lingual/palatal roots overlap. 'Anatomical noise' such as the thick cortical plate in the posterior mandibular region may obscure the area of interest, resulting in difficulty in detecting subtle radiographic changes such as periradicular bone loss in the LR6 in this case. Parallax PRs may provide useful information about the overlapping root canals and localisation of radiographic lesions, but the information is often insufficient for accurate diagnosis and treatment planning.

Can CBCT help in diagnosing vertical root fracture?

CBCT has insufficient sensitivity and accuracy to detect a VRF *within* the root. One of the reasons is that these three-dimensional images do not have sufficient resolution. CBCT images may be impaired by beam hardening due to the presence of radiopaque intracanal materials (i.e. gutta percha, metallic posts, etc.) and/or motion/misalignments. These imaging artefacts will affect the quality of the CBCT images and may result in misdiagnosis. However, there is good evidence that CBCT is more reliable and sensitive than PRs in detecting subtle *periradicular bone loss*, which is often associated to a VRF. With CBCT, the tooth of interest can be assessed in three dimensions without any anatomical noise and distortion.

The European Society of Endodontology CBCT position statement (ESE 2019) and the Joint American Association of Endodontists and American Academy of Oral & Maxillofacial Radiology guidelines (AAE/AAOMR 2015) recommend the use of CBCT when clinical and/or PR findings are inconclusive in cases of suspected VRF. Based on the clinical and conventional PR findings only, the LR6 would have been diagnosed as previously treated symptomatic apical periodontitis, which may have resulted in a decision to attempt root canal retreatment. The isolated periradicular bone loss associated with the LR6 was clearly visualised with CBCT. The CBCT findings confirmed the diagnosis of VRF, thereby impacting clinical decision making.

Diagnosis and Treatment Planning

What is the diagnosis?

The diagnosis for the LR6 was previously treated symptomatic apical periodontitis associated with a VRF.

What are the common clinical and radiographical findings of vertical root fracture?

What are the aetiologies of vertical root fracture?

The exact aetiology of VRF is not well understood, but several risk factors have been suggested (Tables 1.7.1–1.7.3).

What are the treatment options for vertical root fracture?

The treatment objectives for VRF are to prevent the ingress of microorganisms into the tooth through the fracture line and prevent further destruction to the adjacent supporting periodontal tissue. In the majority of cases, extraction of the affected tooth is the only treatment choice for VRF. Treatment should

Table 1.7.1 Clinical features of vertical root fracture (VRF).

- Symptoms and/or signs of apical periodontitis (e.g. tenderness to percussion and/or palpation, swelling, etc.)
- Pain on biting
- Presence of fracture line clinically
- Deep, narrow, isolated periodontal probing depth (may be present on both sides of a root)
- Presence of sinus tract(s) (multiple sinus tracts are pathognomonic features of VRF)
- Increased tooth mobility

Table 1.7.2 Radiographic features of vertical root fracture.

Highly variable, may present with one or more of the following:

- Subtle periradicular and/or crestal bone loss
- Thickening of periodontal ligament along the lateral aspect of the root
- Classic J-shaped radiolucency and/or halo radiolucency often involving furcation region
- Frank separation of root fragments

Table 1.7.3 Risk factors for vertical root fracture in root-filled teeth.

- Minimal remaining tooth structure
- Presence of preexisting (micro)cracks and fractures
- Change in biochemical properties (viscoelasticity, dehydration, etc.) of dentine of root-treated teeth
- Parafunctional habits
- Loss of canine guidance
- Posterior location of teeth, particularly the last standing molar due to occlusal loading
- Diets inclusive of hard food such as betel nut and bones
- Root canal anatomy and morphology such as hourglass-shaped root canal cross-sections or increased root canal curvature
- Excessive removal of pericervical dentine during root canal instrumentation and/or post space preparation
- Excessive force during obturation of root canal treatment (RCT)
- Prolonged usage of intracanal irrigants and/or medicaments
- Absence of cuspal coverage restoration after RCT

be done as soon as VRF is diagnosed to prevent further periradicular bone loss that may impair future prosthodontic treatment, especially if implant placement is planned as well as to minimise acute symptoms.

In multi-root treated teeth where the root fracture is confined to a single root only, root amputation of the affected root or hemi-section may be considered as an alternative option to preserve the tooth. Root canal treatment should be completed prior to the root resection, with the root canal filling removed below the level of root resection and sealed with composite resin or glass-ionomer cement. Root amputation and hemi-section have been reported as treatment options with long-term survival in several studies and systematic reviews, but the results of these studies should be interpreted with caution, as root resections in these studies were mostly done on teeth with perio-endo lesions rather than VRF. Therefore, the teeth included in these studies may not be as structurally compromised as teeth requiring root resection due to VRF.

Other treatment options such as surgical repair of the fractured root with restorative/bioactive materials are not recommended due to the lack of evidence in the literature.

Treatment

Due to the poor prognosis of this tooth, a decision was made to extract the LR6.

Discussion

Although VRFs may occur in teeth with vital pulps, the majority of VRFs are associated with root-filled teeth. VRFs may begin apically or coronally and are more commonly detected in the bucco-lingual plane than in the mesio-distal plane. VRF is classified into incomplete and complete VRF: incomplete if it involves only one side of the root and complete if it extends from one side to the opposite side of the root.

It is often challenging to detect and diagnose VRFs as they may develop slowly without any signs and symptoms at an early stage. In general, teeth with VRFs have poor prognoses. Therefore, it is crucial to prevent or reduce the likelihood of VRF, especially in root-filled teeth with compromised tooth structure.

How can vertical root fractures be reduced or prevented?

- Patient education on parafunction habits and management.
- Reestablishment of canine guidance.
- Occlusal splint.
- Botox to the muscles of mastication.
- Conservative (but pragmatic) access to cavity and root canal instrumentation during endodontic treatment.
- Preservation of pericervical dentine.
- Posts (when indicated) should be passively cemented.
- Timely restoration with a cuspal coverage restoration.

- The use of gold or monolithic all-ceramic materials for cuspal coverage restoration is recommended, as they require only minimal preparation of the residual tooth structure.

The presence of proximal contacts may help to mitigate excessive occlusal loading on root-filled teeth and prevent VRFs. Therefore, in the patient with multiple missing posterior teeth, replacement of the missing teeth should be considered to increase the number of occlusal contacts and distribute the occlusal forces more evenly.

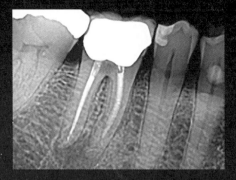

Figure 1.7.1 Periapical radiograph of the LR6.

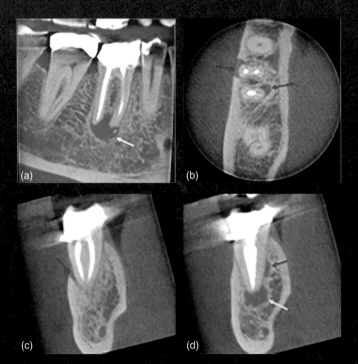

Figure 1.7.2 Small field-of-view cone beam computed tomography of tooth LR6.
(a) Sagittal image revealed periapical radiolucency (yellow arrow) similar to a
periapical radiograph. (b–d) Axial and coronal images revealed separate periradicular
radiolucencies (red arrows) at the buccal aspect of the mesial root and lingual aspect
of the distal root, which were not continuous with the periapical radiolucency
(yellow arrow).

Further Reading

AAE, AAOMR (2015). Special committee to revise the joint AAE and AAOMR position statement on use of CBCT in endodontics. AAE and AAOMR joint position statement: use of cone beam computed tomography in endodontics 2015 update. *Oral Surgery, Oral Medicine, Oral Pathology and Oral Radiology* 120: 508–512.

Byakova, S.F., Novozhilova, N.E., Makeeva, I.M. et al. (2019). The accuracy of CBCT for the detection and diagnosis of vertical root fractures in vivo. *International Endodontic Journal* 52: 1255–1263.

European Society of Endodontology (ESE) (2019). European Society of Endodontology position statement: use of cone beam computed tomography in endodontics. *International Endodontic Journal* 52: 1675–1678.

European Society of Endodontology, Mannocci, F., Bhuva, B. et al. (2021). European Society of Endodontology position statement: the restoration of root filled teeth. *International Endodontic Journal* 54: 1974–1981.

Fuss, Z., Lustig, J., Katz, A., and Tamse, A. (2001). An evaluation of endodontically treated vertical root fractured teeth: impact of operative procedures. *Journal of Endodontics* 27: 46–48.

Patel, S., Bhuva, B., and Bose, R. (2022). Present status and future directions: vertical root fractures in root filled teeth. *International Endodontic Journal* 55 (Suppl. 3): 804–826.

Patel, S., Brady, E., Wilson, R. et al. (2013). The detection of vertical root fractures in root filled teeth with periapical radiographs and CBCT scans. *International Endodontic Journal* 46: 1140–1152.

1.8 Endodontic-Periodontal Infections

Shalini Kanagasingam, Elizabeth Shin Perry, and Nargis Sonde

Objectives

At the end of this case, the reader will be able to evaluate and classify an endodontic-periodontal lesion according to the 2017 World Workshop on the Classification of Periodontal and Peri-implant Diseases and Conditions and gain an understanding of how to manage endodontic-periodontal lesions.

Introduction

A 56-year-old patient was referred to the Endodontic clinic from the Periodontology Department for a symptomatic lower left first molar (LL6). She had no history of periodontal disease, but presented with a localised pocket that was unresponsive to non-surgical periodontal treatment. An opinion was sought regarding the endodontic lesion noted on the corresponding periapical for this tooth.

Chief Complaint

The patient presented with an intermittent dull ache well localised to the LL6. The onset of pain was first noticed when eating and did not require analgesics to manage the symptoms. The patient reported swelling in this area with the occasional episode of a bad taste.

Medical History

Unremarkable.

Pitt Ford's Problem-Based Learning in Endodontology, Second Edition. Edited by Elizabeth Shin Perry, Shanon Patel, Shalini Kanagasingam, and Samantha Hamer.
© 2025 John Wiley & Sons Ltd. Published 2025 by John Wiley & Sons Ltd.

Dental History

The patient was a regular attender to her general dental practitioner, seeing them for six-monthly recalls. She had been referred to the Periodontology Department for an unresolving pocket with a suspected endodontic-periodontal lesion. The symptomatic tooth was restored with a crown only a few months prior to symptoms starting and no endodontic treatment had been done.

Clinical Examination

Extraoral examination was unremarkable. Intraoral soft tissue examination showed mild inflammation of the gingivae on the LL6.

The hard tissue examination showed a well-restored dentition, with missing third molars in all quadrants. Closer examination of the LL6 showed a well-fitting porcelain fused to metal (PFM) crown with no signs of swelling or sinus evident on this tooth, but it was tender to percussion (TTP). No active carious lesions were found and the margins of existing restorations appeared sound. An isolated pocket on the mid-buccal aspect of the LL6 warranted a detailed periodontal assessment. Oral hygiene was good, with minimal plaque deposits evident prior to disclosing.

Pulp testing was performed using electronic pulp testing (EPT) and cold sensitivity testing with Endo-Ice, which elicited a normal positive response from all teeth tested, apart from the LL6.

What did the radiographs reveal?

A periapical radiograph of the LL6 showed less than 25% bone loss on a tooth with a PFM crown (Figure 1.8.1). A periapical lesion was evident and appeared to involve the mesial and distal roots as well as the furcation region. There appeared to be widening of the periodontal ligament space LL7, but a lack of symptoms or evidence of disease warranted no clinical input aside from monitoring.

How did the tooth devitalise in the absence of caries?

Teeth devitalise due to a variety of reasons, though caries is the main factor. Another reason for a tooth devitalising includes thermal injury to the pulp, which can occur from cavity preparation. The LL6 was restored with a PFM crown, which is a less conservative preparation than an all-metal crown. The rates of pulp death over a 10-year period vary depending on the level of preparation, but studies have found this can be as high as 15–20% for PFM crowns. The rates of pulp death decrease where less tooth reduction is undertaken. All teeth planned for an extracoronal restoration should undergo sensibility testing before treatment to limit complications of undertaking endodontic access through a crown. The most common forms of sensibility testing include the use of EPT or temperature testing. Historically ethyl chloride has been widely used to cold test teeth for vitality. However, this is now being replaced with refrigerant sprays such as Endo-Ice and Endo-Frost, which can reach much lower temperatures at −26 and −50 °C, respectively. These lower temperatures allow for more accurate sensibility testing, particularly where a crown is present.

What did the periodontal examination reveal?

Periodontal assessment showed an isolated broad 10 mm pocket on the mid-buccal aspect of the LL6, with no other probing pocket depths exceeding 2 mm (Chart 1.8.1). A Grade I furcation was noted on the buccal aspect of the LL6 (notated as 36 in the periodontal chart). Plaque scores were calculated to be 18% following disclosing and bleeding scores were 15%.

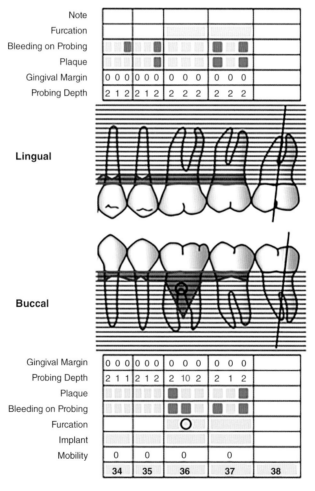

Chart 1.8.1 A section of the detailed pocket chart for the lower left sextant showing a localised pocket on the LL6 with bleeding on probing in this area. Only part of the chart has been included for relevance as no other abnormalities were noted.

How is furcation involvement classified and how does it affect prognosis?

Furcations are present on all multi-rooted teeth and it is imperative that they are explored during a periodontal assessment with a suitably designed probe, such as a Naber's probe. The level of furcation involvement is classified based on how far the probe penetrates:

- Grade I involves the probe being inserted up to a third of the furcation width.
- Grade II has the probe going further than a third of the furcation width, but it does not go all the way through.
- Grade III occurs where the probe can be inserted the full width of the furcation through to the other side.

The presence of a furcation indicates a significant loss of supporting attachment and would be seen in Stage III and IV of periodontitis, which require more complex management. In such cases the prognosis is reduced due to the loss of bone support and the increased likelihood of mobility.

What are the anatomical connections between the dental pulp and the periodontium?

The anatomical connections between the dental pulp and the periodontium are illustrated in Figure 1.8.2. The following features provide a pathway for endodontic-periodontal communication that can lead to combined lesions:

- Apical foramen
- Lateral or accessory canals
- Dentinal tubules
- Perforations
- Fractures
- Resorption

What are the classifications for endodontic-periodontal lesions?

Prior to the introduction of the 2017 Classification, the most widely used system for the classification of endodontic-periodontal infections was Simon's (1972). This is still the most used classification system among endodontists, but relies specifically on the chronology of the disease process, with limited information about the clinical picture in relation to the lesion. The classification of endo-periodontal lesions is much broader since the introduction of the 2017 Periodontal Classification. Endo-periodontal lesions fall into two broad categories under the 2017 Periodontal Classification system: where there is root damage, and where there is not. Root damage can occur in the form of fractures, perforations and resorption and, when evident, will reduce the prognosis of any proposed treatment due to the added complications of such pathology. Where an endo-periodontal lesion exists with the absence of any obvious root damage, it is further separated based on whether the patient has a known history of periodontal disease or not. A patient with active periodontal disease will have a reduced prognosis due to the reduced bony support commonly seen in such patients. A grading system is used thereafter, but its parameters are the same regardless of whether the patient has periodontal disease or not (Table 1.8.1). The grading is as follows:

- Grade 1 – a narrow deep pocket on one tooth surface
- Grade 2 – a wide deep pocket on one tooth surface
- Grade 3 – a deep pocket on more than one tooth surface

Table 1.8.1 A summary of the 2017 Classification of endo-periodontal lesions.

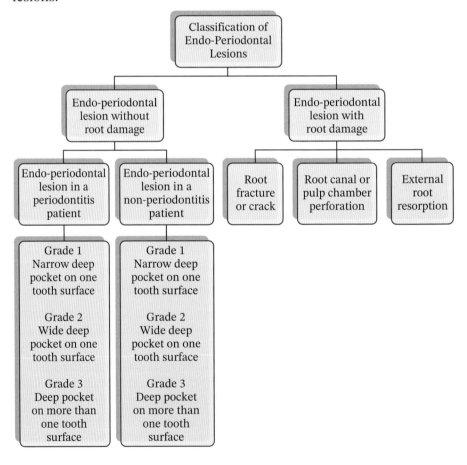

The presence of two distinct disease processes at the same site will complicate whether a site can be declared stable due to the need for both treatment modalities to be successful. The 2017 Classification allows for greater information to be relayed between clinicians on the extent of the endodontic-periodontal infection.

Diagnosis

A diagnosis of a Grade 2 endodontic-periodontal lesion was made on tooth LL6 using the 2017 Classification. However, if utilising Simon's classification it would be a primary endodontic lesion with secondary periodontal involvement. A quick guide to determining the chronology of endo-periodontal lesions can be found in Table 1.8.2.

Table 1.8.2 A summary of the clinical features of endodontic-periodontal lesions.

Diagnosis	Radiographic appearance	Restoration status	Clinical testing
Primary endodontic lesion	Apical radiolucency	Caries + Trauma + Restored +	TTP + Sensibility testing −
Primary periodontal lesion	Radiographic bone loss	Caries ± Restored ±	Sensibility testing + Pocketing + Mobile +
Combined lesion	Apical radiolucency Radiographic bone loss	Caries + Trauma + Restored +	TTP + Sensibility testing − Pocketing + Mobile +
Concomitant lesion	Apical radiolucency Radiographic bone loss Both appear independent of each other	Caries + Trauma + Restored +	TTP + Sensibility testing − Pocketing + Mobile +

What other differential diagnoses should be considered?

The endodontic and periodontal findings associated with endodontic-periodontal lesions are similar to several other pathological entities such as vertical root fractures, periodontal bone loss resulting from complications during endodontic treatment, anatomical defects such as deep grooves and, in rare cases, intra-alveolar malignancies and metastatic diseases. Careful assessment of patient history and meticulous clinical examinations utilising magnification are required to diagnose accurately. In some cases, surgical exposure or biopsy may also be necessary to establish a proper diagnosis.

Treatment Planning

Once the diagnosis was reached and explained to the patient, the treatment options were discussed. When an endodontic-periodontal lesion is diagnosed, the endodontic component is addressed prior to the periodontal element. This is because the periodontal issues are unlikely to resolve if the endodontic issue is left untreated or where endodontic treatment fails. The treatment options discussed for LL6 were:

- Non-surgical root canal treatment followed by non-surgical periodontal therapy should the pocket persist.
- Extraction.
- No treatment to be undertaken, but the patient was warned that the tooth may deteriorate, become increasingly painful and eventually be lost.

The patient was motivated to keep the tooth and opted for endodontic and periodontal treatment.

Treatment

The endodontic treatment was carried out in a single visit. Isolation was achieved with dental dam and clamp, and three canals (mesio-buccal, mesio-lingual and distal) were identified and prepared with rotary instruments. Sodium hypochlorite was used as an irrigant, with a penultimate rinse with ethylenediaminetetraacetic acid (EDTA) before the canals were dried. The canals were obturated with a warm vertical condensation technique and the access cavity restored with composite. The postoperative periapical radiograph showed a well-condensed root filling at working length with slight sealer extrusion evident on the mesial canals

(Figure 1.8.3). The minimal access cavity was achieved through the PFM crown, which can be seen post obturation (Figure 1.8.4).

How soon after the completion of endodontic treatment should periodontal therapy be undertaken?

There remains considerable debate between dental professionals about when the periodontal phase of treatment should be undertaken following endodontic therapy. Typically, in the case of a combined lesion or where primary periodontal disease is suspected, both therapies should be done as close together as possible to limit the chances of reinfection. Where a primary endodontic lesion is suspected, periodontal reevaluation is undertaken two to three months after endodontic treatment has been completed. This is to allow enough time to determine whether endodontic treatment has been effective and the true extent of the periodontal problem remaining. In some cases, the pocket may resolve following completion of root canal treatment and further treatment may be unnecessary. If a period of healing is not observed and debridement is undertaken too soon, there is an increased risk of damage to the periodontal ligament and cementum.

Periodontal review

The periodontal review took place three months after the LL6 was obturated. The patient was asymptomatic and reported no episodes of pain, swelling or bad taste following the completion of endodontic treatment. The mid-buccal pocket depth had reduced to 5 mm, had no suppuration but still bled on probing, so underwent non-surgical periodontal therapy under local anaesthetic using fine ultrasonic tips (Chart 1.8.2). The subsequent three-month review (six months post root canal treatment, RCT) showed a further reduction of the pocket depth to 3 mm with no bleeding on probing and the patient remained symptom free (Chart 1.8.3). There were no other sites of pocketing noted at any of the appointments and oral hygiene was observed to be excellent. She was reviewed once more with the Periodontology Department prior to being discharged with a maintenance plan for the general practitioner.

Endodontic review

A review radiograph was taken at six months showing that the radiolucent area remained but had not increased in size (Figure 1.8.5). In the absence of any symptoms or clinical signs of active disease, a decision was made to monitor the tooth. At the 12-month endodontic review the patient had no complaints. Probing depths were 2 mm, with no bleeding on probing (Chart 1.8.4). A periapical taken at the 12-month review showed a smaller

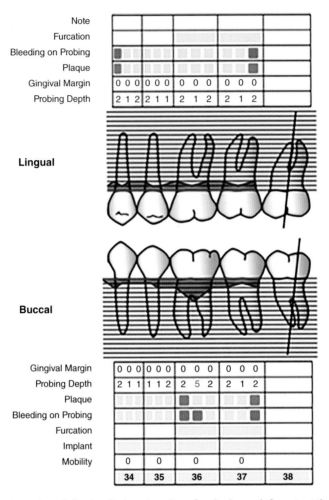

	Note												
	Furcation												
	Bleeding on Probing												
	Plaque												
	Gingival Margin	0	0	0	0	0	0	0	0	0	0	0	0
	Probing Depth	2	1	2	2	1	1	2	1	2	2	1	2

Lingual

Buccal

	Gingival Margin	0	0	0	0	0	0	0	0	0	0	0	0
	Probing Depth	2	1	1	1	1	2	2	5	2	2	1	2
	Plaque												
	Bleeding on Probing												
	Furcation												
	Implant												
	Mobility		0			0			0			0	
			34			35			36			37		38

Chart 1.8.2 A section of the detailed pocket chart for the lower left sextant three months post obturation showing a 5 mm pocket on the LL6 with bleeding. Pocket reduction is evident when compared to baseline charting, but a pocket ≥5 mm would still be considered unstable.

radiolucent area indicative of healing (Figure 1.8.6). Endodontic review was continued on an annual basis for the LL6, showing continued healing and eventually complete resolution of the periapical lesion on the LL6 (Figures 1.8.7–1.8.9). It is important to continue to monitor an area of pathology even where a patient remains asymptomatic until complete healing is seen. This is to ensure that the disease process is resolving and that the correct diagnosis and management were undertaken. Treatment had been deemed successful with a good long-term prognosis for the tooth and so the patient was discharged to the care of her own dentist.

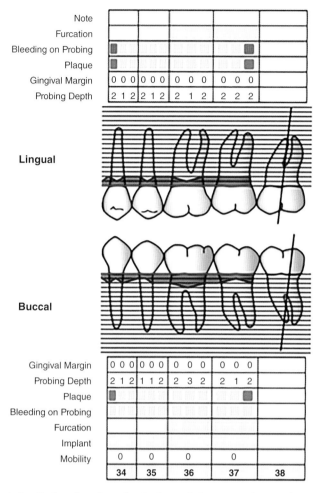

Note				
Furcation				
Bleeding on Probing	▓			▓
Plaque	▓			▓
Gingival Margin	0 0 0	0 0 0	0 0 0	0 0 0
Probing Depth	2 1 2	2 1 2	2 1 2	2 2 2

Lingual

Buccal

Gingival Margin	0 0 0	0 0 0	0 0 0	0 0 0
Probing Depth	2 1 2	1 1 2	2 3 2	2 1 2
Plaque	▓			▓
Bleeding on Probing				
Furcation				
Implant				
Mobility	0	0	0	0
	34	35	36	37	38

Chart 1.8.3 A detailed pocket chart for the lower left sextant six months post obturation showing resolution of the previous mid-buccal pocket on the LL6 with no bleeding.

Discussion

Most endodontic-periodontal lesions have poor prognosis due to extensive bone loss having occurred by the time the correct diagnosis is made. Impeded by inconsistent results of special investigations, for example a positive result to sensibility testing on a multi-rooted tooth, gives the impression that the tooth is vital pointing to a periodontal cause. In reality part of the pulpal tissue may be necrotic and an endodontic lesion may not be visible radiographically at the time. The case discussed was a primary endodontic lesion with secondary periodontal involvement so cannot be deemed a true combined lesion; however, the management in either case would be the same, with the endodontic treatment being done before the periodontal treatment.

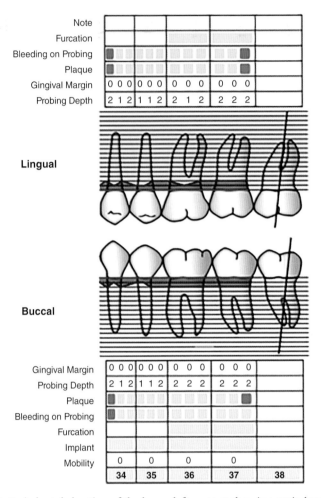

Chart 1.8.4 Periodontal charting of the lower left sextant showing periodontal stability.

It is pertinent for the clinician to keep an open mind about other pathologies when investigating, especially in a case where conventional treatment based on an earlier diagnosis has failed with no clear reason. In cases which exhibit large, J-shaped, tear-drop shaped or halo shaped periapical lesions, clinicians should rule out vertical root fracture. An incorrect diagnosis will lead to the provision of inappropriate or insufficient treatment. The patient was an ideal case for treatment as her level of plaque control was excellent throughout and the endodontic treatment was relatively straightforward on a tooth with an intact existing PFM crown. Good case selection is essential when treatment planning or determining prognosis.

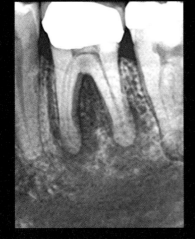

Figure 1.8.1 Pre-operative periapical radiograph of LL6.

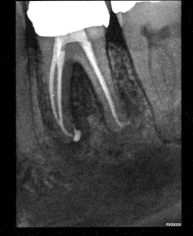

Figure 1.8.3 Post-obturation radiograph of LL6 shows a well-condensed root filling is to length in all canals, with no voids. There is slight sealer extrusion on the mesial canals.

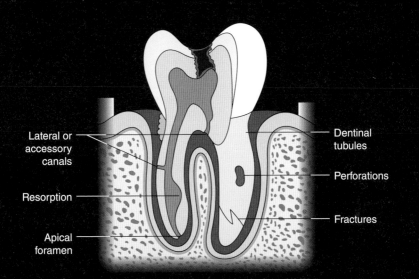

Lateral or accessory canals

Resorption

Apical foramen

Dentinal tubules

Perforations

Fractures

Figure 1.8.2 A diagrammatic representation of the many routes that can lead to the development of an endodontic-periodontal lesion.

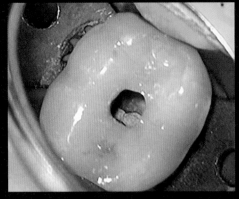

Figure 1.8.4 A conservative access cavity was done through the existing crown as there were no concerns about secondary caries under the crown.

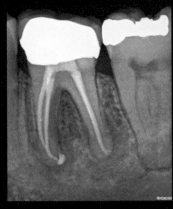

Figure 1.8.5 A periapical taken at six months post obturation review showing no further expansion of the radiolucent lesion.

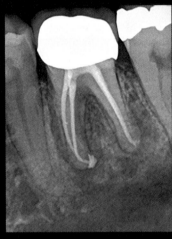

Figure 1.8.6 A periapical radiograph of the LL6 at the 12-month post-operative review.

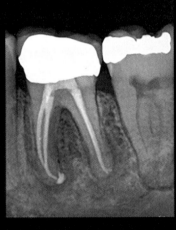

Figure 1.8.7 Periapical radiograph taken at two-year post-operative review.

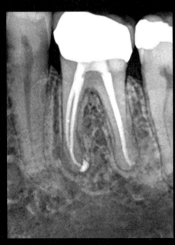

Figure 1.8.8 Three-year post-operative periapical radiograph showing healing.

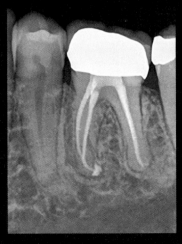

Figure 1.8.9 Four-year review periapical radiograph shows that the pre-operative periapical radiolucency is no longer evident following

Further Reading

Chen, E. and Abbott, P.V. (2009). Dental pulp testing: a review. *International Journal of Dentistry* 2009: 1–12.

Cheung, G.S., Lai, S.C., and Ng, R.P. (2005). Fate of vital pulps beneath a metal-ceramic crown or a bridge retainer. *International Endodontic Journal* 38 (8): 521–530.

De Morais, C.A.H., Bernardineli, N., Lima, W.M. et al. (2008). Evaluation of the temperature of different refrigerant sprays used as a pulpal test. *Australian Endodontic Journal* 34: 86–88.

Hazard, M.L., Wicker, C., Qian, F. et al. (2021). Accuracy of cold sensibility testing on teeth with full-coverage restorations: a clinical study. *International Endodontic Journal* 54 (7): 1008–1015.

Herrera, D., Retamal Valdes, B., Alonso, B., and Feres, M. (2018). Acute periodontal lesions (periodontal abscesses and necrotising periodontal diseases) and endoperiodontal lesions. *Journal of Clinical Periodontology* 45 (Suppl 20): S78–S94.

Lang, N.P. and Tonetti, M.S. (2003). Periodontal risk assessment (PRA) for patients in supportive periodontal therapy (SPT). *Oral Health and Preventive Dentistry* 1: 7–16.

Papapanou, P.N., Sanz, M. et al. (2018). Periodontitis: consensus report of workgroup 2 of the 2017 world workshop on the classification of periodontal and Peri-implant diseases and conditions. *Journal of Periodontology* 89 (Suppl 1): S173–S182.

Rotstein, I. and Simon, J.H. (2006). The endo-perio lesion: a critical appraisal of the disease condition. *Endodontic Topics* 13: 34–56.

Schmidt, J.C., Walter, C., Amato, M., and Weiger, R. (2014). Treatment of periodontal-endodontic lesions – a systematic review. *Journal of Clinical Periodontology* 41: 779–790.

Simon, J.H., Glick, D.H., and Frank, A.L. (1972). The relationship of endodontic-periodontal lesions. *Journal of Periodontology* 43: 202–208.

Tonetti, M.S., Greenwell, H., and Kornman, K.S. (2018). Staging and grading of periodontitis: framework and proposal of a new classification and case definition. *Journal of Clinical Periodontology* 45 (Suppl 20): S149–S161.

1.9 *Cemento-osseous Dysplasia*

Rahul Bose and Simon Harvey

Objectives

At the end of this case, the reader should appreciate the importance of a thorough history and clinical examination to diagnose and manage cemento-osseous dysplasia.

Introduction

A 38-year-old female patient was referred by her general dental practitioner (GDP) to the endodontic unit at Guy's Dental Hospital (London, UK) for investigation of periapical radiolucencies affecting the mandibular incisor teeth.

Chief Complaint

The patient was asymptomatic on presentation to the endodontic unit.

Medical History

Unremarkable.

Dental History

The patient was due to undertake orthodontic treatment to manage relapse of her lower anterior teeth. An orthopantomogram (OPG) taken by the orthodontist revealed an incidental finding of periapical radiolucencies associated with her mandibular central incisor teeth. To further assess the lower incisors, a periapical was taken by her GDP (Figure 1.9.1) and based on the findings a provisional diagnosis of chronic apical periodontitis was made for the LL1 and LR1. However, prior to commencing root canal treatment, the GDP sought a second opinion from the endodontic unit to confirm the

Pitt Ford's Problem-Based Learning in Endodontology, Second Edition. Edited by Elizabeth Shin Perry, Shanon Patel, Shalini Kanagasingam, and Samantha Hamer. © 2025 John Wiley & Sons Ltd. Published 2025 by John Wiley & Sons Ltd.

presence of disease. The patient was unaware of any previous history of traumatic dental injury.

Clinical Examination

Extraoral examination was unremarkable, and the soft tissues were healthy with presence of bilateral mandibular tori (Figure 1.9.2).

The patient had an unrestored dentition, and her oral hygiene and periodontal status were good.

The LL1 and LR1 responded to electric and thermal sensibility tests. The LL1 and LR1 were not tender to palpation or percussion and there was no associated swelling, sinus or mobility. Periodontal probing depths were within normal limits. The adjacent teeth were clinically sound.

What other investigations can be performed to aid in diagnosis?

A small-volume, high-resolution cone beam computed tomography (CBCT) scan (Figure 1.9.3) was taken in line with the European Society of Endodontology (ESE) criteria (detection of radiographic signs of periapical pathosis when the signs and/or symptoms are non-specific and plain film imaging is inconclusive).

The scan revealed presence of a mixed radiolucent and radiopaque lesion at the periapical area of the LL1 and the LR1.

Diagnosis

A diagnosis of periapical cemento-osseous dysplasia was made for the LL1 and LR1.

Why are special tests crucial in diagnosis of cemento-osseous dysplasia?

A thorough history and examination along with special tests are required to avoid a definitive diagnosis made solely on radiographic examination. Teeth presenting with cemento-osseous dysplasia are typically vital, not displaced or resorbed, with no signs of jaw expansion. The size of the lesion is small, usually only up to 5 mm in diameter. Periapical radiolucency may be similar in appearance to a tooth with chronic apical periodontitis, but in fact the appearance is secondary to the early stages of cemento-osseous dysplasia. Misinterpretation of pathosis on a radiograph may lead to inappropriate endodontic or surgical treatment.

Treatment

To treat or not to treat cemento-osseous dysplasia?

This condition is not of infective or inflammatory origin; The development and maturation of the lesion are self-limiting. Hence conservative management and periodic monitoring are recommended. Endodontic or surgical treatment is not indicated and will not have any impact on the progression of the lesion.

In this case, the LL1 and LR1 were monitored and the GDP was advised to review the teeth annually.

Discussion

What is cemento-osseous dysplasia?

Cemento-osseous dysplasia is a benign condition (non-neoplastic process) in which normal bone near the root apices is replaced with a mixture of connective tissue, abnormal bone and cementum. It is associated with the structures of the periodontal ligament (PDL) commonly affecting the mandibular anterior teeth, but can also present in posterior teeth. It is more prevalent in females aged 40+ years and of African/Afro-Caribbean descent.

This condition is also known as fibro-cemento-osseous dysplasia and osseous dysplasia. However, the World Health Organization (WHO) classification of odontogenic tumours prefers the term cemento-osseous dysplasia.

What is the aetiology of cemento-osseous dysplasia?

The aetiology of this condition is unknown and it is regarded as an idiopathic reactive lesion.

What are the various stages involved in cemento-osseous dysplasia and possible associated differential diagnosis?

There are three stages involved in this disease process. The condition can be expressed at an early stage as a radiolucent lesion, which can be deceptively similar to chronic apical periodontitis. Histopathology reveals this to be mainly fibrous tissue. An intermediate stage can arise with progression to a mixed radiolucent-radiopaque state as calcification begins to occur within the fibrous matrix. At the mature stage the lesion can become densely radiopaque with a variable degree of radiolucency (Table 1.9.1).

Table 1.9.1 The main radiographic features of cemento-osseous dysplasia and associated differential diagnosis at varying stages.

Stage	Radiographic appearance	Differential diagnosis
Early stage	Mainly radiolucent	Chronic apical periodontitis
Intermediate stage	Mixed radiolucent–radioopaque	Osteomyelitis, ossifying fibroma
Mature stage	Mainly radioopaque	Hypercementosis, odontomes

Table 1.9.2 Types of cemento-osseous dysplasia.

Type	Structures involved
Periapical osseous dysplasia	Anterior mandible; involving only a few adjacent teeth
Focal osseous dysplasia	Posterior jaw; involving one or a few adjacent teeth
Florid osseous dysplasia	Multi-quadrant

What are the types of cemento-osseous dysplasia?

The WHO classifies three types of cemento-osseous dysplasia: periapical osseous dysplasia, focal osseous dysplasia and florid osseous dysplasia (Table 1.9.2).

Can there be any symptoms and if so, is any treatment indicated?

Symptoms can occur in an extremely small number of cases. Conservative management is recommended in nearly all cases; however, if symptoms are severe, surgical intervention may be required. Surgical treatment of these lesions is nevertheless controversial and there is low-quality and limited evidence for this intervention.

Can this patient undergo orthodontic treatment?

Yes.

Does this case highlight any other important issues?

From a medico-legal aspect, this case underlines the importance of the process a dentist undertakes to reach an appropriate diagnosis. A second opinion can be vital in avoiding misdiagnosis and inappropriate treatment thereafter.

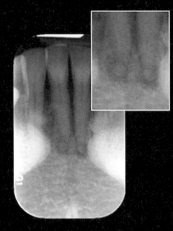

Figure 1.9.1 Periapical radiograph showing bilateral radiopacity overlying the teeth (bilateral mandibular tori); the LL1 and LR1 with intact coronal tooth structure; root canals visible in the coronal to mid-third of the root, with no canals visible in the apical third of the root (fast break), which can often indicate bifurcation of the root canal; periapical radiolucency.

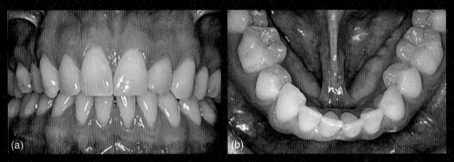

Figure 1.9.2 Clinical photographs: (a) anterior view and (b) occlusal view of the mandibular dentition.

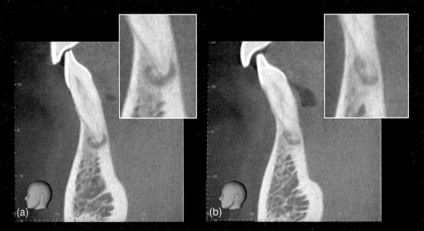

Figure 1.9.3 Cone beam computed tomography scan of the mandibular anterior teeth. (a) Sagittal view of the LL1; (b) sagittal view of the LR1, showing mixed radiolucent and radiopaque lesions at the apices of the LL1 and LR1. LL1 and LR1 both have two canals, as suspected from the fast break seen on the periapical radiograph.

Further Reading

Barnes, L., Eveson, J.W., Reichart, P., and Sidransky, D. (2005). *Pathology and Genetics of Head and Neck Tumours. World Health Organization Classification of Tumours*. Lyon: IARC Press.

Bhasker, S.N. (1966). Periapical lesions—types incidence and clinical features. *Oral Surgery* 21: 657–671.

Ehrmann, E.H. (1977). Pulp testers and pulp testing with particular reference to the use of dry ice. *Australian Dental Journal* 22: 272–279.

Neville, B.W., Damm, D.D., Allen, C.M. et al. (2009). *Oral and Maxillofacial Pathology*, 3e. St. Louis, MO: Saunders.

Patel, S., Brown, J., Semper, M. et al. (2019). European Society of Endodontology position statement: use of cone beam computed tomography in endodontics: European Society of Endodontology (ESE) developed by. *International Endodontic Journal* 52 (12): 1675–1678.

Resnick, C.M. and Novelline, R.A. (2008). Cemento-osseous dysplasia, a radiological mimic of periapical dental abscess. *Emergency Radiology* 15 (6): 367–374.

Smith, S., Patel, K., and Hoskinson, A.E. (1998). Periapical cemental dysplasia: a case of misdiagnosis. *British Dental Journal* 185 (3): 122–123.

Whaites, E. and Drage, N. (2020). *Essentials of Dental Radiography and Radiology*, 6e. New York: Elsevier.

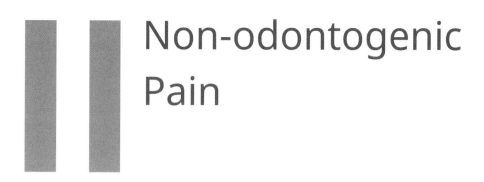

Non-odontogenic Pain

2.1 *Musculoskeletal Pain*

Dermot Canavan

Objectives

On reviewing this case scenario, the reader should appreciate that there are important differences between acute and chronic myofascial disorders in the orofacial region. Most acute muscle or tendon pains can be treated by the general dentist. Chronic musculoskeletal pains tend may have a more complex aetiology and referral to a multi-disciplinary setting may be more appropriate.

Introduction

A 28-year-old Caucasian female patient was referred to the orofacial pain clinic by her general dental practitioner for investigation of persistent dental and facial pain in the left midface area.

Chief Complaint

She described her pain as a persistent nagging discomfort in the upper left posterior teeth, with radiating pain into the left ear at times. Her dental/facial discomfort was present on a continuous basis, but intensity varied between moderate and severe. With higher levels of pain intensity, she also experienced intermittent sharp, stabbing pain that varied in location through the left midface and left hemicranial area. Over a period of time movement of the lower jaw had gradually become painful and restricted. Proprietary analgesics like ibuprofen and acetaminophen (paracetamol) did not alleviate her discomfort. The persistent pain resulted in difficulties in getting to sleep and maintaining sleep.

A review of her history indicated that the patient had been involved in a road traffic accident 12 months earlier. Immediately after the accident she experienced pain in her neck and shoulders bilaterally. But over time, the pain seemed to intensify in the left midface area.

Pitt Ford's Problem-Based Learning in Endodontology, Second Edition. Edited by Elizabeth Shin Perry, Shanon Patel, Shalini Kanagasingam, and Samantha Hamer. © 2025 John Wiley & Sons Ltd. Published 2025 by John Wiley & Sons Ltd.

Previous treatments included root canal treatment on the LL6 and replacement of restorations on the upper left first and second molars, in addition to a course of physiotherapy, anti-inflammatories and muscle-relaxant medications. As her facial pain became more persistent, her tooth site pain became more intense. But the intake of hot or cold drinks did not affect the intensity of her dental discomfort. Likewise, movement of the lower jaw for chewing or talking did not increase her dental pain despite the increase in her facial pain.

Medical History

There was no history of systemic illness prior to the road traffic accident. Subsequent to the accident the patient experienced sleep disruption, anxiety and depression, which she attributed to her chronic pain condition. She had been prescribed the selective serotonin reuptake inhibitor (SSRI) venlafaxine to alleviate these symptoms.

Dental History

This patient was a dental phobic who had a history of infrequent dental attendances, poor oral hygiene and previous extractions of lower left second and third molars under intravenous sedation. When her orofacial pain became intolerable some months after the accident, she sought advice from her general dentist who proceeded to provide root canal therapy on the LL6. He also replaced old restorations on the UL6 and UL7. Despite these dental procedures, her pain continued to increase over time.

Clinical Examination

The diagnosis of persistent orofacial pain complaints must be based on a detailed history and thorough clinical assessment of the head, neck and face (Table 2.1.1). Radiographs are an essential part of the dental assessment, but in themselves are not diagnostic (Figure 2.1.1). Failure to include the head and neck as part of the clinical examination increases the risk of an incomplete diagnosis or misdiagnosis.

What are the key aspects of assessment?

- Cranial nerve examination
- Cervical spine examination
- Musculoskeletal examination
- Intraoral examination

A cranial nerve assessment was carried out with the focus on sensory aspects of the trigeminal nerve. Assessment of the midface areas showed higher levels of responsiveness to the application of cold, light touch and pin prick (extraoral) on the left-hand side. This represents a degree of thermal

Table 2.1.1 Questions relating to a possible diagnosis of chronic myofascial pain in the orofacial region.

Nature of the pain complaint

What words most accurately describe your pain?

Muscular pain is frequently described as 'dull, aching', while words like burning, stinging, sharp shooting more frequently apply to neuropathic pain.

Can you point with one finger to the painful region?

The location of acute muscle pain is usually well defined. In contrast, chronic muscle pain may be more diffuse and difficult to localise, with involvement of several muscle groups.

Is the pain always in the same location or does the location vary?

Pain associated with an acutely inflamed muscle or tendon is usually fixed in location. The intensity and location of chronic myofascial pain are more varied.

How intense is your pain?

Muscle pain tends to remain dull and irritating, often around 3/10 on the 0/10 scale. Headache pain (for example cluster headache) is frequently described as intolerable or excruciating. Neuropathic pain may be severe, but is not always so. Acute toothache may be excruciating but is more easily recognised by dentists. The diffuse dull, recurring pains in the orofacial region are typically more difficult to diagnose.

Can you tell what increases or decreases your pain?

Painful disorders of myofascial tissues will be aggravated by movement or functional activity. This is particularly true in the case of an acute condition. Chronic myofascial pain may also be aggravated by functional movements, but will also be sensitive to changes in mood, anxiety levels, sleep disruption, etc.

Psychosocial factors

What impact is this pain condition having on your life?

Acutely painful disorders of muscle or tendon tissues in the orofacial area will be associated with difficulty chewing, yawning, talking etc. Chronic myofascial pain is also going to be associated with additional factors like disturbance in sleep, changes in mood, inability to concentrate or work or difficulties with personal relationships.

Parafunctional behaviour

Are you conscious of tooth clenching or grinding at night or during the day?

Do you have any other oral habits like fingernail biting, lip/cheek biting or tooth tapping?

Do you have a habit of sucking your thumb or finger?

Do you hold or chew foreign objects with your front teeth like pens/pencils, coins or water bottle caps?

(Continued)

Table 2.1.1 (Continued)

Trauma
Have you ever experienced injury to the face or mouth, for example whiplash injury, sports accidents, a deliberate blow?
Sudden stretching movements like yawning widely can sometimes trigger acute muscle discomfort. Prolonged mouth opening during dental visits may also trigger muscle pain in susceptible patients. Chronic myofascial pain (duration of three months or longer) can also be associated with emotional trauma, as either adult or adolescent.

Jaw movements
Does is hurt to open your mouth, chew hard food, yawn.? Is chewing for a prolonged period of time difficult?
Painful muscles get tired easily. With acute muscle disorders the muscle tiredness is not constant, whereas with chronic myofascial pain patients frequently complain of persistent fatigue/weakness that increases with function.
Does the pain come on immediately when the chewing movement is started or is there a delay between the time of jaw use and the onset of pain?
An immediate onset suggests an inflamed joint, whereas jaw muscle pain tends to hurt more after eating rather than during the meal.

and mechanical sensitivity commonly found in regions of chronic pain (and typically suggestive of central sensitisation). Central sensitisation is a phenomenon whereby intracranial neurons undergo functional change resulting in a lowered threshold for activation, spontaneous impulses or enhanced responses to nociceptive input.

Mobility of the cervical spine was restricted and painful in all dimensions. Palpation of the facet (zygapophyseal) joints on the lateral aspect of the cervical spine elicited significant tenderness at the level of C3/C4 and C4/C5 on the left-hand side.

Muscle palpation in the orofacial region identified widespread tenderness in the masseter and anterior temporalis muscles on the left-hand side (Figure 2.1.2). Increased levels of tenderness were also noted in the superior head of the sternocleidomastoid (SCM) and trapezius muscles. Muscle trigger points were identified in both the superficial aspect of the left masseter and the superior head of the left trapezius muscle. A trigger point is a taut band of muscle that when palpated for more than five seconds provokes a pattern of pain referral into a site beyond the boundary of the muscle being palpated. Palpation of the trigger point in the left masseter provoked a pattern of pain referral into the posterior aspect of the maxilla on the left-hand side (Figure 2.1.3). The patient confirmed that this discomfort was similar to the 'toothache-type' pain she had been experiencing.

Repeated functional testing of the temporomandibular joints showed no evidence of capsular tenderness or discomfort in the posterior attachment tissues. But the unassisted range of mandibular opening was somewhat restricted, with an interincisal distance of 38 mm. The assisted range of opening was 45 mm and this movement provoked pain in the left pre-auricular region. Mandibular movements were stiff, painful (on left only) and showed some asymmetry but no permanent deviation on opening.

The intraoral examination included detailed assessment of the hard and soft tissues. The LL6 was asymptomatic and both electric and cold tests of the maxillary posterior teeth on the left side were within normal limits.

Diagnosis

In this case the lack of positive findings from the dental examination suggests that the symptoms are not odontogenic. Furthermore, the presence of widespread myofascial discomfort distributed through several different dermatomes on the left-hand side and the report of pain for more than six months point to a chronic pain disorder. The objective findings include some limitation of mandibular movement, but there was no evidence of internal derangement on clinical examination. Myofascial pain in the orofacial region will often result in a degree of hesitancy or stiffness with mandibular movement.

The clinical examination also highlighted problems in the upper segment of the cervical spine. Spinal issues are clearly not the remit of dental practitioners, but it is important for dentists to appreciate that the spinal tract of the trigeminal nucleus abuts directly onto the dorsal horn of the spinal cord. The junction between the two is commonly referred as the medullary dorsal horn. The clinical significance is that pain referral may occur from the upper segment of the spinal cord into the mandible posteriorly (dotted line in Figure 2.1.3). This type of pain can mimic toothache.

Based on the clinical findings of widespread muscle tenderness, trigger points with identifiable patterns of pain referral, and muscle fatigue and stiffness, the working diagnosis is chronic (present for more than three months) myofascial pain.

Chronic myofascial pain is typically associated with significant functional impairment and psychosocial distress. Therefore, providing treatment that focuses solely on the patient's physical discomfort is not likely to resolve her difficulties.

What special investigations should be considered for a patient with chronic pain?

- Where possible, magnetic resonance imaging (MRI) of the brain should be ordered for all patients who have chronic orofacial pain to rule out intracranial pathology.
- To help identify underlying systemic illness, blood tests should be ordered. Baseline values looking at a full blood count and liver and kidney function are helpful when monitoring the effects of subsequent medication usage.
- Referral to a clinical psychologist for assessment of factors that may be influencing the pain experience is always prudent. Unfortunately, this level of expertise is not readily available in many clinics.

Treatment Options

A multi-disciplinary approach has been shown to be most effective for conditions like chronic myofascial pain. Successful programmes are generally built around a self-care model that includes the following.

Education and reassurance

This includes promotion of the belief that the patient can and will improve over time.

This component aims to remove the fear factor from the patient's condition, by addressing concerns that may relate to future expectations and their hopes of recovery. The discussion should include strategies aimed at promoting the patient's self-confidence and expectation of a positive outcome. Education also includes providing information that empowers the patient to avoid unhelpful and/or inappropriate therapies.

Exercise

The goal is to improve the patient's general fitness in addition to providing focused therapies for the symptomatic areas. While this is best done under the supervision of a physiotherapist, the emphasis is on engaging the patient and ensuring compliance.

Behaviour modification/stress management programme

Patients can be taught over time about the complex interplay between emotions and pain. A variety of psychological interventions exist that focus on identifying and controlling one's own emotions. A skilled therapist will select an intervention most suited to the patient's needs.

Appropriate use of medication

Commonly used painkilling medications are generally not effective in patients with chronic myofascial pain. In addition, their use may aggravate an underlying problem and cause rebound headache. It is important that patients learn to understand why certain medications have been recommended to them. For example, chronic pain medications like gabapentin, pregabalin or amitriptyline may help to reduce sleep disturbance, anxiety and pain. On the other hand, weight gain and excessive sleepiness are common side effects, among others.

Discussion

In this case the diagnosis is chronic myofascial pain based on criteria outlined in the International Classification of Orofacial Pain (ICOP 2020). While the patient was convinced that her 'toothache' was purely dental in origin, the examination provided clear evidence that her pain was muscular in origin. More specifically, trigger points in the superficial aspect of the left masseter muscle were causing referred pain into the maxilla, which the patient confirmed was similar to her 'toothache'. The examination also confirmed that trigger points in the superior head of the left SCM and trapezius muscles were referring pain to the anterior portion of the left temple and left post-auricular areas.

The underlying mechanism of trigger point referral remains controversial, but there seems little doubt about the clinical reality. Experimental evidence also suggests that persistent severe odontogenic pain may lead to pain/discomfort in adjacent muscle tissue. There is some evidence that dry needling or trigger point injection with local anaesthetic may be useful therapeutically. But the traditional approach of stretching the affected muscle tissue in conjunction with the application of hot/cold packs has continued to be the therapy of first choice.

Chronic muscle pain is typically described as dull or aching (Table 2.1.2). However, pain quality may change as intensity increases and occasionally patients may complain of superimposed stabbing pains. These sharper pains tend to be randomly distributed throughout the head and face. These pains would be somewhat similar to the 'jabs and jolts' of migraine. This is in contrast to the lancinating pains of trigeminal neuralgia, which tend to be consistent in location.

From a clinician's perspective the priority is to recognise this condition as a chronic disorder. Patients like this should be referred where possible to multi-disciplinary clinics. The type of treatment required is generally outside the scope of a dental practitioner. Furthermore, disorders of the

Table 2.1.2 Comparison of acute and chronic myofascial pain.

	Acute myofascial pain	Chronic myofascial pain
Clinical exam of head, neck and face	Localised areas of tenderness	Areas of tenderness tend to be more widely distributed
Cranial nerve screening	Normal	Normal
Aggravated by physical activity	Responds strongly to physical activity	Mild to moderate responses to physical activity
Aggravated by stress/ anxiety	Mild to moderate increases in pain levels	Significant increases in pain levels in response to stress
Response to physical therapies	Responds well to physical therapies	Mild to moderate responses to physical therapies
Response to common analgesics	Responds well to analgesics	Little or no response to analgesics
Response to chronic pain medications	No response to chronic pain meds	Responds well to chronic pain meds

trigeminal nervous system often co-exist, thus it is not unusual for the patient's problem list to include myofascial pain, headache and temporomandibular joint dysfunction.

Given that a chronic pain profile may change over time, it makes it increasingly difficult for a dentist to manage this type of orofacial pain. Specialists in orofacial pain management will more easily recognise the symptom variability and manage the patient more appropriately.

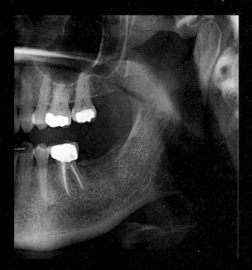

Figure 2.1.1 Left sectional orthopantomogram (OPG).

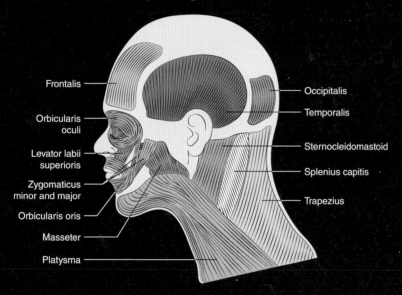

Frontalis

Orbicularis
oculi

Levator labii
superioris

Zygomaticus
minor and major

Orbicularis oris

Masseter

Platysma

Occipitalis

Temporalis

Sternocleidomastoid

Splenius capitis

Trapezius

Figure 2.1.2 Major muscles of the head neck and face.

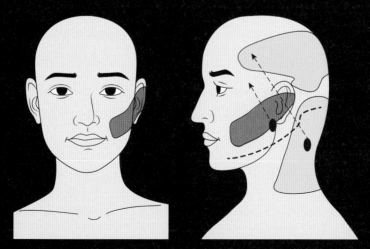

Figure 2.1.3 Trigger points in the left masseter and superior head of the left trapezius muscle, with pain referral beyond the boundary of the muscle palpated.

Further Reading

International classification of orofacial pain (ICOP), 1st edition (2020). *Cephalalgia* 40 (2): 129–221.

Welte-Jzyk, C., Pfau, D.B., Hartmann, A. et al. (2018). Somatosensory profiles of patients with chronic myogenous temporomandibular disorders in relation to their pain DETECT scores. *BMC Oral Health* 18: 138.

Zakrzewska, J.M. (2013). Differential diagnosis of facial pain and guidelines for management. *British Journal of Anaesthetics* 111: 95–104.

2.2 Neuropathic Pain

Dermot Canavan

Objectives

At the end of this case the reader should appreciate that persistent neuropathic pain in the orofacial area is easily misdiagnosed as toothache.

Trigeminal neuralgia (TN) is perhaps the best known of the neuropathic disorders, and due to extensive research we now have a much clearer understanding of this complex disorder.

Introduction

A 57-year-old female patient was referred to the orofacial pain clinic with concerns regarding persistent pain and sensitivity around the lower left first molar tooth (LL6). The patient's endodontist sought an opinion following completion of root canal treatment on the LL6.

Chief Complaint

The patient complained of persistent pain in the left midface area. She described episodic dull, aching discomfort in the mandible and maxilla on the left side that lasted for hours at a time. Pain intensity was mild to moderate on average and from the patient's perspective it felt like 'toothache coming from the lower left molar tooth'. She was also experiencing superimposed sharp shooting (lancinating) pain of increasing severity. These severe pains were relatively brief but almost 'unbearable'. They were triggered by speech, eating, movement of the tongue and touching the lower lip on the left side. Her pain was unresponsive to ibuprofen, acetaminophen (paracetamol) and codeine. The sharp pains regularly woke the patient at night. On occasion she noticed that her left eye was tearing, she had some swelling (oedema) of the eyelids on the left side and redness of the eye (conjunctival injection).

Pitt Ford's Problem-Based Learning in Endodontology, Second Edition. Edited by Elizabeth Shin Perry, Shanon Patel, Shalini Kanagasingam, and Samantha Hamer.
© 2025 John Wiley & Sons Ltd. Published 2025 by John Wiley & Sons Ltd.

Medical History

Her current medication regime included levothyroxine 50 mg/day for her underactive thyroid condition and esomeprazole 20 mg/day for gastric discomfort. She had suffered from recurrent migraine attacks with significant frequency during her late 20s and early 30s. The headaches gradually resolved as she got older and at the time of assessment she was headache free.

There was a positive family history of episodic migraine (her mother suffered from migraine as a young woman).

Dental History

The patient had a history of recurring toothache-like pain in the lower left posterior quadrant when in her early 40s. Despite repeated dental visits and procedures, the toothaches continued and eventually led to the extraction of the lower second molar (LL7). Following this extraction, the episodic toothache seemed to resolve. Tooth LL6 had been root treated recently by a specialist endodontist, however the patient complained of persistent intermittent pain and sensitivity around this tooth. All of her wisdom teeth had been removed under general anaesthesia at the age of 27.

What are the important questions to ask in this scenario?

- *Is there a history of trauma to the orofacial region?* Traumatic injury to the orofacial area may lead to the onset of trigeminal neuropathic pain weeks, months or even years after the injury.
- *When the pain is active in the symptomatic area does it extend into areas outside the orofacial region? For example, is it also experienced in the ipsilateral parietal and suboccipital areas?* The trigeminal neuropathic pain disorders (including trigeminal neuralgia) are typically experienced within the area normally innervated by the trigeminal nerve. If the orofacial complaint is associated with simultaneous pain in the parietal, occipital or posterior neck area, then a broader differential diagnosis needs to be considered. Possible causes would include intraoral disease, headache disorders and cervicogenic pathology.
- *Are the sharp shooting pains experienced in a fixed location or do they move to other areas in the face or head? For example, are the lancinating pains experienced in the tongue, throat or ear?* Lancinating pain in the ipsilateral border of the tongue is a common feature of TN. The sharp shooting pains of TN are typically unilateral and do not extend outside the trigeminal region. More widely distributed sharp shooting pains may be associated with headache complaints or myofascial disorders.
- *Are the sharp shooting pains ever triggered by certain smells or tastes?* Nonnoxious stimuli like certain smells or tastes will rarely trigger pain, but there are exceptions. The lancinating pains of TN may be triggered by foods that are spicy or bitter. Strong pungent smells like paint, diesel or perfume may be quite repulsive to patients experiencing headache disorders.

Clinical Examination

A screening assessment of cranial nerve function was within normal limits. Sensory testing of the skin in the mandibular and maxillary region on the left side showed no evidence of sensory loss or motor weakness. However, a small area of exquisite sensitivity was identified on the vermillion border of the upper lip on the left side. Touching this area provoked lancinating pain through the mandible and maxilla on the left side. Assessment of the cervical spine was also within normal limits. The temporomandibular joint examination was within normal limits, although repeated movement of the lower jaw seemed to provoke the sharp shooting pains on the left side. Intraorally there was no evidence of pathology that might explain the patient's pain. The recently root filled LL6 responded normally to mechanical pressure (Figures 2.2.1–2.2.3).

Diagnosis and Treatment Planning

Although the differential diagnosis for this type of pain complaint is theoretically quite extensive, findings from the history and clinical examination were consistent with a diagnosis of trigeminal neuralgia. TN is described as 'a disorder characterised by recurrent unilateral brief electric shock-like pains, abrupt in onset and termination, limited to the distribution of one or more divisions of the trigeminal nerve and triggered by innocuous stimuli' (International Classification of Orofacial Pain, January 2020). The same classification system states that 'there may or may not be concomitant continuous pain of moderate intensity within the affected division(s)'. There is often a clinical dilemma, as acute or chronic pulpitis may mimic TN very closely. Thus, it is imperative that the presence of odontogenic pain is ruled out before the diagnosis of TN is confirmed.

There are two primary investigations that should be carried out prior to initiating treatment. Where possible, both magnetic resonance imaging (MRI) of the brain and routine blood tests should be done. The brain MRI will help to identify the presence of neurological disease and it may also confirm the presence or absence of vascular compression of the trigeminal nerve root. Atrophy or compression of the trigeminal nerve root is considered to be a common cause of TN. Routine blood tests may also help to rule out systemic illness and baseline values for liver and kidney function are useful when considering trials of medication.

Carbamazepine is still the gold standard for treatment of this condition, but side effects may be problematic. Oxcarbazepine is a more modern version of this drug with fewer side effects. However, there are many different anticonvulsant drugs with good membrane-stabilising qualities that may be equally effective (see Table 2.2.1). The gabapentoids (gabapentin and pregabalin) are useful when medication needs to be prescribed quickly and blood test results are not available. These medications may not be as efficacious, but they have good safety profiles, minimal drug interactions and few side effects.

Table 2.2.1 Medications known to be effective in the management of trigeminal neuralgia.

Medication	Typical dose range	Side effects	Drug interactions
Carbamazepine	200–800 mg/day	Common Patients need close supervision	This drug is a hepatic enzyme inducer. This drug will interact with many others
Oxcarbazepine	900–1800 mg/day	May be problematic, but side effects less than carbamazepine	As with carbamazepine, close supervision and frequent blood tests required
Gabapentin	900–1800 mg/day	Few side effects, but not as effective as carbamazepine	Few drug interactions Less need for blood tests
Pregabalin	100–200 mg/day	Few side effects	Few drug interactions Less need for blood tests
Baclofen	30–80 mg/day	Side effects may occur, but typically not severe May be useful in conjunction with carbamazepine if required	Less frequent drug interactions than carbamazepine
Lamotrogine	50–200 mg/day	Side effects are typically less severe than carbamazepine	Drug interactions are common and patients need to be closely monitored with blood tests

Education and reassurance are an essential part of the treatment programme, as the disorder often triggers significant anxiety/distress due to the intensity of the pain. Pharmacological therapy is effective for most patients, but unfortunately over time the disorder may be progressive. For those patients unresponsive to medication a number of surgical options exist. The most effective of these is CyberKnife therapy (radiotherapy directed at the trigeminal ganglion) or microvascular decompression surgery (where the artery or vein displacing the nerve root is decompressed).

Discussion

Most dentists are familiar with the basic features of TN, but there are many misconceptions. It is often assumed that TN does not wake patients at night. Toothache-type pain that wakes patients at night is often misdiagnosed as odontogenic pain. In fact, it is well documented that TN does in fact wake patients, particularly when pain intensity is high or pain is poorly controlled with medication. The persistent background pain (typically described as dull aching) with TN can last for days or weeks before the condition goes into remission. Its presence is often misdiagnosed as odontogenic pain.

More recent studies confirm that this background persistent discomfort occurs in 35–45% of patients. Unfortunately, the quality of this pain closely mimics irreversible pulpitis. TN is a condition that is most often seen in patients that are in their mid-50s or older, and females are affected slightly more than males. It has recently been established that there is a link between migraine and TN. Patients who have been diagnosed with migraine are more likely to experience TN. It has been noted that dull aching discomfort in the symptomatic area may be a precursor to the development of lancinating pain at a later stage.

In addition, studies have shown that trigger zones are present in the vast majority of patients with TN. A trigger is an area of acute sensitivity that may be stimulated by innocuous stimuli like light touch or skin movement, to provoke an acute attack of pain. This feature is unique among pain disorders. Trigger zones may be found with careful clinical examination, or the patient may have already identified their location. Recognition of the trigger zone largely confirms the diagnosis. Their presence may vary over time, but typically they are located in the infraorbital and perioral areas. A trigger zone located within the oral cavity may be a tooth or an area of soft tissue.

The pain triggered by stimulation of the trigger zone tends to be explosive and severe. From the patient's perspective it is often the worst pain they have experienced. Once the pain has been triggered, there is a brief period of latency during which the pain cannot be triggered again. This latent period may last for two or three minutes while the nerve is 'recharging'. If the trigger zone is a tooth, the severe pain experienced on touching the tooth may suggest periapical inflammation. However, a true trigger zone will demonstrate a period of latency, whereas periapical inflammation will be repeatedly painful with stimulation.

Conclusion

While the full nature of TN is not yet understood, protocols for its management are well established. Some patients may be easily managed 'in-house' within a general practice, but many present with complex medical, psychosocial and neurological issues that are best addressed in a specialist clinic.

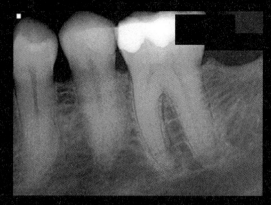

Figure 2.2.1 Pre-operative periapical radiograph of the LL6.

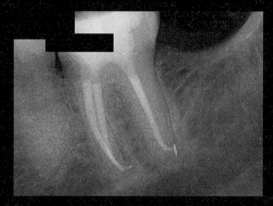

Figure 2.2.2 Post-operative radiograph of the LL6.

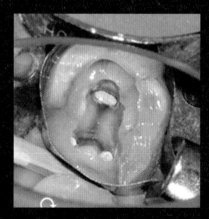

Figure 2.2.3 Intraoral view of the LL6 following completion of endodontic treatment.

Further Reading

Christofofrou, J. (2018). Neuropathic orofacial pain. *Dental Clinics of North America* 62: 565–584.

Haviv, Y., Khan, J., Zini, A. et al. (2016). Trigeminal neuralgia (part I): revisiting the clinical phenotype. *Cephalalgia* 36 (8): 730–746.

Maarbjerg, S., Di Stagano, G. et al. (2017). Trigeminal neuralgia – diagnosis and treatment. *Cephalalgia* 37 (7): 648–657.

Vital Pulp Therapy and Regeneration

3.1 *Apexogenesis*

Elizabeth Shin Perry

Objectives

Apexogenesis is a vital pulp therapy procedure that encourages the continued physiological development of the immature root. At the end of this case, the reader should understand the importance of preserving the vitality of the pulp in immature teeth and identify clinical situations that would benefit from this treatment.

Introduction

A 9-year-old female patient presented for evaluation of the upper right central incisor after the onset of discomfort of a previously traumatised tooth.

Chief Complaint

The patient reported 'My tooth started hurting two to three weeks ago. It stings.'

Medical History

Unremarkable.

Dental History

The patient was a regular attender and visited her dentist every six months. The patient experienced a traumatic injury one year previously when a playground trapeze bar hit her on the upper right central incisor (UR1) and the incisal edge fractured. There was no pulp exposure at the time and her dentist restored the tooth without complications. The tooth remained asymptomatic until recently.

Pitt Ford's Problem-Based Learning in Endodontology, Second Edition. Edited by Elizabeth Shin Perry, Shanon Patel, Shalini Kanagasingam, and Samantha Hamer.
© 2025 John Wiley & Sons Ltd. Published 2025 by John Wiley & Sons Ltd.

Clinical Examination

Extraoral examination was unremarkable and intraoral examination revealed a mixed dentition with good oral hygiene. An incisal composite restoration was present on the UR1. The UR1 was tender to percussion and palpation. All four maxillary incisors had a positive response to thermal testing (cold). The UR1 responded normally to pulp sensibility testing.

What did the radiograph reveal about the UR1?

- A restoration across the incisal edge of the crown.
- Large root canal space with an open apex and immature root anatomy (Figure 3.1.1).

Diagnosis and Treatment Planning

Diagnosis of the UR1 was reversible pulpitis associated with the prior incidence of trauma. The tooth had an immature root anatomy with a large root canal space.

What are the treatment options for the UR1?

- No treatment
- Apexogenesis with vital pulp therapy
- Root canal treatment
- Extraction

In the young patient with immature root anatomy, apexogenesis with vital pulp therapy is the preferred option. By maintaining the vitality of the pulp, the physiological development of the root continues. Achieving closure of the root apex and thickening and lengthening of the root anatomy gives the patient a stronger tooth with a better long-term prognosis. In these patients, removal of the pulp should only be performed if the pulp appears to be irreversibly inflamed, vital pulp therapy is not successful and the pulp becomes necrotic, or if the patient exhibits symptoms that are not resolving.

Conversations with the patient's parents should include the possibility that root canal treatment may be necessary in the future, but that vital pulp therapy gives the tooth the best chance for maturation of the root and long-term survival. In addition, due to the nature of traumatic dental injuries, the neighbouring teeth should be assessed periodically for clinical and radiographic changes.

Treatment

Local anaesthetic was administered and dental dam isolation was performed. The external surface of the tooth was disinfected with sodium hypochlorite. The pulp appeared to be inflamed and bled easily (Figure 3.1.2). The coronal pulp was removed stepwise using a sterile round diamond bur in a high-speed dental handpiece with water coolant until haemostasis could be achieved. Placement of a cotton pellet moistened with 2.5% sodium hypochlorite gently over the exposed pulp was done for several minutes to control the bleeding in healthy non-inflamed pulp tissue. In this case the pulp tissue had to be removed to the level of the cemento-enamel junction before healthy non-bleeding tissue was observed (Figure 3.1.3). Subsequently, 3 mm of a calcium silicate material was placed directly over the exposed pulp, followed by glass ionomer and composite to seal the access opening (Figures 3.1.4 and 3.1.5). Mineral trioxide aggregate (MTA) was used in this case as other calcium silicate materials were not yet available. Currently, however, Biodentine or bioceramic putty is preferred due to the tendency for MTA to cause discolouration of dentine.

The patient was monitored post treatment and the discomfort resolved. Clinical examination one month later revealed the tooth to be non-tender to percussion and palpation and responsive to pulp sensibility tests. A five-month review revealed formation of a calcific bridge adjacent to the MTA (Figure 3.1.6). The tooth was monitored at regular intervals and continued thickening of the calcific bridge, apical closure and root maturation were observed (Figures 3.1.7 and 3.1.8). Eight years after treatment, the patient returned with a slight grey discoloration of the cervical area of the crown (Figure 3.1.9). The restorative material and the MTA were removed to reveal a hard dentine layer in the floor of the chamber (Figure 3.1.10). Internal bleaching was performed to restore the appearance of the crown (Figure 3.1.11). Eight-year follow-up examination revealed continued vitality of the pulp and complete root end closure and maturation of the root (Figure 3.1.12).

What are the goals of vital pulp therapy of an immature tooth?

- Resolution of symptoms
- Preservation of the vitality of the pulp
- Continued development of the root in length and width of the root canal walls
- Maturation and closure of the root apex

What are the main prognostic factors for apexogenesis?

- Vital pulp
- No irreversible inflammation is present
- Pulpotomy can be performed to reveal healthy non-bleeding tissue

When would a tooth require further endodontic treatment?

- Persistence of symptoms
- Irreversible inflammation or necrosis of the pulp occurs
- Symptoms of infection develop (swelling, sinus tract formation)
- Periapical radiolucency develops

What are the different vital pulp therapies that can be used to achieve apexogenesis?

- Pulp capping
- Partial pulpotomy
- Full pulpotomy

The amount of inflammation on the surface of the coronal pulp is the determining factor for the pulp tissue to be removed. If the exposure is small and haemostasis is achieved, a pulp cap can be performed by placement of an appropriate vital pulp dressing directly over the exposed pulp. Pulpotomy involves the removal of the coronal portion of the pulp, either partially or completely, to the level of the cemento-enamel junction, to preserve the vitality of the radicular pulp. The pulp is removed incrementally until haemostasis can be achieved, followed by placement of a vital pulp dressing that facilitates formation of reparative dentine and maintenance of the vitality of the pulp.

Discussion

Vital pulp therapy is an important treatment for immature teeth and can provide predictable long-term results for the young patient. The prognosis for the treatment described in this case is good and illustrates the benefits of apexogenesis achieved by maintaining the vitality of the pulp. The continued development with increased length and width of the dentine in the root is critical for structural integrity and resistance to fracture. In addition, the maintenance of pulp vitality allows for continued proprioception and support of the defensive role of the pulp–dentine complex.

Careful clinical examination and diagnosis are paramount to case selection. An intact neurovascular supply that can maintain the vitality of the pulp is necessary to support further development of the root. In addition, the health of the pulp must be determined, as a necrotic or irreversibly inflamed pulp is not a candidate for vital pulp therapy. Symptoms such as tenderness to percussion and sensitivity to temperature can be present in teeth with reversible inflammation of the pulp and these symptoms can resolve while keeping the vitality of the pulp intact. After removal of the necrotic or inflamed coronal pulp tissue, if haemostasis can be achieved and healthy pulp tissue is observed, vital pulp therapy should be considered as the first line of treatment. Sodium hypochlorite is the irrigant of choice for disinfection and haemostasis of the remaining exposed pulp tissue. It is essential to remove any blood clots to allow for direct placement of the pulp capping material.

Historically, vital pulp therapy procedures have been performed with calcium hydroxide before the introduction of calcium silicate cement materials (MTA, Biodentine, EndoSequence® BC RRM™ putty [Brasseler USA,

Savannah, GA, USA]). The advantage of these materials over calcium hydroxide has allowed for improved biocompatibility and sealing ability to dentine and a less porous dentinal bridge formation. MTA was the first bioceramic material to be used in dentistry and has yielded excellent results; however, because of the staining of dentine by MTA (due to the bismuth oxide radiopacifier), the use of newer-generation materials such as Biodentine and bioceramic putty is recommended.

Successful outcome of vital pulp therapy can be confirmed with clinical and radiographic follow-up. Clinically, an absence of symptoms and a positive response to sensibility testing are factors that indicate a successful treatment outcome. Radiographically, increased length and width of the dentine in the root as well as maturation of the root apex are indicators of a successful outcome (Table 3.1.1). Formation of a dentinal bridge adjacent to the pulp capping material may be present and is the direct result of the stimulation of progenitor/stem cells within the dental pulp.

Thoughtful treatment planning for the immature tooth with pulp exposure is essential for long-term retention of the tooth. Thus, preservation of the vitality of the pulp should always be the treatment of choice in immature teeth when possible.

Table 3.1.1 Parameters of successful vital pulp therapy for the immature tooth.

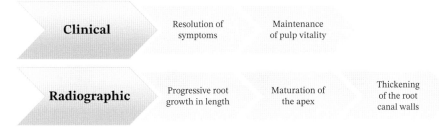

Clinical	Resolution of symptoms	Maintenance of pulp vitality	
Radiographic	Progressive root growth in length	Maturation of the apex	Thickening of the root canal walls

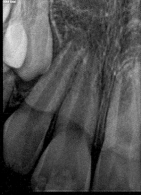

Figure 3.1.1 Pre-operative radiograph of the upper right central incisor with immature root formation, large root canal and open apex.

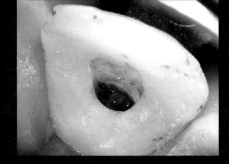

Figure 3.1.2 Initial access revealed inflamed and hyperaemic pulp tissue in the pulp chamber.

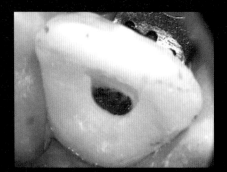

Figure 3.1.3 Partial pulpotomy was performed with a sterile high-speed diamond bur to remove the inflamed pulp tissue. Dilute sodium hypochlorite (2.5%) on a cotton pellet was applied with gentle pressure to control haemorrhage of the pulp.

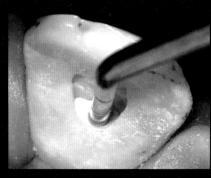

Figure 3.1.4 Bioceramic material was placed directly over the vital pulp tissue. MTA was used in this case; however, Biodentine or bioceramic putty is preferred due to the tendency for MTA to cause discolouration of dentine.

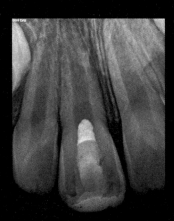

Figure 3.1.5 Immediate post-operative radiograph showing 3 mm MTA placed over the remaining vital pulp followed by composite.

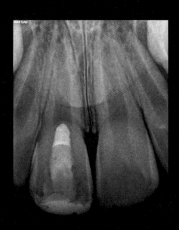

Figure 3.1.6 Five-month follow-up radiograph showing dentine bridge formation over the vital pulp.

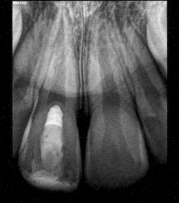

Figure 3.1.7 Two-year follow-up radiograph showing increased thickness in the dentine bridge over the vital pulp, apical closure and increased length and width of the root canal walls.

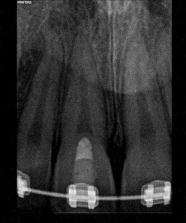

Figure 3.1.8 Follow-up radiograph after 4.5 years showing continued root development.

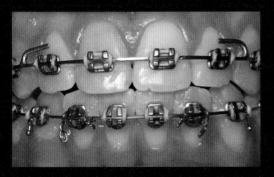

Figure 3.1.9 Eight-year follow-up. The patient is completing orthodontic treatment and there is obvious grey discolouration of the upper right central incisor.

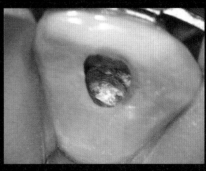

Figure 3.1.10 Removal of the restorative material and MTA revealed a significant dentine layer over the pulp.

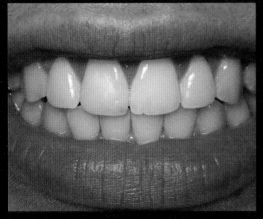

Figure 3.1.11 Eight-year follow-up after orthodontic treatment was completed and internal bleaching was performed.

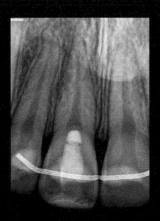

Figure 3.1.12 Eight-year follow-up radiograph shows continued root development and no endodontic pathology. Sensibility tests indicate that the pulp is vital.

Further Reading

American Association of Endodontists (2021). AAE position statement on vital pulp therapy. Chicago, IL: American Association of Endodontists. https://www.aae.org/wp-content/uploads/2021/05/VitalPulpTherapy PositionStatement_v2.pdf.

Arguilar, P. and Linsuwanont, P. (2011). Vital pulp therapy in vital permanent teeth with cariously exposed pulp: a systematic review. *Journal of Endodontics* 37: 581–587.

Cvek, M. (1978). A clinical report on partial pulpotomy and capping with calcium hydroxide in permanent incisors with complicated crown fractures. *Journal of Endodontics* 4: 232–237.

Cvek, M. (1993). Partial pulpotomy in crown-fractured incisors-results 3–15 years after treatment. *Acta Stomatologica Croatica* 27: 167–173.

Ricucci, D., Siqueira, J.F. Jr., Li, Y., and Tay, F.R. (2019). Vital pulp therapy: histopathology and histobacteriology- based guidelines to treat teeth with deep caries and pulp exposure. *J Dent* 86: 41–52.

Smith, A.J. (2012). Dentin formation and repair. In: *Dental Pulp* (ed. K.M. Hargreaves, H.E. Goodis, F.R. Tay, et al.). Chicago, IL: Quintessence.

3.2 Apexification

Elizabeth Shin Perry

Objectives

Apexification is the induction of a calcified barrier in a root with an open apex or the continued apical development of an incompletely formed root in a tooth with a necrotic pulp. At the end of this case, the reader should understand the management of a non-vital tooth with immature root anatomy and open apex with the current protocols for apexification and be able to identify clinical situations that would benefit from this treatment.

Introduction

A 7-year-old girl presented with discoloration and tenderness associated with her upper left central incisor (UL1). Three months previously the patient had experienced a traumatic dental injury when she fell and hit her central incisors on the corner of a table. The teeth were palatally displaced and she was seen immediately by her dentist, who repositioned the teeth and splinted them with a flexible wire splint for two weeks.

Chief Complaint

The patient's tooth was discoloured (grey) and was tender to touch.

Medical History

Unremarkable.

Dental History

Regular attender at her dentist and visited the hygienist every six months.

Pitt Ford's Problem-Based Learning in Endodontology, Second Edition. Edited by Elizabeth Shin Perry, Shanon Patel, Shalini Kanagasingam, and Samantha Hamer.

Clinical Examination

Extraoral examination was unremarkable. Intraoral examination revealed a mixed dentition. Oral hygiene status was good.

The UL1 appeared grey (Figure 3.2.1a) and was tender to percussion. The UL1 did not respond to thermal (cold) or electric vitality testing. The UR1 responded within normal limits to sensibility testing and was not tender to percussion. Both central incisors were incompletely erupted.

What did the radiograph reveal about the UL1?

- Periapical radiolucency.
- Incomplete root anatomy with thin canal walls and open apex.
- Arrested or slower root development compared to the UR1 (Figure 3.2.1b).

It is not uncommon for immature teeth to have periapical radiolucent areas in the region of the developing root apices. In this case, the radiolucent area associated with tooth UL1 was larger than the radiolucent area around the apex of UR1, indicating that an area of pathology may be present.

Diagnosis and Treatment Planning

What was the diagnosis and treatment plan?

The diagnosis was pulpal necrosis with symptomatic apical periodontitis.

What were the potential treatment options for this patient?

- Apexification (endodontic therapy) with root end closure
- Regenerative endodontics
- Extraction
- No treatment

As with all types of endodontic treatment, the objective of treatment is prevention of periapical periodontitis in teeth with irreversible pulpitis and resolution of periapical periodontitis in teeth with infected, necrotic root canal spaces. Apexification with root end closure allows for the formation of a calcific barrier at the apical extent of teeth with incomplete root development.

Today regenerative endodontics is an exciting treatment option for teeth with immature root development (see Case 3.3). However, when there is a concern for regenerative endodontic treatment or follow-up, apexification is a viable option to save a necrotic tooth with incomplete root formation. Extraction of a tooth in a young child is never a desirable option, as this commits the patient to a lifetime of prosthodontic procedures to replace the missing tooth.

What are the challenges in the treatment of teeth with immature root anatomy?

Teeth with immature root anatomy present unique challenges for treatment. These teeth have wide root canals with open apices and thin, divergent canal walls. The large root canal space does not allow for traditional mechanical instrumentation, as the large canal diameter can exceed the size of root canal instruments. In addition, dentine preservation of the already delicate root structure is important. The open apex presents a challenge for obturation with traditional methods, as the canal has minimal or no resistance form for compaction of root canal materials. In addition, application of any irrigants or medicaments must be carefully controlled to prevent extrusion into the periapical tissues.

Treatment

Endodontic treatment was carried out with local anaesthetic and dental dam isolation. The root canal was accessed, and the canal was irrigated with sodium hypochlorite and a pre-measured syringe tip. The working length was measured on the pre-operative radiographs and confirmed with a working length radiograph (Figure 3.2.2). The canal was minimally instrumented with large files and irrigated with sodium hypochlorite to remove the necrotic pulp remnants. The canal was dried with paper points and dressed with calcium hydroxide for two weeks.

When the patient returned for the second visit, her symptoms had resolved. The tooth was anaesthetized and was isolated with the dental dam. The canal was accessed, irrigated with sodium hypochlorite and dried with paper points. Mineral trioxide aggregate (MTA) was placed in the apical 4–5 mm of the root canal and was compacted with gentle pressure and pre-measured endodontic pluggers. The MTA placement was confirmed radiographically (Figure 3.2.3a). The remaining portion of the root canal was obturated with gutta percha and endodontic sealer. The access opening was sealed with a dual-cure resin-modified glass ionomer followed by composite (Figure 3.2.3b).

Follow-up at one year showed reestablishment of the trabecular bone around the apex of the tooth (Figure 3.2.4a). Follow-up at nine years showed resolution of the periapical radiolucency as well as increased root length beyond the MTA apical barrier and the establishment of the periodontal ligament around the apex of the tooth. The development of the right central incisor was observed to be complete (Figure 3.2.4b).

What are the goals of apexification?

The primary goal of successful apexification includes the resolution of clinical symptoms and the resolution of the apical radiolucency. The secondary goal is the formation of a biological hard tissue barrier and even continued root development at the apex of a non-vital tooth with immature root anatomy and open apex (Table 3.2.1).

Table 3.2.1 Parameters of successful apexification.

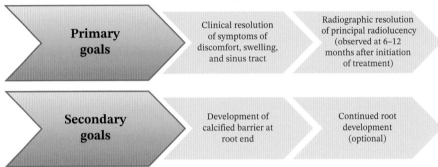

| Primary goals | Clinical resolution of symptoms of discomfort, swelling, and sinus tract | Radiographic resolution of principal radiolucency (observed at 6–12 months after initiation of treatment) |
| Secondary goals | Development of calcified barrier at root end | Continued root development (optional) |

What are the ways in which apexification can be achieved?

Historically, apexification was performed with the long-term placement of calcium hydroxide in the root canal, allowing Hertwig's epithelial root sheath to form an apical barrier. In these cases, the calcium hydroxide is replaced approximately every 3 months and apexification is completed in 12–24 months. When the hard tissue barrier is evident radiographically and clinically, the root canal is obturated using traditional methods. Although calcium hydroxide apexification is predictable, studies have shown that long-term calcium hydroxide can weaken the already fragile canal walls, making the tooth more prone to fracture.

Since the introduction of the calcium silicate cement MTA, it has been used for placement in the root canal apex as an artificial apical barrier in apexification procedures. The properties of biocompatibility, antimicrobial activity, excellent sealing ability and ability to set in the presence of moisture (blood) make MTA an ideal material to provide an apical seal. Apexification with MTA can be completed in one or two visits over a short period of time and offers an excellent alternative over apexification with long-term calcium hydroxide (Table 3.2.2). Studies have shown that MTA apexification offers equivalent or better outcomes when compared to calcium hydroxide apexification. Recent studies have shown that other calcium silicate cements such as bioceramic root repair material (EndoSequence® BC RRM™, Brasseler USA, Savannah, GA, USA) and Biodentine are as effective as MTA. Apexification with calcium silicate cements offers a predictable and efficient treatment option over regenerative endodontic procedures (see Case 3.3) when follow-up of the patient may be a challenge.

What are the advantages to using calcium hydroxide as an intracanal medication?

The main advantage to using calcium hydroxide as an intracanal medication is its antimicrobial properties, mostly attributed to its high pH of 12.5–12.8. It is chemically classified as a strong base and dissociates into calcium and

Table 3.2.2 Comparing calcium hydroxide and calcium silicate apexification.

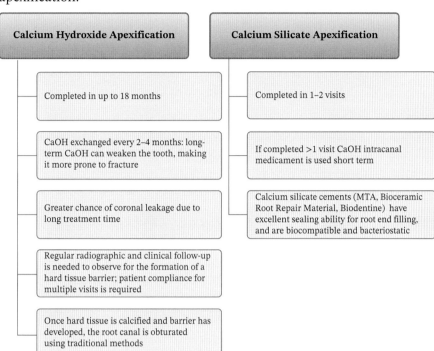

Calcium Hydroxide Apexification	Calcium Silicate Apexification
Completed in up to 18 months	Completed in 1–2 visits
CaOH exchanged every 2–4 months: long-term CaOH can weaken the tooth, making it more prone to fracture	If completed >1 visit CaOH intracanal medicament is used short term
Greater chance of coronal leakage due to long treatment time	Calcium silicate cements (MTA, Bioceramic Root Repair Material, Biodentine) have excellent sealing ability for root end filling, and are biocompatible and bacteriostatic
Regular radiographic and clinical follow-up is needed to observe for the formation of a hard tissue barrier; patient compliance for multiple visits is required	
Once hard tissue is calcified and barrier has developed, the root canal is obturated using traditional methods	

hydroxyl ions on contact with an aqueous solution. The main actions of calcium hydroxide can be attributed to the effect that these ions have on vital tissue. The hydroxyl ions are responsible for the highly alkaline nature of calcium hydroxide, and bacteria within the infected root canal are eliminated on direct contact with these ions. In addition, calcium hydroxide can induce hard tissue formation and can be used to control exudate or bleeding within the root canal.

What are calcium silicate cements and how do they work?

MTA was the first calcium silicate cement to be used in dentistry. It is principally composed of di- and tricalcium silicate, tricalcium aluminate, and tetracalcium aluminoferrite, with the addition of bismuth oxide for radiopacity. When mixed with water, MTA forms a highly alkaline (pH 13) paste that then sets through a hydration reaction to produce a calcium silicate hydrate gel and calcium hydroxide. The high pH is due to the sustained release of calcium hydroxide, which is maintained over time and allows for the antimicrobial property of MTA. When set, MTA has excellent sealing ability, is biocompatible and bioactive, and has the ability to induce cementum-like hard tissue formation.

Since the introduction of MTA, additional calcium silicate materials such as bioceramic root repair material and Biodentine have been developed and have been recommended for use in apexification procedures for their handling properties. These calcium silicate cements vary in composition, but share the same principal ingredients of calcium and silicate. The formation of the hydroxyapatite layer when these calcium silicate materials come into contact with tissue results in their biocompatible, osteoinductive and osteoconductive ability.

Discussion

Treatment of a necrotic tooth with immature root anatomy and open apex presents many challenges. In this case, the ability to save the traumatised necrotic tooth on the 7-year-old patient was critical for her dental health and confidence as she matured. Apexification allowed for the immediate outcome of elimination of the disease and also allowed for continued root development and long-term success of the tooth. The nine-year follow-up of this tooth showed an excellent long-term outcome and a significant increase in root length of the treated tooth. Apexification with calcium silicate cements offers a valuable treatment alternative for patients in need of treatment of a necrotic immature tooth.

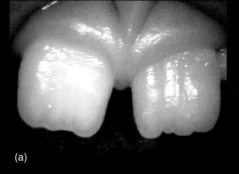

(a)

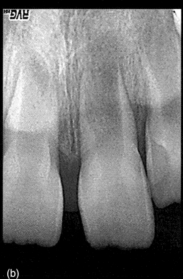

(b)

Figure 3.2.1 (a) Clinical photograph shows grey discolouration and incomplete eruption of left central incisor. (b) Periapical radiograph shows central incisors with incomplete root development and open apices. Trabecular bone around the apex of the left central incisor exhibits a radiolucency suggestive of periradicular inflammation.

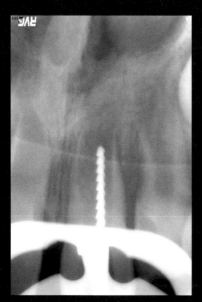

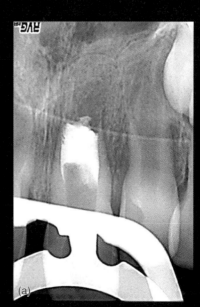

(a)

Figure 3.2.2 Endodontic treatment was initiated. The working length radiograph shows the very thin canal walls in relation to the file.

Figure 3.2.3 (a) Canal debridement was initiated, and an MTA apical barrier was placed followed by obturation with gutta percha.

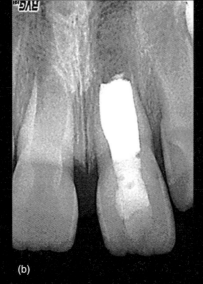

Figure 3.2.3 (Continued) (b) Immediate post-operative radiograph. The access opening was sealed with glass ionomer and composite.

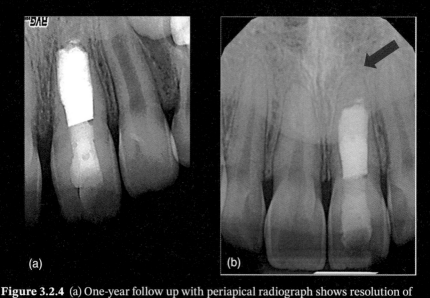

(a)

(b)

Figure 3.2.4 (a) One-year follow up with periapical radiograph shows resolution of the periapical radiolucency, the increased root length beyond the MTA apical barrier, and the establishment of the periodontal ligament around the apex of the left central incisor. (b) Nine-year follow up of MTA apexification. Note the resolution of the periapical radiolucency, the increased root length beyond the MTA apical barrier, and the establishment of the periodontal ligament around the apex of the left central incisor (arrow). The development of the right central incisor is observed to be complete.

Further Reading

Andreasen, J.O., Farik, B., and Munksgaard, E.D. (2002). Long-term calcium hydroxide as a root canal dressing may increase risk of root fracture. *Dental Traumatology* 18: 134–137.

Chala, S., Abouqal, R., and Rida, S. (2011). Apexification of immature teeth with calcium hydroxide or mineral trioxide aggregate: systemic review and meta-analysis. *Oral Surgery, Oral Medicine, Oral Pathology, Oral Radiology, and Endodontology* 112: e36–e42.

Chugal, N., Mallya, S.M., Kahler, B., and Lin, L.M. (2017). Endodontic treatment outcomes. *Dental Clinics of North America* 61 (1): 59–80.

Rafter, M. (2005). Apexification: a review. *Dental Traumatology* 21: 1–8.

Shabahang, S. (2013). Treatment options: apexogenesis and apexification. *Journal of Endodontics* 39: S26–S29.

Torabinejad, M. and Parirokh, M. (2010). Mineral trioxide aggregate: a comprehensive literature review – Part II: Leakage and biocompatibility investigations. *Journal of Endodontics* 36: 190–202.

3.3 *Regenerative Endodontics*

Elizabeth Shin Perry

Objectives

Regenerative endodontics describes the 'biologically based procedures designed to physiologically replace damaged tooth structures including dentin and root structures, as well as cells of the pulp-dentin complex' (American Association of Endodontics Glossary). Regenerative endodontic procedures offer an alternative treatment of the necrotic immature permanent tooth.

At the end of this case, the reader should understand the biological basis for regenerative endodontic procedures and should be able to identify cases in which this treatment would be appropriate.

Introduction

An 8-year-old girl presented with discolouration of the maxillary right central incisor. She had a history of trauma six months previously when she had a bicycle accident and chipped her tooth.

Medical History

Unremarkable.

Dental History

The patient had a bicycle accident during a holiday weekend six months previously. At that time, she chipped her tooth and she was taken to her paediatric dentist. She was monitored for signs of alveolar fracture and the condition of the adjacent teeth. The chip was repaired and she was feeling well. She returned for a routine dental visit and her dentist noticed a change in the colour of the tooth and took a radiograph. She was subsequently referred for endodontic specialty care.

Pitt Ford's Problem-Based Learning in Endodontology, Second Edition. Edited by Elizabeth Shin Perry, Shanon Patel, Shalini Kanagasingam, and Samantha Hamer.
© 2025 John Wiley & Sons Ltd. Published 2025 by John Wiley & Sons Ltd.

Clinical Examination

Clinical examination revealed tenderness to palpation in the anterior buccal vestibule over the upper right central incisor (UR1). The tooth was not mobile or tender to percussion. Periodontal probing depths were within normal limits. The tooth did not respond to thermal or electric sensitivity tests and was discoloured (grey).

What did the radiographic examination reveal?

- UR1 with an immature root development with an open apex and apical radiolucency.
- UL1 appeared to be more developed than UR1 (apically, it appears to have thicker dentine walls and a more closed apex compared to UR1) (Figure 3.3.1a).

Diagnosis and Treatment Planning

The diagnosis was symptomatic periapical periodontitis associated with an infected necrotic pulp of an immature permanent tooth.

Treatment options discussed with the patient's parents were:

- Regenerative endodontic treatment – If root maturation can be achieved, the root would have increased structural integrity, which may improve fracture resistance. The patient and her parents were informed of the possibility that the tooth may require root canal therapy in the future.
- Root canal therapy with apexification.
- Internal bleaching would be performed to address the discoloration following either the regenerative endodontic procedure or root canal therapy with mineral trioxide aggregate (MTA) apexification.

The patient and her parents were interested in saving the tooth and treating the infection and discolouration. Due to the benefits of continued root maturation, they decided to treat with regenerative endodontic treatment.

What is the aim of regenerative endodontic procedures?

The objectives of regenerative endodontic procedures are twofold:

- Removal of necrotic tissue and bacteria from the root canal system to facilitate elimination of apical periodontitis.
- Induction of further root maturation with increased width of the root walls and apical closure as well as increased root length in an immature permanent necrotic tooth.

Treatment

The first visit involved local anaesthesia with 2% lidocaine with 1 : 100 000 epinephrine, followed by dental dam placement and access into the root canal. Minimal instrumentation of the canal was performed. The canal was copiously and slowly irrigated with 1.5% sodium hypochlorite (20 ml, five minutes) followed by irrigation with 17% ethylenediaminetetraacetic acid (EDTA; 20 ml, five minutes), with the irrigating needle measured for delivery at least 1 mm from the root end to minimise cytotoxicity to the periapical tissues. The canal was dried with paper points. A double antibiotic paste of ciprofloxacin and metronidazole was placed in the canal as an intracanal antimicrobial dressing and a Cavit™ (3M, St. Paul, MN, USA) temporary restoration was placed in the access opening (Figure 3.3.1b).

Four weeks later the patient returned for the second appointment. At that time, clinical symptoms were assessed. The palpation tenderness had resolved and the patient was feeling well. Local anaesthesia with 3% mepivacaine without vasoconstrictor was administered followed by dental dam placement and the canal was accessed. Copious gentle irrigation with 20 ml of 17% EDTA was performed. The canal was dried with paper points. Bleeding into the canal was initiated by over-instrumentation through the open apex into the periapical tissues using a sterile endodontic file (e.g. size 40 Hedström). The canal was allowed to fill with blood 2 mm below the gingival margin, and 15 minutes was allowed for a blood clot to form. A resorbable matrix was placed using CollaPlug® (Zimmer Biomet, Warsaw, IN, USA) and the collagen matrix was allowed to soak with blood to avoid formation of a void. An intracanal barrier of white MTA was placed below the cemento-enamel junction followed by glass ionomer (Figure 3.3.1c). Due to the dentine staining caused by MTA, other bioceramic materials are recommended today.

Internal bleaching was performed immediately following, with a temporary restoration (Figure 3.3.1d). Two weeks later the patient returned and resolution of the discolouration was observed. The internal bleaching paste was removed and a permanent composite restoration was placed in the access (Figure 3.3.1e).

Follow-Up

Clinical and radiographic examination revealed (Figure 3.3.2):

- No pain, soft tissue swelling or sinus tract; resolution of symptoms was observed between the first and second appointments.
- Resolution of apical radiolucency observed at 4 months.
- Apical closure observed at 14 months.
- Increased width of root walls observed at 2 and 3 years.
- 7 and 9 year followup showed continued successful regenerative endodontic treatment.
- Yearly follow-up recommended.

Discussion

The treatment of necrotic immature teeth presents treatment challenges due to multiple factors. Open apices can be difficult to manage, and thin root walls make risk of fracture a concern. In 2001, a new treatment alternative for immature permanent teeth with necrotic pulp and apical periodontitis was described by Iwaya et al. and was termed *revascularisation*. The case report described a treatment technique that promoted further root maturation with thickening of the canal walls, increased root length and apical closure. The potential for strengthening of the root by the deposition of new mineralised tissue addressed the limitations of traditional apexification (Table 3.3.1). Since that time, many published reports of these procedures have demonstrated the efficacy of regenerative endodontic protocols and have described the parameters for successful treatment (Table 3.3.2).

Table 3.3.1 Regenerative endodontics as compared to apexification.

Regenerative Endodontics	Apexification

• **Pros**
   • Root maturation progresses with increased root wall thickness and increased root length
   • Potentially less risk of root fracture
 • **Cons**
   • Follow up is essential and is recommended at 6, 12, and 24 months
   • May require root canal therapy with apexification if primary goals of treatment are not met
	• **Pros**
	   • Apexification with calcium silicate cements can be completed in one or two visits
	   • Once apexification is complete and the canal is obturated, follow up is not essential
	 • **Cons**
	   • Root maturation usually does not progress
	   • Risk of root fracture due to the thin root walls
	   • Apexification with CaOH is not complete for many months and may result in weakening of the root walls due to long term exposure of the dentine to CaOH

Table 3.3.2 Parameters of successful regenerative endodontics.

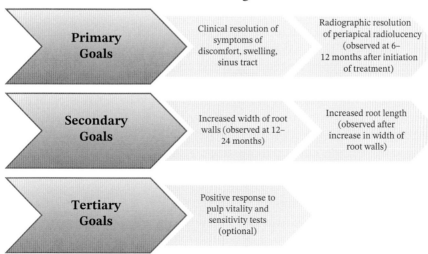

Primary Goals	Clinical resolution of symptoms of discomfort, swelling, sinus tract	Radiographic resolution of periapical radiolucency (observed at 6–12 months after initiation of treatment)
Secondary Goals	Increased width of root walls (observed at 12–24 months)	Increased root length (observed after increase in width of root walls)
Tertiary Goals	Positive response to pulp vitality and sensitivity tests (optional)	

American Association of Endodontists (AAE) guidelines recommend that the first visit should involve disinfection of the root canal space with 1.5% sodium hypochlorite followed by irrigation with saline or EDTA. The lower concentration of sodium hypochlorite minimises cytotoxicity to stem cells in the apical tissues. An antimicrobial dressing is then placed in the canal followed by a temporary restoration. Early protocols recommended a low-concentration triple antibiotic paste composed of minocycline, ciprofloxacin and metronidazole. Due to the staining capacity of minocycline, subsequent recommendations include a double antibiotic paste of ciprofloxacin and metronidazole or a triple antibiotic paste substituting other antibiotics for minocycline (clindamycin, amoxicillin).

Studies have shown that antibiotic pastes may have a negative effect on stem cell viability due to the difficulty to control levels of concentration. Calcium hydroxide has been shown to be effective on bacterial reduction while promoting stem cell survival and proliferation, and thus may be a better choice for an intracanal medicament in regenerative endodontic procedures and is currently recommended by the European Society of Endodontology. Calcium hydroxide has also been recommended as an option along with the antibiotic pastes by the AAE in its current recommendations.

At the second appointment, anaesthesia without a vasoconstrictor is used. The canal is copiously irrigated with 17% EDTA. EDTA releases growth factors from the dentine matrix and exposes specific binding sites in the root dentine. Bleeding into the canal is induced by over-instrumenting through the open apex into the periapical tissues, with the goal of filling the canal to the level of the cemento-enamel junction. Stem cells from the apical papilla and progenitor cells are introduced into the canal to facilitate further root maturation. An alternative to creation of a blood clot is the use of platelet-rich plasma (PRP), platelet-rich fibrin (PRF) or autologous fibrin matrix (AFM). A resorbable matrix such as CollaPlug, Collacote® (Integra Life Sciences, Plainsboro, NJ, USA) or CollaTape® (Zimmer Biomet) followed by a 2–3 mm barrier of a calcium silicate cement (MTA, EndoSequence® BC RRM™ [Brasseler USA, Savannah, GA, USA] or tricalcium silicate cement) is placed over the blood clot and the access cavity is restored with glass ionomer and composite resin. Bioceramic or tricalcium silicate cements such as Biodentine or EndoSequence BC RRM putty should be considered in teeth where there is an aesthetic concern, as there is a risk of tooth discoloration associated with MTA. Follow-up is recommended at 6, 12 and 24 months, followed by yearly follow-up thereafter.

Historically, regenerative endodontic procedures have been described with different terminology, including 'revascularisation', 'revitalisation' and 'pulp regeneration'. Histological studies have shown that the newly derived tissue is not pulp-like, but appears to be similar to cementum, connective tissue and bone and is likely derived from the periodontium. Therefore, regenerative endodontics represents a tissue engineering procedure that facilitates the development of dental hard tissues. These procedures offer a valuable treatment alternative to patients with a necrotic immature permanent tooth. Careful treatment planning and discussion with the patient and parent are essential and regular follow-up of the treatment of these teeth is recommended.

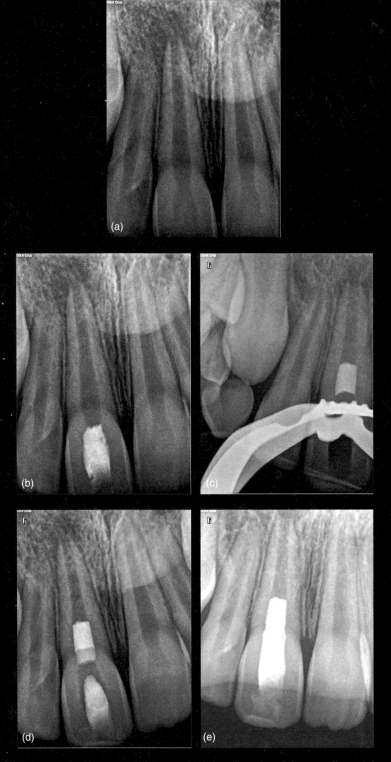

Figure 3.3.1 (a) Pre-operative periapical radiograph shows the apex of the maxillary right central incisor with an open root apex and a periapical radiolucency, consistent with pulpal necrosis and chronic apical periodontitis. (b) Double antibiotic paste intracanal medication placed, Cavit temporary restoration. (c) MTA placement over a collagen matrix. (d) Post-operative regenerative endodontic procedure. MTA followed by glass ionomer was placed. Internal bleaching initiated followed by temporary restoration. (e) Post-regenerative endodontic procedure and internal bleaching with composite restoration.

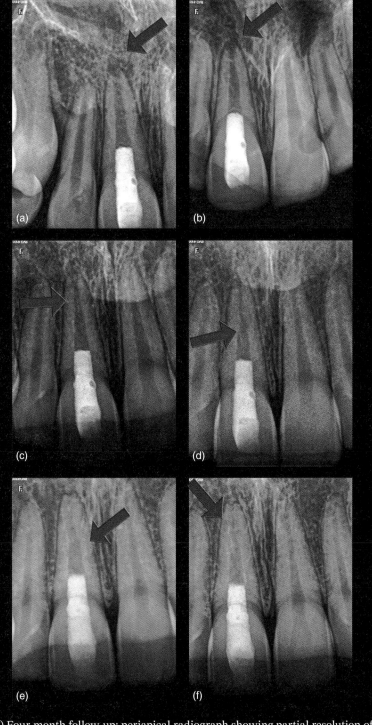

Figure 3.3.2 (a) Four-month follow-up: periapical radiograph showing partial resolution of the periapical radiolucency around the right central incisor, consistent with resolution of clinical symptoms. Overall, the appearance is indicative of healing of the periapical inflammation. (b) The 14-month follow-up periapical radiograph showing resolution of the periapical radiolucency with evidence of osseous healing and reestablishment of the periodontal ligament space and lamina dura around the apex of the right central incisor. Note minimal changes in the width of the apical foramen. (c) Two-year follow-up showing closure of the root end and thickening of the canal walls in the apical third. (d) Three-year follow-up confirms closure of root apex, with no periapical rarefaction, confirming successful regenerative endodontic treatment. There is thickening of the root wall apical to MTA that was placed into the coronal one-third of the canal. (e) Seven-year follow-up demonstrates continued successful regenerative endodontic treatment. (f) Nine-year follow-up reveals continued successful regenerative endodontic treatment. The tooth is responsive to pulp testing.

Further Reading

Althumairy, R.I., Teixeria, F.B., and Diogenes, A. (2014). Effect of dentin conditioning with intracanal medicaments on survival of stem cells of apical papilla. *Journal of Endodontics* 40: 521–525.

American Association of Endodontists (2016). AAE clinical considerations for a regenerative procedure. Chicago, IL: AAE. https://www.aae.org/uploadedfiles/publications_and_research/research/currentregenerativeendodonticconsiderations.pdf.

Banchs, F. and Trope, M. (2004). Revascularization of immature permanent teeth with apical periodontitis: new treatment protocol? *Journal of Endodontics* 30: 196–200.

Diogenes, A., Henry, M.A., Teixeira, F.B. et al. (2013). An update on clinical regenerative endodontics. *Endodontic Topics* 28: 2–23.

Diogenes, A., Ruparel, N.B., Shiloah, Y. et al. (2016). Regenerative endodontics. A way forward. *Journal of the American Dental Association* 147: 372–380.

Galler, K.M., Krastl, G., VanGorp, G. et al. (2016). European Society of Endodontology position statement: revitalization procedures. *International Endodontic Journal* 49: 717–723.

Geisler, T.M. (2012). Clinical considerations for regenerative endodontic procedures. *Dental Clinics of North America* 56: 603–626.

Iwaya, S., Ikawa, M., and Kubota, M. (2001). Revascularization of an immature permanent tooth with apical periodontitis and sinus tract. *Dental Traumatology* 17: 185–187.

Kim, S.G., Malek, M., Sigurdsson, A. et al. (2018). Regenerative endodontics: a comprehensive review. *International Endodontic Journal* 51: 1367–1388.

Nagy, M.M., Tawfik, H.E., Hashem, A.A. et al. (2014). Regenerative potential of immature permanent teeth with necrotic pulps after different regenerative protocols. *Journal of Endodontics* 40: 192–198.

Ruparel, N.B., Teixeira, F.B., Ferraz, C.C., and Diogenes, A. (2012). Direct effect of intracanal medicaments on survival of stem cells of the apical papilla. *Journal of Endodontics* 38: 1372–1375.

IV Endodontic Treatment

4.1 *Access Cavity Preparation*

Shanon Patel

Objectives

Access cavity preparation is the first and most important aspect of endodontic treatment. A well-executed access cavity is essential for successful instrumentation and subsequent obturation of the root canal system. At the end of this chapter the reader should have an appreciation of the rationale and design principles of access cavity preparation.

Introduction

A 45-year-old male presents with pain associated in the upper left molar region.

Chief Complaint

The patient complains of a low-grade intermittent ache when trying to chew on the UL7; the symptoms last for several minutes. The symptoms were also spontaneous, but the tooth was not temperature sensitive. The symptoms have been present for two months and are getting progressively worse.

Medical History

Patient has anxiety issues after losing his job and a recent divorce, both of which occurred within a few months of each other. He has been prescribed antidepressants by his doctor.

Dental History

Regular attender.

Pitt Ford's Problem-Based Learning in Endodontology, Second Edition. Edited by Elizabeth Shin Perry, Shanon Patel, Shalini Kanagasingam, and Samantha Hamer.
© 2025 John Wiley & Sons Ltd. Published 2025 by John Wiley & Sons Ltd.

Clinical Examination

The dentition was minimally restored. The soft tissues were healthy and the periodontal probing depths were less than 2 mm.

The UL7 was tender to finger pressure. No other signs of endodontic or periodontal disease could be elicited from the neighbouring teeth. The UL5, UL6 and UL8 responded normally to sensibility testing, the UL7 did not respond to sensibility testing.

What does the periapical radiograph reveal?

- Good bone levels.
- Tooth UL7 restored with what initially appeared to be a shallow plastic restoration; however, on closer inspection a deeper restoration was present beneath this restoration.
- Teeth UL6, UL7 and UL8 showed reduction in pulp chamber volume with pulp chamber sclerosis.
- Teeth UL6 and UL7 have acute curvatures in the mesio-buccal roots (Figure 4.1.1).

Diagnosis and Treatment Planning

The diagnosis for the UL7 was symptomatic periapical periodontitis associated with an infected necrotic root canal system.

The following treatment options were discussed with the patient:

- Root canal treatment, followed by cuspal coverage restoration.
- Extraction, including possible fixed and removable prosthodontic options.
- Leave alone.

The patient decided to go ahead with root canal treatment and subsequent restoration of the tooth.

Preparation of the Tooth for Root Canal Treatment

Once the patient has consented for root canal treatment, the first step of treatment is to determine the restorability of the tooth; that is, whether treatment is going to be viable.

The angulation and any rotation of the tooth should be appreciated, as these will influence the access cavity design. Anatomical landmarks, such as the cemento-enamel junction and furcation, are useful landmarks indicating the level of the floor of the pulp chamber.

*What information may be gained from a diagnostic radiograph
to aid in access cavity preparation?*

A diagnostic periapical radiograph is essential to appreciate the extent
(depth) of any restorations and decay, position of the pulp horns as well
as the roof of the pulp chamber, and size and depth of the pulp chamber.

As patients get older, and also as teeth get more tired and/or irritated, the
pulp chamber and also the root canal system gradually close up; that is,
secondary dentine is deposited that reduces the volume of the pulp chamber.
This may also result in loss of the 'dentine map' on the floor of the pulp
chamber, which may make locating canal entrances more challenging. In
this case, a darker groove can be seen linking the canal entrances. The often
described 'classic' dentine map of dark grooves against a lighter dentine
background is usually only seen in younger teeth in which there has been
less secondary and tertiary dentine deposition.

Over the life of a tooth, tertiary dentine in response to specific noxious
stimuli such as caries, microleakage or tooth surface loss may have a
significant effect on the size of the pulp chamber, further obscuring the
canal entrances.

What are the aims of access cavity preparation?

- To remove the pulp tissue contents from the pulp chamber, allowing
  the floor of the pulp chamber to be visualised and the canal entrance
  to be located.
- To create straight-line access into the coronal portion of the root
  canal(s), thus allowing unhindered and smooth instrumentation of
  the root canals.

These aims are the same regardless of the tooth type or whether carrying out
primary or secondary (re-root canal) endodontic treatment. A well-designed
access cavity minimises canal aberrations and also reduces the stress exerted
on the endodontic files, which therefore minimises the likelihood of instrument fracture.

The existing restoration, if present, and all decay must be removed to allow
the remaining tooth structure to be assessed. It may then be necessary to
restore the tooth with a (provisional) restoration before commencing. Time
spent on this stage of the procedure will make the rest of the treatment more
efficient. As well as confirming restorability, assessing the volume and location of remaining dentine will help determine what type of post-endodontic
restoration will be required. The number and nature of hairline cracks on
one or more axial walls will influence the endodontic prognosis and the
design of the post-endodontic restoration.

A new trend of minimally invasive access cavity preparation is emerging in endodontics and a variety of 'novel' preparations have been purported to improve clinical outcomes. The aim is to preserve more sound dentine than conventional access cavity design. By preserving more of the pulp chamber roof and conserving more sound dentine, the fracture resistance of teeth after root canal treatment is increased (Table 4.1.1 – 4.1.2 and Figure 4.1.2).

What are the perceived issues with a more minimally invasive approach?

- May compromise debriding and disinfecting of the complex root canal system.
- Prevents and/or makes locating root canal entrances more challenging.
- Places undue stress on instruments, resulting in canal aberrations and/or instrument fracture.
- Compromises obturation.
- Leaves pulp tissue debris in the pulp chamber leading to discoloration, poor adhesion of root canal sealers and composite resin restorations.

Table 4.1.1 Essential armamentarium for access cavity preparation.

- Front surface mirror
- DG16 endodontic probe
- Long shank excavator, endodontic ultrasonic tips & access burs
- Magnification and good illumination (loupes or dental operating microscope)

Table 4.1.2 Comparison of access cavities.

Traditional access cavity	• Complete removal of pulp chamber roof and straight-line access into all canal entrances.
Conservative access cavity	• More centred, with diverging axial walls from coronal to floor of pulp chamber, thus partially preserving lateral borders of the pulp chamber roof.
Ultra-conservative (Ninja) access cavity	• A more minimal version of a conservative access cavity preserving more of the pulp chamber roof
Truss access cavity	• Retention of entire thickness of coronal dentine between the individual smaller mesial and distal access cavities
Caries/ restorative-driven access cavity	• The pulp chamber is accessed via the existing plastic restoration and/or caries, preserving as much sound dentine as practicably possible.

Treatment

The tooth was treated in a single visit. Four canals were identified and sealed with gutta percha and sealer. The access cavity was restored with a direct plastic restoration. In this case there were subtle grooves on the floor of the pulp chamber indicating the location of the root canal entrances (Figures 4.1.3 and 4.1.4).

What were the potential challenges in treatment of this tooth?

The position and mesial inclination of the tooth made canal negotiation challenging; stainless steel scout files (08, 10) had to be pre-curved to allow unimpeded access into the root canals. Controlled memory nickel titanium instruments were selected as they are more flexible with increased resistance to cyclic fatigue, thus making them suitable for complex curvatures. Moreover, as the file could be pre-bent it could be easily inserted into the mesio-buccal canals.

Discussion

At first glance, the UL7 appeared to have a superficial restoration; however, a more detailed assessment revealed a much deeper restoration that was in very close proximity to a pulp horn. This case highlights the importance of a pragmatic access cavity preparation to allow access to the root canal system, but minimal enough to avoid a cuspal coverage restoration.

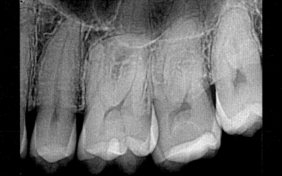

Figure 4.1.1 Pre-operative radiograph of UL7.

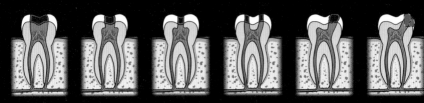

Figure 4.1.2 Access cavity designs (left to right): Traditional, Conservative, Ultra-conservative (Ninja), Truss, Caries, Restorative driven.

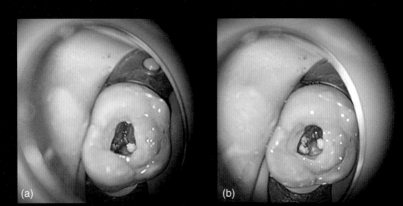

Figure 4.1.3 (a, b) Magnified intra-operative photographs of obturated canals.

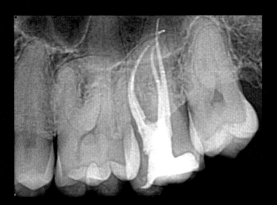

Figure 4.1.4 Post-operative radiograph of obturation and restoration of UL7.

Further Reading

Clark, D. and Khademi, J. (2010). Modern molar endodontic access and directed dentin conservation. *Dental Clinics of North America* 54: 249–273.

Gluskin, A.H., Peters, C.I., and Peters, A.O. (2014). Minimally invasive endodontics: challenging prevailing paradigms. *British Dental Journal* 216: 347–353.

Moore, B., Verdelis, K., Kishen, A. et al. (2016). Impacts of contracted endodontic cavities on instrumentation efficacy and biomechanical responses in maxillary molars. *Journal of Endodontics* 42: 1779–1783.

Pinto, K.P., Ferreira, C.M., Belladonna, F.G. et al. (2020). Current status on minimal access cavity preparations: a critical analysis and a proposal fora universal nomenclature. *International Endodontic Journal* 53: 1618–1635.

4.2

Glide Path
Frédéric Bukiet, Benoit Ballester, and Maud Guivarc'h

Objectives

This case aims to discuss the importance of glide path preparation in endodontics. It should help the reader to better understand why and when glide path preparation is indicated and how to achieve glide path during the endodontic procedure.

Introduction

A 21-year-old female patient presented with intermittent pain and biting sensitivity from the upper right first molar (UR6). During the endodontic consultation, the patient mentioned that she had not received any previous dental intervention on this tooth. However, she described previous infectious episodes treated by antibiotics.

Chief Complaint

Several previous infectious episodes requiring antibiotics.

Medical History

Unremarkable.

Dental History

The discomfort started five months ago with slight biting sensitivity related to the right maxillary first molar that increased over time. The relevant history included two consecutive infectious episodes with maxillary sinus involvement. The patient was prescribed antibiotics. After visiting a general practitioner, she was referred to the endodontic department.

Pitt Ford's Problem-Based Learning in Endodontology, Second Edition. Edited by Elizabeth Shin Perry, Shanon Patel, Shalini Kanagasingam, and Samantha Hamer.
© 2025 John Wiley & Sons Ltd. Published 2025 by John Wiley & Sons Ltd.

Clinical Examination

Extraoral examination was unremarkable. Intraoral examination revealed satisfactory oral health with acceptable oral hygiene and the periodontal probing depths were all less than 2 mm. Tooth UR6 showed an occlusal carious lesion and was tender to percussion. The adjacent teeth were intact with no evidence of caries or restorations present and responded normally to pulp sensitivity tests, while tooth UR6 did not respond. No abnormal mobility was noticed. A pre-operative periapical radiograph was taken (Figure 4.2.1).

The periapical radiograph revealed:

- Good bone level.
- Deep occlusal carious lesion.
- Large periapical radiolucency around the palatal and disto-buccal (DB) root.
- Initial coronal curvature and apical curvature of the mesio-buccal (MB) canal(s).

Taking into consideration the dental history, the anticipated anatomy of the mesio-buccal root, the extent of the radiolucency and the suspected maxillary sinus involvement, pre-operative cone beam computed tomography (CBCT) was taken.

The pre-operative CBCT revealed (Figure 4.2.2):

- The extent of the carious lesion (blue arrow).
- The root canal curvatures. An abrupt apical curvature was seen in the apical third of the DB root.
- The presence of an MB2 canal only detectable in the coronal third (white arrow).
- A wide accessory canal in a buccal direction located at the junction between the middle and apical third of the palatal root (green arrows).
- A wide radiolucency surrounding the three roots indicating extensive osseous destruction (red arrows).
- The persistence of a thin bone layer between the periapical radiolucency and the maxillary sinus.
- Localised thickening of the sinus membrane (pink arrows).

Diagnosis and Treatment Planning

The diagnosis of the UR6 was pulpal necrosis with symptomatic apical periodontitis.

What were the potential treatment options for the patient?

- No treatment (not suitable)
- Root canal treatment
- Extraction

After discussion with the patient, the decision was made to proceed with root canal treatment on tooth UR6. The purpose of endodontic treatment was to alleviate the symptoms, resolve the infection/inflammation, maintain the tooth and regenerate the bone support.

Treatment

The root canal treatment required two visits.

First visit

Under local anaesthesia, the dental dam was placed and the carious tissue was excavated. The endodontic access cavity was performed taking into consideration the root canal anatomy previously observed on the pre-operative periapical radiograph and CBCT. Initial negotiation of the root canals was performed with a stainless steel (SS) K file size 10 to passively explore and evaluate the initial patency of the root canals. The MB1, MB2 and DB canals were negotiable but narrow with regular to severe curvatures. The coronal third of the root canals was shaped with a reciprocating nickel titanium (NiTi) single file. After NaOCl irrigation, it was possible to gently introduce a SS K file size 10 into the apical third of the palatal and MB1 canals and to establish the apical patency. However, despite the coronal enlargement, the SS K file size 10 could not be introduced into the apical third of the MB2 and DB canals. A resistance to file penetration was felt especially in the DB canal. It was decided to shape the middle third of all the root canals with the same reciprocating NiTi single file to create enough space to maintain the apical pre-curvature of a SS K file size 08. Small amplitudes with clockwise rotations were implemented to direct the file tip in different inclinations until the path to the apical third was found and apical patency was established in MB2 and DB. Working lengths were determined with the electronic apex locator in all canals.

In the MB2 and DB canals, a manual pre-enlargement was carried out with a pre-curved SS K file size 08 until a size 10 file could be inserted to working length. The same procedure was repeated with the size 10 until it was 'super loose' in the root canal and manual endodontic glide path preparation was achieved.

This procedure was performed with copious NaOCl irrigation and the apical patency was rechecked with the SS K file size 08 to avoid debris accumulation in the last millimetre of the apical third.

Taking into consideration the previous difficulties and to prevent procedural errors, mechanical glide path enlargement in MB2 and DB with a flexible automated glide path NiTi file (12.5/04) was performed after establishing the manual glide path (10/02).

Shaping was completed in all canals with a reciprocating NiTi single file. After root canal shaping, the root canals were irrigated again with 3% NaOCl, dried and medicated with calcium hydroxide.

Second visit

The patient reported no intermittent symptoms between the visits. A 17% ethylenediaminetetraacetic acid (EDTA) solution was used to remove calcium hydroxide and smear layer followed by final NaOCl activation/rinse. The root canal system was obturated using a thermo-plasticised obturation technique with an epoxy resin-based sealer, after which a provisional restoration was placed. The post-operative radiograph showed a satisfactory obturation despite an inadvertent sealer extrusion (Figure 4.2.3). The patient was scheduled the following week to place a computer-aided design/manufacturing (CAD/CAM) overlay to protect the remaining dental structures from the risk of fracture.

Follow-up

At one-year review, the patient was asymptomatic and the tooth was functional. A periapical radiograph revealed obvious signs of bone healing (Figure 4.2.4). This was confirmed by the one-year review CBCT that showed:

- Significant bone regeneration.
- Overfilling of the accessory canal located in the palatal root.
- Clear improvement of the periapical mucositis with a substantial decrease of the sinus mucosa thickness (the only treatment performed was the root canal therapy of the UR6) (Figure 4.2.5).

Discussion

The endodontic glide path is still a matter of debate in the endodontic community. This discussion aims to summarise the clinical strategies to establish the glide path.

What are the basic concepts of the endodontic glide path?

The term 'glide path' refers to a smooth, uninterrupted patent canal from its entrance to the apical constriction. Its aim is to prevent procedural errors during root canal instrumentation and to preserve the original root canal anatomy.

Glide path preparation reduces the torsional stress/cyclic fatigue on the ensuing NiTi instruments and decreases debris extrusion and the risk of canal blockages and deviations. The endodontic glide path is achieved when the practitioner is able to introduce a 'super-loose' K file size 10 at the apical constriction; that is, without encountering resistance from the dentine walls. This is the minimal enlargement required at working length before root canal shaping with NiTi files.

When and how to establish the glide path in primary root canal treatment

After access cavity, root canal exploration with a pre-curved K file size 08 or 10 (also known as a scouting file) is recommended to evaluate the initial patency (Table 4.2.1). Introduction of the scouting file directly into the apical third is not recommended, because it may lead to blocking the canal or to extruding microorganisms and pulp debris through the apical foramen.

If necessary, a gentle manual pre-enlargement with the same file is performed without seeking to penetrate deeper than the initial penetration. This is carried out with EDTA lubricant gel or with NaOCl.

Then shaping of the coronal third is implemented with a flexible reciprocating or rotating NiTi file. The crown-down pressureless technique introduced in the 1980s is still highly relevant. It is well known that this approach aims to facilitate access to the apical third and limits procedural errors during root canal preparation. It has been demonstrated that

Table 4.2.1 Clinical strategy for endodontic glide path management. NiTi, nickel titanium; SS, stainless steel; WL, working length.

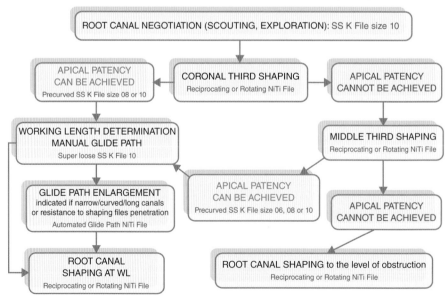

shaping the coronal third improves the accuracy of working length determination and also reduces debris extrusion.

It must be pointed out that the practitioner can encounter initial difficulties to negotiate the coronal third of the root canal with SS K files (MB2, for instance). It can be helpful to directly use an automated heat-treated NiTi file, taking advantage of the flexibility and cutting ability. Features of the most recent NiTi files allow better preservation of the pericervical dentine and respect of the first curvature. Obviously, the size of the rotating or reciprocating NiTi file for this purpose is selected according to the specifications of each case.

Several situations can be encountered after coronal shaping:

- Apical patency can be easily and passively achieved with a K file size 10 already being 'super loose': the working length can be determined, the glide path naturally exists, and no glide path enlargement is needed before further shaping.
- Apical patency can be achieved with a K file size 10, but a slight resistance with the dentine walls is felt: the working length can be determined, and a manual pre-enlargement is performed until the file becomes 'super loose'. The manual glide path preparation is now achieved, and root canal shaping can be conducted while maintaining the apical patency and irrigating throughout the procedure.
- Apical patency cannot be achieved with a K file size 10. However, the apical patency is reached with a pre-curved K file size 08 (Figure 4.2.6). Once the latter can penetrate at working length in a repeatable manner without resistance, the K file size 10 can be used until it becomes 'super loose'. The manual glide path preparation is now achieved. In case of a narrow or severely curved canal, the same procedure can be done by starting with a pre-curved SS K file size 06, then 08 and 10.

It must be noted that apical patency should not be forced and shaping the middle third of the root canal can also help the practitioner to establish apical patency.

The use of automated reciprocating or rotating glide path NiTi instruments for glide path enlargement is recommended when dealing with severely curved, long and/or narrow canals. They are generally used once the manual glide path preparation has been achieved and prior to root canal shaping, making the overall preparation of the root canal more gradual and safer. Despite shaping of the coronal and middle thirds, some canals can be non-negotiable in the apical third (i.e., no apical patency). In these cases, more emphasis is put on the chemical action/activation of root canal irrigants and the obturation strategy.

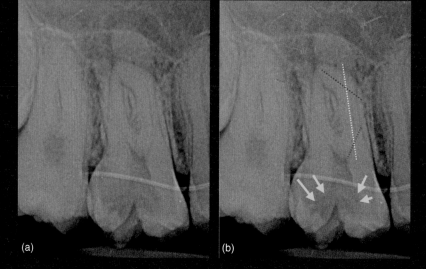

Figure 4.2.1 Pre-operative radiograph showing a deep carious lesion (blue arrows) and a large periapical radiolucency (red arrows). Notice the curvatures of the mesio-buccal canal(s) illustrated by the red and yellow dotted lines.

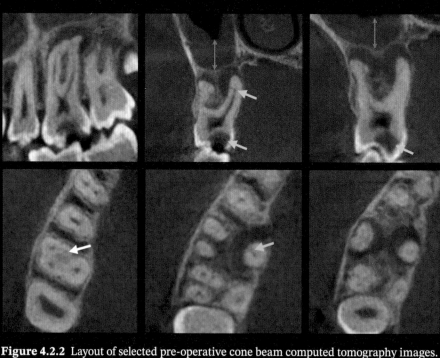

Figure 4.2.2 Layout of selected pre-operative cone beam computed tomography images. Extent of the carious lesion (blue arrow). Presence of an MB2 canal only detectable in the coronal third (white arrow). A wide accessory canal in a buccal direction located at the junction between the middle and apical third of the palatal root (green arrows). A wide radiolucency surrounding the three roots indicating extensive osseous destruction (red arrows). Localised thickening of the sinus membrane (pink arrows).

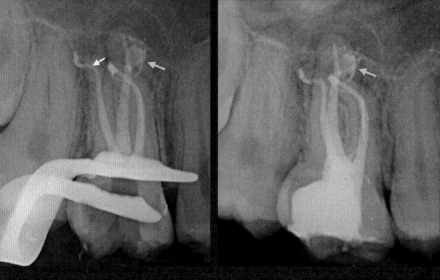

Figure 4.2.3 Post-operative radiographs showing the abrupt apical curvature of the disto-buccal canal (yellow arrow), the separated MB2 and the inadvertent sealer extrusion through an accessory canal (green arrows).

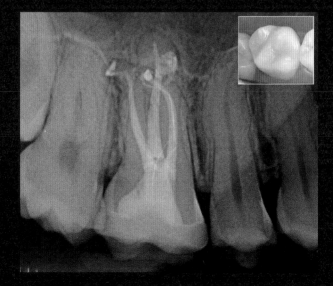

Figure 4.2.4 One-year review radiograph showing the reduction of the radiolucency and the protection of the remaining dental structure with a computer-aided design/manufacturing (CAD/CAM) overlay.

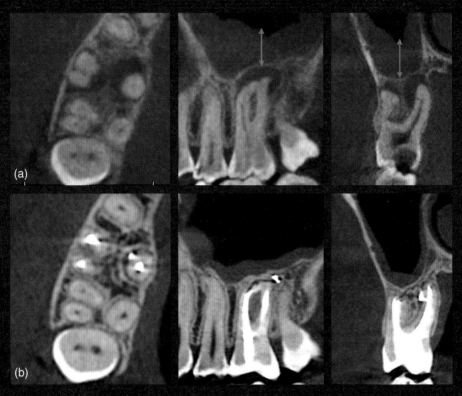

Figure 4.2.5 Comparison between (a) pre-operative and (b) one-year review cone beam computed tomography showing the bone regeneration and the reduction of the sinus mucosal thickness following the endodontic procedure.

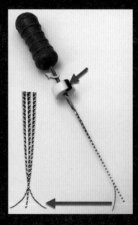

Figure 4.2.6 In case of apical curvature, a pre-bent K file can be used. The black landmark of the stop (blue arrow) is used to locate the direction of the root canal curvature.

Further Reading

Hartmann, R.C., Peters, O.A., de Figueiredo, J.A., and Rossi-Fedele, G. (2018). Association of manual or engine-driven glide path preparation with canal centring and apical transportation: a systematic review. *International Endodontic Journal* 51: 1239–1252.

Plotino, G., Nagendrababu, V., Bukiet, F. et al. (2020). Influence of negotiation, glide path, and preflaring procedures on root canal shaping-terminology, basic concepts, and a systematic review. *Journal of Endodontics* 46: 707–729.

Tsotsis, P., Dunlap, C., Scott, R. et al. (2021). A survey of current trends in root canal treatment: access cavity design and cleaning and shaping practices. *Australian Endodontic Journal* 47 (1): 27–33.

West, J. (2010). The endodontic glidepath: secrets to rotary success. *Dentistry Today* 29: 90–93.

4.3 Working Length Determination

Bhavin Bhuva and Shanon Patel

Objectives

At the end of this case, the reader should understand the importance of accurate working length determination during root canal treatment. Accurate working length determination is critical to ensure the root canal system has been chemo-mechanically prepared and filled to full length, to minimise iatrogenic complications such as under-/over-preparation. The reader should be aware of the methods available to determine working length, as well as the advantages and disadvantages of each technique.

Introduction

A 43-year-old female patient presented complaining of sensitivity and acute pain on the right side of the mouth.

Chief Complaint

Spontaneous radiating intense pain on the right-hand side; the pain was poorly localised and would last for several hours.

Medical History

Unremarkable.

Dental History

The patient gave a history of acute pain that had been relapsing and remitting in nature for the previous two days. Prior to the acute pain, there had been sensitivity to hot and cold foods and liquids that had progressively worsened.

Pitt Ford's Problem-Based Learning in Endodontology, Second Edition. Edited by Elizabeth Shin Perry, Shanon Patel, Shalini Kanagasingam, and Samantha Hamer.
© 2025 John Wiley & Sons Ltd. Published 2025 by John Wiley & Sons Ltd.

Clinical Examination

The patient had a moderately restored dentition. The lower right first and second molar teeth (LR6 and LR7) were restored with ceramic onlay restorations. The LR6 was tender to percussion, whilst no other teeth in the upper or lower right quadrants elicited a similar response. There were no probing depths greater than 3 mm associated with either the LR6 or LR7.

The LR6 gave a pronounced and prolonged response to both thermal and electric sensibility testing. The LR5, LR7 and LR6 all responded normally to both thermal and electric testing.

A pre-operative radiograph of the lower right molar region was taken and did not reveal any periapical changes associated with either the LR6 or LR7 (Figure 4.3.1). There were moderately deep restorations evident in both teeth.

Diagnosis and Treatment Planning

A diagnosis of symptomatic irreversible pulpitis was reached for the LR6.

The treatment options for the LR6 were:

- No treatment.
- Root canal treatment of LR6 followed by cuspal coverage restoration.
- Extraction.

Following discussion of the treatment options, the patient elected to have root canal treatment and definitive cuspal coverage restoration.

Treatment

Prior to carrying out root canal treatment, it is important to have at least one periapical radiograph taken with a beam-aiming device. Two radiographs taken with different horizontal (parallax) angulation may be useful to assess the anatomy of teeth with multiple roots (Figure 4.3.2). A good-quality pre-operative radiograph facilitates treatment planning in advance of the endodontic procedure, and provides important information to the clinician, for example the working length(s) of the canal(s) may be estimated (Table 4.3.1).

What is the working length of a root canal?

The working length of a root canal is the distance from a designated coronal reference point (for example, incisal edge) on the tooth crown to the end point of root canal preparation (Figure 4.3.3).

Table 4.3.1 Essential information provided by pre-operative radiograph.

- Periapical status
- Number of roots and anatomy
- Length of root canals (estimated working length)
- Curvature of root canals
- Depth and size of pulp chamber
- Canal obstructions
- Caries
- Depth and quality of existing restoration

What are the drawbacks of conventional radiography?

With two-dimensional (2D) radiographs, estimated working length(s) may be measured directly from the radiograph. With digitally acquired images, a measurement facility is provided with the accompanying software, which can be used to estimate the root canal length(s).

Conventional radiographic techniques produce a compressed 2D image that can only provide limited clinical information with respect to three-dimensional (3D) anatomy. For example, a radiograph will not demonstrate root curvatures in the bucco-lingual plane. Even with the use of a beam-aiming device, periapical radiography has poor geometrical accuracy and is susceptible to image distortion. Therefore, the length(s) derived from these images will always be subject to a degree of error. All periapical radiographic images are magnified by up to 5%.

Problems with positioning of the film or digital sensor may also occur, reducing the quality of the image further. For example, when taking radiographs of the upper posterior teeth, the film may bend, leading to image distortion. A further problem may be encountered with lower molar teeth as the patient may have difficulty tolerating the image receptor when it is placed into the lingual sulcus. This may lead to an image which does not capture the root apices and surrounding periapical tissues.

Bisecting angle radiographs should, if possible, be avoided as they are susceptible to even greater distortion and inaccuracy. These images are also very difficult to reproduce. Superimposition of various anatomical structures and image distortion may result in limited diagnostic yield from conventional radiography. For example, superimposition of the root apices of the upper molar root teeth with the floor of the maxillary sinus or zygomatic arch may commonly occur during periapical radiography in this region.

What additional information does a pre-treatment cone beam computed tomography scan give?

Small field-of-view cone beam computed tomography (CBCT) has been shown to be highly reliable for determining the pre-operative working length, as it provides geometrically accurate images and overcomes the issue of superimposition of anatomical structures. This technique may be employed to assess both periapical status and root canal anatomy/length when 2D imaging does not provide the necessary information. CBCT may be utilised in cases of complex root canal anatomy.

The pulp chamber was accessed, and the root canal orifices were located and coronally flared. Following this, the length of each of the root canals was determined and root canal treatment was completed. One year review demonstrated healthy periapical tissues (Figure 4.3.1).

What are the important apical anatomical landmarks?

The apical region of the root canal has been studied in great detail and descriptions of the anatomy of this area are well documented. Changes in the apical anatomy occur throughout life as the effects of destructive resorption and reparative cementum deposition occur.

The main anatomical landmarks of the apical region of the tooth are as follows (Figure 4.3.4):

- The root or anatomical apex (A) is the most apical point of the root; it may be several millimetres from the apical foramen.
- The apical foramen is the opening of the root canal onto the external root surface of the tooth. The apical foramen consists of a major apical foramen (B), which is the opening on the external surface of the root surface, and a minor apical foramen (C), which is also called the apical constriction.
- The apical constriction (C) is the narrowest point of the apical root canal (see the description that follows).

The cemento-dentinal junction or CDJ (D) represents the true histological junction of the root canal space with the periodontal tissues. Therefore, in theory, the CDJ is the most desirable end point of root canal preparation. However, in reality the anatomy of the apical CDJ is highly variable. Furthermore, the effects of resorption and cementum deposition throughout life will continually alter the position of the CDJ. The CDJ represents the exact delineation of the pulp and periodontal tissues, but as it is a histological landmark it cannot be determined clinically or radiographically.

What is the most desirable end point for root canal preparation?

The apical constriction is the narrowest point of the apical root canal and has been suggested as the ideal end point for root canal preparation. Most product specifications for electronic apex locators refer to the apical constriction as the point that they most accurately detect. However, it is more likely that they detect a point somewhere between the apical constriction and major apical foramen.

The radiographic apex is an important reference point that is defined as the most apical point of the root as seen on a radiograph. However, the apical foramen may exit the root laterally, buccally or lingually, some way from the anatomical and radiographic apices.

What methods are available for determining the working length intra-operatively?

Electronic apex locator

The electronic apex locator provides an accurate, reliable and safe method of determining the working length of a root canal, overcoming many of the limitations of radiographs.

An electronic apex locator works on the principle of electrical impedance (a measure of resistance to an alternating current). Apex locators consist of a display that may be digital or analogue, and two electrodes (Figure 4.3.5). The first electrode is a lip hook, which is positioned at the corner of the patient's mouth in contact with the oral mucosa. The second electrode attaches or makes contact with the endodontic instrument within the root canal (Figure 4.3.6). As the instrument approaches the apex of the tooth, the electrical impedance (resistance) gradually reduces until the apical foramen is reached ('zero' reading). At the point where the instrument makes contact with the periodontal ligament, the impedance reaches the same fixed value irrespective of the patient, the age or the type of tooth.

Modern apex locators are very accurate and can work in the presence of moisture and fluid within the root canal. They are capable of measuring to within 0.5 mm of the apical foramen in over 90% of cases. If a tolerance of 1 mm is accepted, the accuracy approaches 100%. No other method of root canal length determination is as accurate.

A further advantage of an electronic apex locator is that it reduces the need for working length radiographs during root canal treatment, thereby decreasing the overall exposure for the patient.

Occasionally, an apex locator may give an erroneous reading (Table 4.3.2), such as when the file makes contact with a metallic restoration in a tooth

Table 4.3.2 Reasons for erroneous apex locator readings.

- Excessive fluid in pulp chamber
- Contact with a metallic restoration (e.g. amalgam filling, gold crown)
- Contact with caries
- Iatrogenic perforation of the pulp chamber floor or root canal
- Purulent discharge within canal
- Perforation due internal or external resorptive processes
- Teeth with significant apical resorption
- Teeth with large apical foramina
- Lateral canal

(Figure 4.3.7). This situation may become apparent initially when the reading is not consistent with the estimated working length obtained from the pre-operative radiograph. Alternatively, a false reading may be suspected if the length obtained is not consistent with the other canal lengths.

Once the working lengths of each canal have been determined using the electronic apex locator, a working length (diagnostic) radiograph may be taken for verification.

Working length radiograph

The working length (diagnostic) radiograph (Figure 4.3.1) is taken during root canal treatment to establish or confirm the length of a root canal. This radiograph is taken with a small file (for example, ISO size 10 or 15). In a multi-rooted tooth, different types or sizes of files (for example a K file and a Hedström file) can be used to differentiate the file position in each specific canal. Working length radiographs should be taken with a beam-aiming device (for example, Endoray II) to optimise the geometrical accuracy and minimise the distortion of the radiograph. Working length radiographs taken with the bisecting angle technique provide limited accuracy.

Paper points

Paper points have been used to establish the working length of a root canal. With this technique, the root canal is dried, after which a pre-measured paper point is advanced slightly beyond the estimated working length. The paper point is removed after a few seconds and assessed to see whether the tip has absorbed moisture (i.e. tissue fluid or blood) (Figure 4.3.8). The working length is calculated according to the length of the paper point that remains dry. The process needs to be repeated to ensure the reproducibility of the measurement. It is important that the canal is dry prior to using the technique; it will not work where there is continual exudate or bleeding from the periapical tissues. In addition, it is important not to keep the paper point in the canal for too long, as the exudate or bleeding will be absorbed further up the paper point, giving a less accurate measurement.

The paper point technique may be useful in teeth with wide apical foramina, where an apex locator may not give an accurate reading. However, this technique should only be used in conjunction with a working length radiograph.

Tactile sensation

Tactile sensation may be a useful technique for the more experienced practitioner to initially determine where the apical constriction is located. This technique should be used only as an adjunct to a more reliable technique and never in isolation; and it is only useful when the apical constriction is small and has not been damaged through resorption or previous instrumentation.

What are the consequences of incorrect length determination during root canal treatment?

The rationale behind instrumentation to the level of the apical constriction is to ensure the complete cleaning and shaping of the root canal space. Incorrect length determination during root canal instrumentation may have significant consequences on the preparation and subsequent obturation of the root canal, which in turn may adversely impact the outcome of treatment (Table 4.3.3).

Table 4.3.3 Consequences of inaccurate working length determination.

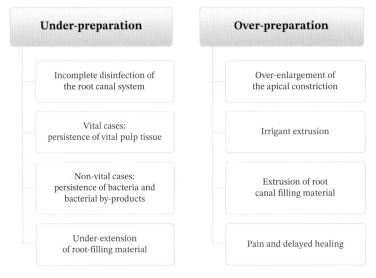

Under-preparation	Over-preparation
Incomplete disinfection of the root canal system	Over-enlargement of the apical constriction
Vital cases: persistence of vital pulp tissue	Irrigant extrusion
Non-vital cases: persistence of bacteria and bacterial by-products	Extrusion of root canal filling material
Under-extension of root-filling material	Pain and delayed healing

If the 'working' length is underestimated, the full length of the root canal will not be accessed and disinfected. In the case of an infected tooth, this will lead to the persistence of bacteria and bacterial by-products in the root canal.

The consequence of over-instrumentation may be increased post-operative pain, and delayed healing as a result of direct tissue trauma and extrusion of bacteria. The enlargement of the apical constriction increases the probability of extrusion of root canal filling material into the periapical tissues.

Discussion

The desirable end point for root canal instrumentation is the apical constriction. Theoretically, the apical constriction delineates the junction between the root canal system and the periapical tissues. It is important to remember that this landmark may be several millimetres from the anatomical or radiographic apex.

Accurate working length determination is critical to the success of endodontic treatment. By ensuring that the full length of the root canal(s) have been instrumented (and disinfected), the biological objectives of root canal treatment can be achieved. In addition, confining instrumentation to the root canal prevents irritation of the periapical tissues and delayed healing. Outcome studies clearly demonstrate the poorest healing rates for root-filled teeth with over-extended root canal filings, followed by those that have been filled more than 2 mm short of the apical constriction. Teeth with root canal obturation within 2 mm of the apical constriction have the best prognosis for successful healing.

The use of an apex locator in conjunction with a good-quality paralleled pre-operative radiograph(s) should be considered best practice. A pre-operative small-volume CBCT scan may be justified when anatomical superimposition prevents accurate assessment of root canal anatomy or where conventional periapical radiographs cannot be taken.

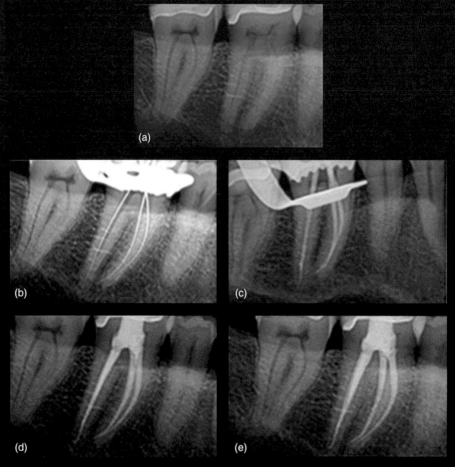

Figure 4.3.1 (a) Pre-operative radiograph of LR6 showing a moderately deep restoration and healthy periapical tissues. (b) Working length (diagnostic) radiograph of LR6. Note that a Hedström file has been placed in the mesio-buccal canal, whilst a K-Flexofile has been used in the mesio-lingual canal so that the two canals can be distinguished from each other. The file in the distal canal is approximately 2 mm under-extended; the working length is rechecked with the electronic apex locator and the canal reprepared accordingly. (c) Master cone radiograph of LR6 demonstrating good length extension of the gutta percha master cones in all three canals prior to obturation. (d) Post-operative radiograph of completed root canal treatment. (e) One-year review demonstrating healthy periapical tissues.

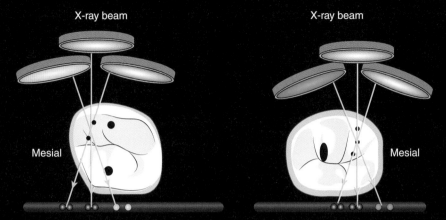

X-ray beam   X-ray beam

Mesial   Mesial

Figure 4.3.2 Parallax technique. Note how horizontal shift of the radiograph can aid in separation of the root canals.

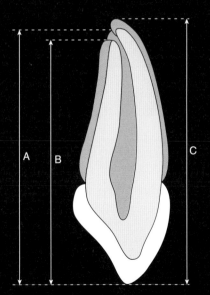

A   B   C

Figure 4.3.3 Working length estimation. A = distance from incisal tip to apical foramen, B = distance from incisal tip to apical constriction, C = distance from incisal tip to radiographic apex. The diagnostic radiograph only reveals the position of the radiographic apex. The radiographic apex does not accurately represent the position of the apical constriction or foramen. Therefore it is desirable to use an electronic apex locator.

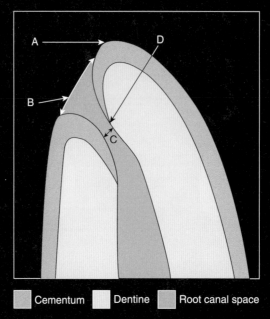

| ■ Cementum | ■ Dentine | ■ Root canal space |

Figure 4.3.4 Diagrammatical representation of the apical region. A = the tooth or anatomical apex, B = the major apical foramen, C = the apical constriction, D = the cemento-dentinal junction. On the basis of studies on extracted human teeth, the distance from the apical foramen to the apical constriction is on average 0.5–0.8 mm. There is a trend for this distance to increase with age.

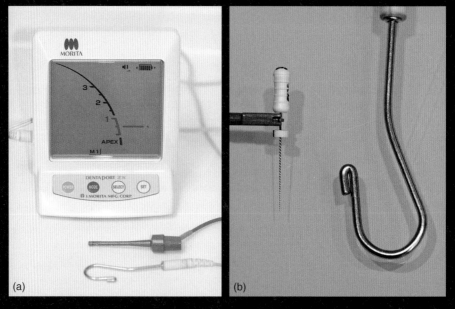

Figure 4.3.5 (a) Electronic apex locator. (b) Apex locator electrodes, consisting of a 'clip' for the endodontic file within the canal and a lip hook.

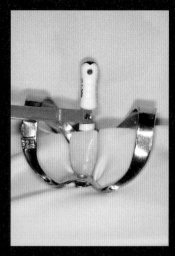

Figure 4.3.6 Endodontic file in position for apex locator reading. The rubber stop on the file is positioned at the level of a reproducible landmark on the tooth surface (in this case, the incisal edge).

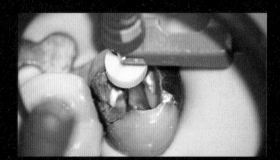

Figure 4.3.7 An erroneous apex locator reading may be obtained when the endodontic file makes contact with a metallic restoration in the tooth. This may occur when the access cavity is made through a metal crown or amalgam restoration.

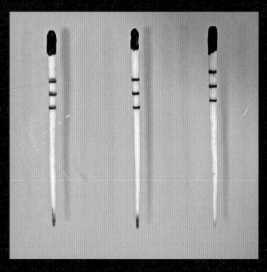

Figure 4.3.8 A series of pre-measured paper points have been used to determine the position of the periapical tissues.

Further Reading

Connert, T., Hülber, J.M., Godt, A. et al. (2014). Accuracy of endodontic working length determination using cone beam computed tomography. *International Endodontic Journal* 47: 698–703.

Dummer, P.M., McGinn, J.H., and Rees, D.G. (1984). The position and topography of the apical constriction and apical foramen. *International Endodontic Journal* 17: 192–198.

Kuttler, Y. (1955). Microscopic investigation of root apexes. *Journal of the American Dental Association* 50: 544–552.

McDonald, N.J. (1992). The electronic determination of working length. *Dental Clinics of North America* 36: 293–307.

Ng, Y.L., Mann, V., Rahbaran, S. et al. (2008). Outcome of primary root canal treatment: systematic review of the literature – Part 2. Influence of clinical factors. *International Endodontic Journal* 41: 6–31.

Patel, S., Brown, J., Pimentel, T. et al. (2019). Cone beam computed tomography in endodontics – a review of the literature. *International Endodontic Journal* 52: 1138–1152.

4.4 Disinfection of the Root Canal System

Ali Hilmi

Objectives

At the end of this case, the reader should understand the importance of disinfection in root canal treatment, the role of irrigation and the clinical procedures for effective disinfection of the root canal system.

Introduction

A 45-year-old female presented as a new patient complaining that one of her mandibular right molar teeth does not feel right. What is the cause of her dental problem and how will you treat it?

Chief Complaint

The patient reported occasional tenderness of their lower right first molar (LR6) when chewing on it.

What further details do you need to know about the patient's complaint?

The first step in the management of any patient is an accurate history. This informs what aspects of the clinical examination are most relevant, which in turn will inform which special investigations are most appropriate.

If it is an endodontic problem, it will help you to work out whether it is a pulpal and/or periapical problem. It is also necessary to determine what type of dental treatment (if any) has been recently carried out in the lower and upper right quadrants.

Typical questions that should be asked include:

- Where is the pain? Can the symptoms be localised to a specific tooth or region, or are they diffuse (poorly localised)?
- When and how did the symptoms start, and has the character of these symptoms altered over this period?

Pitt Ford's Problem-Based Learning in Endodontology, Second Edition. Edited by Elizabeth Shin Perry, Shanon Patel, Shalini Kanagasingam, and Samantha Hamer.
© 2025 John Wiley & Sons Ltd. Published 2025 by John Wiley & Sons Ltd.

- How would you describe the symptoms – dull, sharp or throbbing?
- When the symptoms are at their worst, how severe are the symptoms on a scale of 1–10?
- Once triggered, how long do the symptoms last for: seconds, minutes or hours?
- How are the symptoms affected by cold, hot or chewing?
- Does anything trigger or worsen the symptoms?
- Does anything relieve the symptoms (for example, analgesics)?
- Can the symptoms be spontaneous and/or have they woken you up during the night?
- Have you had any recent dental treatment on this side of your mouth, and do you remember what type of treatment was carried out?

From the answers to these questions, you find out that the patient has had an occasional low-grade intermittent dull ache for approximately six months, localised to the mandibular right first molar. She has had two acute episodes of pain (flare-ups) in this time that eventually subsided after she took a course of antibiotics prescribed by her previous dentist. The patient noticed that the pain was more common when she was run-down or tired. She occasionally took non-steroidal anti-inflammatory analgesics when the pain became too uncomfortable, which helped with her symptoms. The patient advised you that when she initially developed her symptoms from this tooth, she occasionally woke up in the middle of the night with a dull, throbbing pain localised to this tooth.

Medical History

Unremarkable.

Dental History

The patient was a regular attender at her dentist for annual check-ups.

Up to her early 20s, the patient drank two or three cans of cola a day. She changed to bottled water after her dentist advised her of the effects of excessive consumption of carbonated drinks on her teeth.

Clinical Examination

Extraoral examination was unremarkable. Intraoral examination revealed that the oral hygiene status was good. The patient had 2–3 posterior teeth restored in each quadrant; these restorations appeared to be sound. The LR6 had been restored with a disto-occlusal composite restoration that appeared sound. The LR6 was in functional occlusion with the UR6, which was minimally restored.

What clinical investigations would be most appropriate?

- Assessment of the structural and strategic value
- Palpation
- Presence of a sinus tract
- Mobility
- Percussion
- Periodontal probing

The clinical examination revealed that the LR6 was slightly tender to percussion and buccal palpation only. The tooth was not mobile, and examination of the adjacent mucosa did not reveal a sinus tract. There were no periodontal probing depths greater than 2 mm. The margins of the existing restoration appeared to be sound. Examination of the upper right quadrant did not reveal any abnormalities.

What special investigations would you carry out?

- *Sensitivity (vitality) test*: Cold, heat and/or electric pulp testing should be carried out to assess the pulpal status. It is essential to test neighbouring and contra-lateral teeth for comparison (controls). The response can be described as immediate/delayed, normal/exaggerated/reduced/no response, and reference made to whether it reproduced the patient's symptoms.
- *Radiographs*: A periapical and/or bitewing radiograph and cone beam computed tomography (CBCT) scan can reveal clues to the status of the pulp and periradicular tissues (Figures 4.4.1 and 4.4.2a–d). Features that may indicate an unhealthy pulp include dystrophic calcification, gross caries and restorations in close proximity to the pulp. Infection of the root canal system may be inferred from widening of the periodontal ligament, periapical radiolucency and previous (inadequate) root canal treatment.

The LR6 did not respond to electric or cold sensitivity testing; the LR5, LR7, UR5, UR6 and UR7 responded within normal limits.

What did the radiograph and cone beam computed tomography scan reveal about the lower right first molar?

- Minimal horizontal bone loss.
- Secondary caries.
- Calcification of the pulp and canals.
- Periapical radiolucency associated with the mesial and distal roots.
- Isthmus between mesial canals (Figure 4.4.2a, arrow).
- Wide, elliptical cross-section of distal canal (Figure 4.4.2c, arrow).

Diagnosis and Treatment Planning

What is the diagnosis?

A diagnosis of symptomatic periapical periodontitis associated with an infected necrotic root canal system was reached for the LR6.

The potential treatment options that should be discussed with the patient are:

- Root canal treatment
- Extraction
- Leave alone

Treatment decisions are informed by the particular array of prognostic factors and treatment complexities. In this case, root canal treatment and subsequent restoration of the tooth, if adequately executed, is very likely to result in periapical healing and tooth survival. The treatment is of moderate complexity owing to the root canal anatomy (calcification, curvatures, and ramifications) and deep distal restorative margin. In light of this, root canal treatment is the preferred option as the tooth appears to have a good overall prognosis, and is of functional and strategic value. Extraction would also eliminate the patient's symptoms; however, she would also lose a functionally strategic tooth, and the resulting unopposed maxillary first molar tooth would become non-functional and may over-erupt. You may also want to briefly discuss with the patient the costs and risks of replacement options for this tooth.

Although the patient could leave the tooth alone (i.e. have no treatment), this is not advisable as her existing symptoms will continue as will her occasional flare-ups, for which repeated courses of antibiotics are not appropriate. In addition, she may eventually suffer from an acute apical abscess that, in severe cases, may result in pyrexia, malaise and even obstruction of her airway. Similarly, a prolonged delay in initiating treatment may result in a reduced endodontic prognosis, as well as risk further structural deterioration of the tooth.

Endodontic treatment was carried out in a single visit under dental dam. The existing restoration and carious tissue were removed, and the restorability was reassessed. As the tooth was deemed restorable, a pre-endodontic restoration was placed prior to access cavity preparation. On accessing the pulp, no cracks or fracture lines were detected. The working length was determined using an apex locator and confirmed with a radiograph. Mechanical preparation was carried out, with frequent irrigation with sodium hypochlorite throughout the procedure. The canals were subsequently obturated with gutta percha and root canal sealer using a warm vertical compaction technique. The access cavity was restored with a composite restoration.

What was the most likely cause of this endodontic problem?

The mouth contains an abundance of microbial species, most of which are opportunistic pathogens. If there is an interruption in the integrity of the protective enamel surface, such as caries or a crack, this can allow microbes to colonise the dentine, and ultimately affect the pulp. Unfortunately, the pulp has a limited capacity to protect itself against an advancing microbial front, particularly where it is sustained by nutrients and additional microbes from the oral environment.

Regarding the tooth LR6, the cumulative effect of caries and cycles of restorative treatment most probably resulted in the root canal system becoming infected and subsequently necrotic. An infected, necrotic root canal system provides a protected and nutrient-rich environment for a microbial population to proliferate. The spread of bacteria and/or their by-products via portals of exit, such as the apical foramen or lateral canals, can result in inflammation and/or infection of the periradicular tissues (apical periodontitis).

The aim of root canal treatment is to prevent, or in this case allow healing of, apical periodontitis by disinfecting and sealing the root canal system.

What are the challenges of disinfecting the root canal system?

Disinfection of the root canal system is a formidable task (Table 4.4.1), and most cases of apical periodontitis persisting after root canal treatment are due to inadequate disinfection. The challenges to disinfection arise from the complex anatomy, infection in the form of a microbial biofilm, the presence of organic and inorganic debris and the immediate proximity to the surrounding tissues that are easily damaged (Table 4.4.2).

Table 4.4.1 Diagram of the mesial root illustrating the some of the challenges to disinfection. (a) Adherent biofilm (b) Complex canal configurations (c) Dentine Tubules (d) Dentine and pulp debris (e) Lateral canals (f) Canal ramifications and isthmuses (g) Canal curvatures (h) Narrow diameters (i) Closed end.

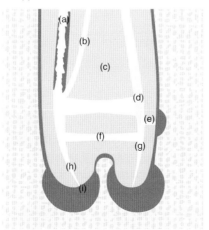

Table 4.4.2 Challenges of canal disinfection.

	Challenges	Effect on disinfection
Canal anatomy	Complex configurations Canal ramifications Closed-ended Narrow diameter Dentine tubules Lateral canals Elliptical shape	The root canal system is complex and mechanical instrumentation will leave 30–50% of canal walls untouched Irregularities, narrow diameters, cul-de-sacs and dentine tubules allow accumulation of debris in inaccessible areas and resist fluid movement and exchange
Microbial biofilm	Adherent Multi-layered Diverse community Synergism Protection	Bacteria function in complex communities embedded in a multi-layered adherent biofilm, often in isthmuses or ramifications, making them highly resistant to disinfection and able to survive in hostile environments
Canal contents	Pulp remnants Debris from instrumentation	The infected debris accumulating during preparation provides protection and substrate for bacteria, can cause blockages, rapidly exhausts the activity of the disinfectant and can prevent the obturating material forming a seal with the canal wall
Adjacent tissues	Various potential paths of communication to bone, periodontal ligament and soft tissues	Can restrict the safe delivery, potency and extent of disinfection

How was disinfection of the root canal system achieved?

Thorough disinfection can only be achieved through effective irrigation with an antimicrobial irrigant. Irrigation performs a number of functions that are prerequisites for disinfection (Table 4.4.3) and arguably make it the most important step of root canal treatment. For disinfection to be effective, the irrigant must reach the entire root canal system with sufficient force, potency, volume, and frequency. The pulp and canals need to be accessed

Table 4.4.3 The functions of irrigation.

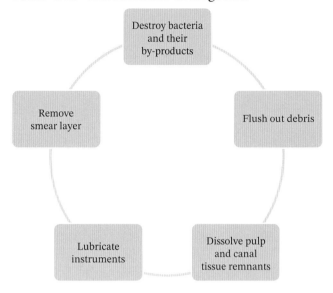

for this to be achieved, but as coronal and radicular preparation weakens the tooth structure (thereby compromising long-term survival), this should only be undertaken to the extent required for sufficient delivery and exchange of irrigant to the apical region. An apical preparation to a size 30 has been shown to be sufficient for use with a 30G needle.

How can the effectiveness of the irrigant be safely improved?

Improving the effectiveness of irrigation requires an understanding of the fluid dynamics of a closed-end system, as well as the physical and chemical interactions occurring. Attempts to improve effectiveness must be balanced with the corresponding risks or drawbacks (Table 4.4.4). Simple techniques such as using a smaller or more flexible irrigation syringe allow delivery of the irrigant to a greater depth, but require greater injecting pressure to deliver irrigant with sufficient flow and shearing forces. Frequent replenishment, higher concentration and longer duration aim to maintain the presence of active irrigant, but rely on diffusion to ensure chemically active molecules continually reach the reacting surfaces. Similarly, a side-vented needle has a lower risk of irrigant extrusion through the apex, but the irrigant does not extend significantly beyond the irrigation tip.

The extent to which the irrigant reaches passively in the canal is called the *stagnation plane* and is a consequence of a closed-ended system (Table 4.4.5). This is an important consideration, as beyond this level there is no fluid exchange. The stagnation plane can be extended further apically or overcome completely by regular recapitulation with a small file and *activation* of the irrigant. Activating forces include ultrasonic, sonic, rotary, laser or

Table 4.4.4 Techniques for effective irrigation.

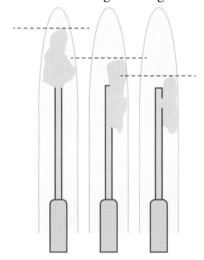

Table 4.4.5 Effect of needle design on stagnation plane (red line).

manual pumping of a non-binding gutta percha point to working length (Table 4.4.6). Activation improves the penetration and activity of the irrigant by creating turbulence and microenvironments of alternating positive and negative pressure. This results in enhanced fluid shear forces, replenishment of irrigant, flushing of debris and greater penetration into dentine tubules and accessory canal anatomy. Ultrasonic and laser activation appear to demonstrate the greatest potential for this purpose due to their ability to generate acoustic cavitation and streaming forces. It is important to note, however, that the evidence of improved patient outcomes associated with a single technique or a combination of activation techniques is limited.

Activated irrigation is most effective following completion of mechanical preparation, where the canals are at their widest and canal contents

Table 4.4.6 Advantages and disadvantages of irrigation techniques.

Technique	Advantages	Disadvantages
Smaller needle	More apical delivery	Less volume and force of flow
Side-vented needle	Safer delivery with lower risk of extrusion	Stagnation plane is 1 mm from needle tip
Greater injecting forces	Greater penetration and shear force of fluid	Greater risk of extrusion
Higher concentration	Tissue dissolution and antibacterial effect	Greater risk of damage to tissues
Frequent replacement	Consistent active irrigant and flushing effect	Extends treatment time
Heating	Improves reactivity	Short-lasting effect and risk of noxious fumes
Activation	Greater penetration and flushing of irrigant	Risk of extrusion and iatrogenic event

largely removed and allow the irrigant to exert its antimicrobial effectiveness. Adopting a combination of measures to improve the effectiveness is recommended.

What irrigants are available and which is best to use?

Various irrigants are available, such as sodium hypochlorite, ethylenediaminetetraacetic acid (EDTA), saline, chlorhexidine and iodine (Table 4.4.7). Each has its advantages and drawbacks, and the clinician should consider which irrigant or combination of irrigants is best suited to the clinical context. Sodium hypochlorite is most suited for root canal disinfection and dissolution of pulp tissue through its ability to release free chlorine ions. EDTA is an effective irrigant for removal of the smear layer, and may also aid in disrupting biofilm integrity. However, its presence in the canal can reduce the activity of sodium hypochlorite. Sodium hypochlorite should not be used in conjunction with chlorhexidine due to the formation of an orange-brown precipitate which may occlude dentinal tubules, and compromise the seal from root canal obturation. This insoluble precipitate was previously thought to contain parachloroanaline, a carcinogen, however, this has since been disputed by recent studies.

What is the smear layer?

Instrumentation results in a layer of organic and inorganic debris (including bacteria), coating the instrumented portions of the root canal wall (Figure 4.4.3), called the smear layer.

Table 4.4.7 Characteristics of different endodontic irrigants.

	NaOCl	**EDTA**	**CHX**	**Iodine**	**Saline**
Antibacterial effectiveness	+++	–	Substantivity	+	–
Tissue dissolution	+++	–	–	–	–
Biocompatible	–	–	+	+	+++
No interactions	*CHX	*NaOCl	*NaOCl	+	+++
Smear layer removal	–	+++	–	–	+
Low risk of allergy	+++	+++	–	–	+++
No discoloration	+++	+++	–	–	+++
Low cost	+++	++	–	–	+++

CHX, chlorhexidine; EDTA, ethylenediaminetetraacetic acid.
Efficacy of action of irrigants in ascending order: +, ++, +++; no effect: –.

Table 4.4.8 The negative effects of the smear layer.

It harbours bacteria and may act as a source of nutrition for bacteria	It hinders irrigant/medicament penetration	If/when it disintegrates, it compromises the seal of the root filling	It may compromise the bond of certain sealers

What are the advantages of removing the smear layer?

Removal of the smear layer appears to be beneficial not only because it contains bacteria, but also because its removal results in a cleaner root canal wall, thus improving the adaptation of the root-filling material (Table 4.4.8). As well as containing bacteria, the smear layer may also be a source of nutrition for residual bacteria that may remain in the root canal after disinfection.

How is the smear layer removed?

EDTA may be used. As a mild acid, it chelates heavy metal ions found within the organic component of the dentine debris, resulting in removal of the smear layer from the *instrumented* parts of the root canal wall. EDTA is typically used as a penultimate irrigant following completion of mechanical canal preparation, followed by final activated irrigation with sodium hypochlorite.

What is an example of an effective irrigation protocol?

See Table 4.4.9.

Table 4.4.9 An example of an effective irrigation protocol.

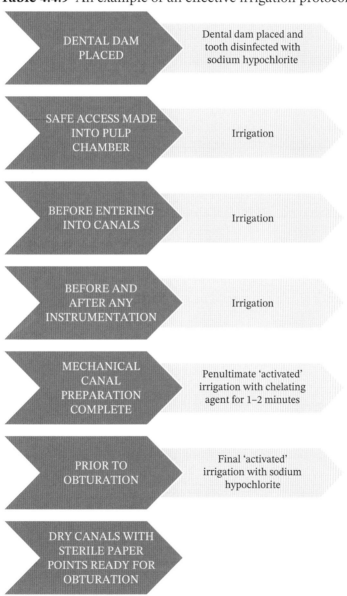

DENTAL DAM PLACED	Dental dam placed and tooth disinfected with sodium hypochlorite
SAFE ACCESS MADE INTO PULP CHAMBER	Irrigation
BEFORE ENTERING INTO CANALS	Irrigation
BEFORE AND AFTER ANY INSTRUMENTATION	Irrigation
MECHANICAL CANAL PREPARATION COMPLETE	Penultimate 'activated' irrigation with chelating agent for 1–2 minutes
PRIOR TO OBTURATION	Final 'activated' irrigation with sodium hypochlorite
DRY CANALS WITH STERILE PAPER POINTS READY FOR OBTURATION	

What is the prognosis for the treatment and is there any further advice you would give your patient?

The endodontic prognosis was excellent as all canals were identified, thus allowing the complex root canal system to be adequately prepared, disinfected and sealed with a root filling to the ideal working length (Figure 4.4.4).

The patient should be advised that it is not uncommon to have some discomfort for one to two weeks after root canal treatment has been carried out. It is also desirable to review the patient in a year to confirm, clinically and radiographically, that there are signs of healing. Importantly, the patient should be informed that the survival of the tooth is largely dependent on its structural integrity, and efforts should be made to avoid unfavourable forces, such as biting hard objects or bruxism.

Discussion

The ultimate aim of root canal treatment is to prevent or allow healing of chronic periapical periodontitis. It is essentially an exercise in infection control of the complex canal anatomy, and successful treatment is dependent on effective irrigation. Successful endodontic treatment is dependent on thoroughly disinfecting not only the instrumented aspects of the root canal system, but also of the complex webs, isthmi, accessory canals and anastomoses that are present in almost every root canal system.

The success rate for endodontic treatment in this case should be in the region of 85%. If this tooth did not have a periapical radiolucency, an even higher success rate (in the region of 95%) would be expected. The 5–10-year survival rate of this tooth would be expected to be 80–90%.

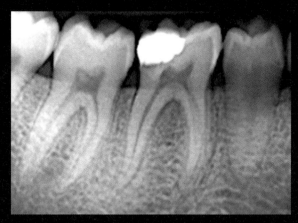

Figure 4.4.1 Pre-operative periapical radiograph.

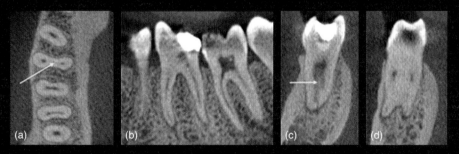

Figure 4.4.2 Pre-operative cone beam computed tomography scan. (a) Axial view; (b) sagittal view; (c) coronal view of distal root; (d) coronal view of mesial root.

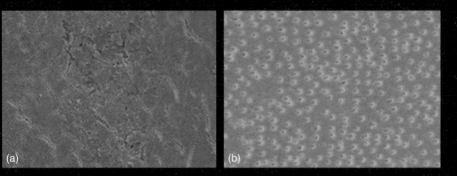

Figure 4.4.3 (a) Scanning electron microscopic (SEM) image of smear layer on a root canal surface. (b) SEM after removal of the smear layer. Note the patent dentinal tubules and clean root canal surface.

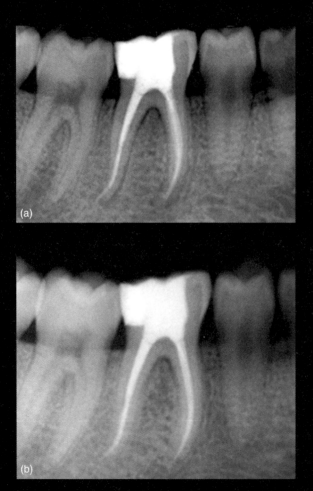

Figure 4.4.4 (a) Post-treatment radiograph. (b) One-year review radiograph. Note the complete resolution of the pre-treatment periapical radiolucency.

Further Reading

Boutsioukis, C. and Arias-Moliz, M.T. (2022). Present status and future directions – irrigants and irrigation methods. *International Endodontic Journal* 55 (Suppl 3): 588–612.

Boutsioukis, C., Lambrianidis, T., Verhaagen, B. et al. (2010). The effect of needle-insertion depth on the Irrigant flow in the root canal: evaluation using an unsteady computational fluid dynamics model. *Journal of Endodontics* 36: 1664–1668.

Byström, A. and Sundqvist, G. (1981). Bacteriologic evaluation of the efficacy of mechanical root canal instrumentation in endodontic therapy. *Scandinavian Journal of Dental Research* 89 (4): 321–328.

Byström, A. and Sundqvist, G. (1983). Bacteriological evaluation of the effect of 0.5% sodium hypochlorite in endodontic therapy. *Oral Surgery, Oral Medicine, Oral Pathology* 55 (3): 307–312.

Gulabivala, K., Ng, Y. L., Gilbertson, M., and Eames, I. (2010). The fluid mechanics of root canal irrigation. *Physiological measurement*, 31(12), R49–R84.

Haapasalo, M., Endal, U., Zandi, H., and Coil, J.M. (2005). Eradication of endodontic infection by instrumentation and irrigation solutions. *Endodontic Topics* 10 (77): 102.

Siqueira, J.F. and Rôças, I.N. (2008). Clinical implications and microbiology of bacterial persistence after treatment procedures. *Journal of Endodontics* 34 (11): 1291–1301.e3.

van der Sluis, L.W., Versluis, M., Wu, M.K., and Wesselink, P.R. (2007). Passive ultrasonic irrigation of the root canal: a review of the literature. *International Endodontic Journal* 40: 415–426.

Virdee, S.S., Farnell, D.J.J., Silva, M.A. et al. (2020). The influence of irrigant activation, concentration and contact time on sodium hypochlorite penetration into root dentine: an ex vivo experiment. *International Endodontic Journal* 53: 986–997.

4.5 Root Canal Instrumentation 1

Jianing He

Objectives

On completion of this chapter, the reader should be able to describe the goals and principles of root canal instrumentation and perform the steps of instrumentation on routine cases.

Introduction

A 35-year-old Asian male patient was referred by his general dentist for evaluation and possible root canal treatment due to throbbing pain in the lower right quadrant.

Chief Complaint

The patient complained of sensitivity from the lower right side, mostly to cold. This started after his dentist placed a new filling and has been getting worse. The patient has not been able to chew on the tooth.

Medical History

The patient is generally healthy, and does not take any medications. He has no known drug allergies.

Dental History

Routine dental care. Good dental hygiene. Composite on the lower right first molar (LR6) was placed about two weeks ago.

Pitt Ford's Problem-Based Learning in Endodontology, Second Edition. Edited by Elizabeth Shin Perry, Shanon Patel, Shalini Kanagasingam, and Samantha Hamer. © 2025 John Wiley & Sons Ltd. Published 2025 by John Wiley & Sons Ltd.

Clinical Examination

LR6 had a disto-occlusal (DO) composite resin restoration with intact margins. The tooth had no pain to buccal palpation, but was tender to percussion with digital pressure. Endo-Ice elicited intense pain that lingered for more than 10 seconds.

The lower right second premolar (LR5) and second molar (LR7) were intact with no caries or restorations. Both teeth responded to Endo-Ice and had no pain to percussion or palpation.

Radiograph interpretation: the DO composite on LR6 appeared to be of good quality, but may be approximating the mesial pulp corn (Figure 4.5.1). The disto-lingual (DL) root (radix entomolaris) appeared to be shorter than the other roots with a moderate curvature. Periapical tissue appeared normal.

Diagnosis and Treatment Planning

Diagnosis for LR6 was symptomatic irreversible pulpitis with symptomatic apical periodontitis.

Treatment options:

- No treatment.
- Non-surgical root canal treatment was recommended for LR6 followed by a full-coverage crown.
- Extraction and replacement.

The non-surgical root canal treatment was planned to be completed in a single visit.

What are some of the potential difficulties of this case?

Potential difficulties related to the case included achieving profound anaesthesia due to the presence of pulpal inflammation. Another potential challenge is the management of the complex root canal anatomy (radix entomolaris).

Treatment

Local anaesthesia was achieved with inferior alveolar nerve block followed by buccal infiltration. Soft tissue and pulpal anaesthesia were confirmed by the lack of response to probing and cold test with Endo-Ice. Upon dental dam isolation, an access cavity was created through the existing composite using a high-speed carbide fissure bur. Once the pulp was exposed, unroofing of the pulp chamber was achieved with a safe-ended Endo Z bur, and the access cavity was further refined with an ultrasonic instrument. Two orifices on the mesial and two orifices on the distal were located.

What are the objectives and principles of root canal instrumentation?

Root canal instrumentation combined with chemical irrigation is a critical step in non-surgical root canal treatment to remove the aetiology of endodontic disease and provide a foundation for root canal obturation. The main goal of mechanical instrumentation is to create a space with sufficient diameter and taper to allow adequate penetration of the irrigants to remove pulp tissue and bacteria. An important consideration during instrumentation is to respect the original canal anatomy and to avoid unnecessary removal of tooth structure whenever possible.

In the last decade, vertical root fracture has been identified as a major cause of extraction for endodontically treated teeth. Preserving more root dentine, especially in the pericervical region, is critical to maintaining the mechanical strength of the roots and reduce the likelihood of root fracture. Accordingly, aggressive canal shaping with large-tapered instruments is no longer advocated. The improved properties and design of instruments combined with active irrigation have allowed a more conservative and biologically based root canal preparation without negatively affecting the efficacy of root canal disinfection.

What are the considerations before starting instrumentation?

Appreciation of root canal anatomy along with a careful assessment of the pre-operative radiographs is critical in accurately assessing the complexity of the root canal system. The assessment should include an estimate of the number of canals, the configuration of the canal system, the location and severity of the curvature, and any potential obstruction. This knowledge can help the clinician to select the appropriate instruments and strategy and prepare for any potential challenges encountered during treatment.

In this case of the LR6, based on data reported in the literature and the pre-operative radiographs, it appears that there was one mesial root with two canals and two separate distal roots. The two mesial canals may or may not join apically. The DL root is also known as the radix entomolaris. The incidence of radix entomolaris varies from 0.9% to 22.4% depending on the geographical location, with a higher prevalence among patients of East Asian descent. The radix is often thinner and shorter than the other roots and has a greater curvature towards the buccal. The orifice of the radix is typically located more lingual than the mesio-lingual (ML) canal and more mesial than the disto-buccal (DB) canal. Due to these characteristics of the radix, more conservative preparation of this canal is recommended.

The roots appeared to be longer than average. There was a moderate curvature located in the apical third of both the mesial and distal canals.

What are the steps of instrumentation?

While there are a wide variety of instruments and techniques available to mechanically prepare the root canal systems, the following basic steps are recommended for a case with moderate difficulty such as this LR6:

- *Coronal flaring*: The aim of coronal flaring is to remove the coronal restrictive dentine to create a straight-line access to the apical portion of the canal. This step allows easier placement of subsequent instruments into the canal space, and reduces stress on the instruments and the risks of instrument separation. It also allows more accurate tactile sensation and more effective canal scouting and gauging. Coronal flaring can be achieved using Gates Glidden drills or orifice shapers, which are nickel titanium (NiTi) rotary instruments with shorter cutting flutes, a smaller tip diameter and larger tapers. Examples of orifice shapers include ProTaper® SX (Dentsply Sirona, Charlotte, NC, USA), EdgeTaper™ SX (EdgeEndo, Albuquerque, NM, USA) and ESX™ 20/08 files (Brasseler USA, Savannah, GA, USA). These instruments are typically side cutting. They should not be placed deeper than one-third of the canal length and should be used to cut on the outstroke and directed away from the furcation in multi-rooted teeth to minimise the risk of strip perforation.

- *Canal scouting*: A small hand file (e.g. no. 8 or no. 10K file) should be used to confirm the patency of the canal. The tactile feedback from the file helps the clinician to get an estimate of the size and curvature of the canal space. The file should be pre-bent in the apical 3 mm with a gentle curve to allow the file to follow and negotiate the apical curvature better (Figure 4.5.2).

- *Working length (WL) determination*: The ideal terminus of root canal instrumentation has been a topic of debate. The general consensus is to limit root canal instrumentation to the level of the apical constriction, which is on average 0.5–1 mm from the radiographic apex. Electronic apex locators such as Root ZX (J. Morita, Irvine, CA, USA) have been shown to be highly accurate and reliable in determining WL. A periapical radiograph with the WL files or gutta percha cones in place can be taken to verify the measurements (Figure 4.5.3). The main advantage of taking WL measurement after coronal flaring is the improved accuracy once the coronal restriction and curvature have been eliminated.

- *Establishing a glide path*: A glide path refers to a smooth pathway from the orifice of the canal to the apical constriction. It can be created by using a series of hand files, typically to a size no. 15 prior to rotary instrumentation. Engine-driven instruments such as PathFile or WaveOne® Gold Glider (Dentsply Sirona), EndoSequence® Scout Files (Brasseler USA), ProTaper Ultimate Slider and EdgeGlidePath™ (EdgeEndo) can also be used for glide path preparation. These files typically have a small tip size (no. 10–20) and a small taper (02 to 04). The proposed benefit of creating a glide path first is to reduce torsional stress of the files and minimise the risk of file separation, especially in calcified canals during the subsequent rotary instrumentation.

- *Crown-down preparation*: This technique is sometimes also referred to as the 'step-down' preparation. In this technique, the coronal two-thirds of the canal is prepared first by using instruments of the same tip size with decreasing taper or instruments of the same taper but with decreasing tip sizes to gradually approach the apical third (Table 4.5.1). This technique allows earlier penetration of the irrigant, more efficient removal of soft and hard tissue debris and more unimpeded placement of files into the apical third. By removing constrictions in the coronal portion and reducing file engagement with the canal walls, this technique reduces the stress on the files as they approach the apical portion, therefore lowering the risks of file separation and other procedural errors. The risk of extruding bacteria or tissue debris into the periapical tissue is also reduced. Examples of files used for crown-down preparation include ProTaper Gold S1 and S2 files or WaveOne Gold (Dentsply Sirona), TF Adaptive™ files (Kerr Dental, Uxbridge, UK) and EdgeTaper S1 and S2 files (EdgeEndo).

- *Apical enlargement*: Once the coronal portion of the canal has been cleaned and shaped into a continuously tapered space, the apical third of the canal can be further enlarged with files of increasing tip diameter to remove tissue debris and infected dentine, thus facilitating deeper

Table 4.5.1 Schematic drawing showing two crown-down preparation methods. Source: Adapted from original illustration by Dr. Alex Fleury.

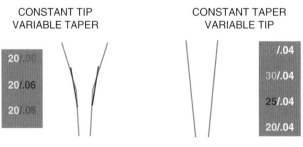

CONSTANT TIP
VARIABLE TAPER

CONSTANT TAPER
VARIABLE TIP

20/.08
20/.06
20/.06

35/.04
30/.04
25/.04
20/.04

CROWN-DOWN PREPARATION

irrigant penetration. Apical preparation size is another subject of disagreement among clinicians and scholars and has evolved over time. The final apical size of the preparation is typically determined by the initial apical size, canal anatomy and pulpal status. Initial apical size can be estimated during the initial canal gauging, which may not always be accurate and tends to under-estimate the initial apical diameter. It is traditionally believed that the final preparation should be at least three sizes larger than the initial apical size in infected canals with necrotic tissue. This will allow the removal of infected dentine, as studies have shown bacteria penetration up to $150\,\mu m$ into the dentine tubules. A minimal size of 30/04 has also been proposed, which will allow adequate irrigant exchange in the apical third. However, this may not always be possible in constricted canals or canals with significant curvature.

Aggressive apical enlargement also may not be necessary in canals with a vital pulp, as minimal bacteria presence is expected. With the development of active irrigation such as sonic, ultrasonic, multi-sonic and laser-assisted irrigation, effective irrigant penetration and exchange in the apical portion of the canal may be achieved without excessive mechanical apical enlargement.

In this case of the LR6 with a vital pulp, a 30/04 final apical preparation size for the mesial canals and 30/04 or 35/04 for the DB canal were considered appropriate. The DL canal was prepared to 25/04 due to the canal curvature.

Numerous file systems are available for apical enlargement. Examples include ProTaper Gold Finishing files and Vortex Blue™ files (Dentsply Sirona), EdgeTaper Finishing files and EdgeSequel Sapphire™ files (EdgeEndo), EndoSequence CM files (Brasseler USA) and HyFlex® CM files (Coltene Holding, Altstätten, Switzerland).

Some general clinical tips for instrumentation are listed in Table 4.5.2.

Completion of root canal treatment and follow-up

Once the canal instrumentation was completed, the canal space was further disinfected with copious irrigation with NaOCl followed by a final rinse with 17% ethylenediaminetetraacetic acid (EDTA). The canals were dried with paper points and obturated with a sealer-based technique using gutta percha and EndoSequence BC sealer. The tooth was temporised with a sterile cotton pellet and intermediate restorative material (IRM) and referred back to the general dentist for core build-up and crown (Figure 4.5.4). At the 12-month follow-up visit, the tooth had been fully restored with a full-coverage crown. The patient was asymptomatic. Periapical radiograph showed normal periapical tissue with no radiolucency noted (Figure 4.5.5).

Table 4.5.2 General clinical tips for instrumentation.

- Irrigate between each instrument.
- Ensure the canal is always flooded with irrigant to facilitate debris removal and reduce friction.
- Never force an instrument; allow the instrument to follow the natural canal anatomy. When resistance is encountered, step back and use a smaller file.
- Clean debris off the flutes of the instrument after each use.
- Inspect the instrument often for 'unwinding', 'stripping' and other signs of file fatigue. Discard the file once damage is observed.
- Recapitulate often between rotary instruments.
- Use reference points that allow accurate and reproducible working length measurements.

Discussion

Recent advances in instrumentation systems

Since NiTi rotary instruments were introduced in the 1990s, they have largely replaced stainless steel (SS) hand files in carrying out the main task of mechanical preparation due to their improved efficiency and safety. However, SS hand files remain critical for canal scouting, gauging, recapitulating or instrumenting severely curved canals. In the last decade, there has been considerable advancement made in the field of NiTi instruments. These changes and innovations can be categorised into three main areas:

- *Improved metallurgic properties*: various proprietary heat treatment methods modify phase transformation temperature and give the alloy increased flexibility and better fatigue resistance. Examples include the M-wire from Dentsply, R-phase alloy from Kerr, FireWire from EdgeEndo, HyFlex CM files and MaxWire from Brasseler USA. The heat treatment also modifies the shape memory of the alloy and allows the files to be pre-bent and stay bent, which helps the files to maintain the original canal curvature and reduces transportation.

- *Improved file design*:
  - *Variable taper*: many new systems have a variable taper or regressive taper design instead of the traditional 04 or 06 constant taper. The regressive taper means the taper becomes smaller moving from the tip of the file towards the shank (Figure 4.5.6). This design allows the preservation of the valuable cervical dentine. Examples of files with such design include WaveOne Gold, ProTaper Gold Finishing files, TRUShape, TruNatomy® (Dentsply Sirona) and V Taper files. The ProTaper Gold Shaping files have a variable taper design in the

opposite direction – the taper increases from the tip towards the coronal direction to perform the crown-down preparation while maintaining the flexibility at the tip.

- *Off-set design*: another relatively new design feature is the off-set design, which means the geometrical cross-sectional centres of these instruments are displaced from the instruments' centres of rotation. This design reduces the contact between the file surface and the canal walls, therefore reducing friction and facilitating debris removal, further lowering the risk of file separation. Examples of files with this offset design include ProTaper Next and TruNatomy files.
- *'Expandable' files*: the unique longitudinal design gives these files an S-curve. As the file rotates, its orbit 'expands' to allow better and more even contact with the canal walls. The main advantage of these files is the better cleaning of oval-shaped canals without excessive removal of root dentine. Examples of this type of files include TRUShape and XP-3D™ Shaper (Brasseler USA).

- *Reciprocating movement*: a number of instrumentation systems have been created to be used in a reciprocating motion instead of the traditional rotary motion. These files perform the cutting action while rotating in a counterclockwise direction, which is followed by a smaller clockwise rotation to release the files from engagement. This reciprocating motion reduces file engagement and the risks of file separation. Examples include WaveOne and WaveOne Gold files, Reciproc® and Reciproc Blue (VDW, Munich, Germany) and EndoSequence Reciprocating (ESR) files.

Considerations for Instrument Selection

There are numerous NiTi rotary instrumentation systems on the market with new ones continuously being developed and added to the ever-growing list. These different systems with different metal properties, design and motion can make file selection a daunting task. An ideal file system should have good cutting efficiency, flexibility, fatigue resistance and be easy to use. Different systems have their own advantages and limitations. The design features, advantages and disadvantages of some of the commonly used contemporary file systems are listed in Table 4.5.3.

Existing scientific evidence does not support the superiority of one file system over the other. Clinicians typically combine files from different commercial systems to form their own customised hybrid system (Figure 4.5.7). Optimal outcomes can be achieved as long as the principles of instrumentation are followed, regardless of the specific file system the clinician chooses to use. Recent advances in alloy treatment and file design can potentially help clinicians to achieve the goals of root canal instrumentation in a safer and more efficient manner while preserving more root dentine.

Table 4.5.3 Design features, advantages and disadvantages of commonly used contemporary nickel titanium systems.

Category	Examples	Features	Advantages	Disadvantages
Rotary	ProTaper Gold EdgeTaper Gold EndoSequence CM Vortex Blue EdgeSequel Sapphire HyFlex CM TF	Convex triangular cross-section Active cutting Variable or constant taper Heat treated	High cutting efficiency Flexible	ProTaper and EdgeTaper Gold files have aggressive taper and remove more coronal root dentine; may be more prone to strip perforation and canal transportation
Reciprocating	WaveOne Gold Reciproc ESR TF adaptive	Rectangular or modified triangular cross-section Regressive variable taper or constant taper Used in reciprocating motion Heat treated	Flexible Reduced risk of file separation High cutting efficiency Allows completion of instrumentation using a single file	May pack debris apically Requires special reciprocating motor May need additional files to complete apical preparation Higher cost
'Expandable'	TRUShape XP-3D Shaper	S-curve Small taper Heat treated	Better and more even contact with canal walls Better cleaning of oval-shaped canals Preserve more root dentine Use fewer files	Learning curve Higher cost

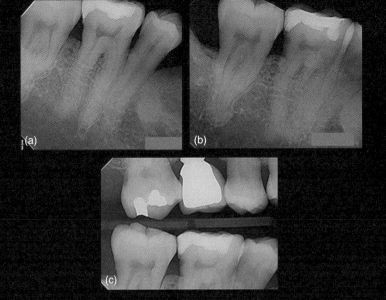

Figure 4.5.1 (a) Pre-operative periapical radiographs of the lower right first molar (LR6) and (b) parallax radiograph. (c) Pre-operative bitewing radiograph.

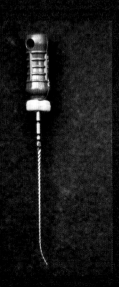

Figure 4.5.2 Pre-curved hand file for canal scouting and gauging.

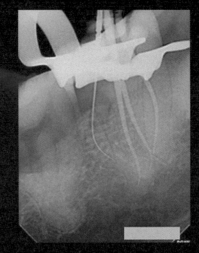

Figure 4.5.3 Working length/cone fit radiograph.

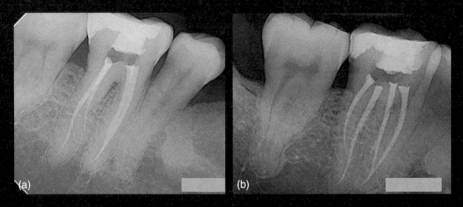

(a)　　　　　　　　　　　　　　　　　(b)

Figure 4.5.4 (a) Post-operative periapical radiographs and (b) parallax view.

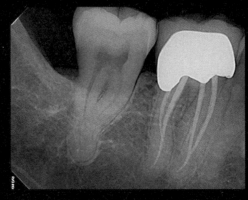

Figure 4.5.5 12 month follow-up radiograph.

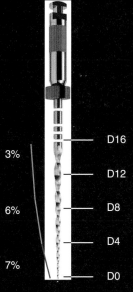

3% — D16

D12

6% — D8

D4

7% — D0

Figure 4.5.6 An example of a regressive taper design.

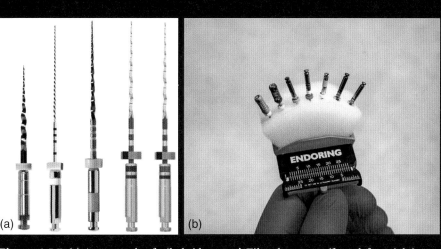

Figure 4.5.7 (a) An example of a 'hybrid system'. Files shown are (from left to right) orifice shaper: EdgeTaper SX; glide path file: PathFile no. 16; crown-down preparation: WaveOne Gold Small; apical enlargement: EndoSequence CM 25/04 and 30/04. (b) Showing the set-up of hand files and a mix of rotary files from different systems in an EndoRing.

Further Reading

Hülsmann, M., Peters, O.A., and Dummer, P.M.H. (2005). Mechanical preparation of root canals: shaping goals, techniques and means. *Endodontic Topics* 10 (1): 30–76.

Peters, O.A., de Azevedo Bahia, M.G., and Pereira, E.S. (2017). Contemporary root canal preparation: innovations in biomechanics. *Dental Clinics of North America* 61 (1): 37–58.

Tomson, P.L. and Simon, S.R. (2016). Contemporary cleaning and shaping of the root canal system. *Primary Dental Journal* 5 (2): 46–53.

Young, G.R., Parashos, P., and Messer, H.H. (2007). The principles of techniques for cleaning root canals. *Australian Dental Journal* 52 (1 Suppl): S52–S63.

Zanza, A., D'Angelo, M., Reda, R. et al. (2021). An update on nickel-titanium rotary instruments in endodontics: mechanical characteristics, testing and future perspective-an overview. *Bioengineering (Basel)* 8 (12): 218.

4.6 Root Canal Instrumentation 2

Luis Ferrandez

Objectives

At the end of this chapter, the reader should understand the aims of root canal instrumentation, have knowledge about the properties and indications of hand and rotary instruments and be able to formulate a strategy to treat curved root canals.

Introduction

A 68-year-old male patient was referred by his general dentist to a specialist endodontic practice for root canal treatment of his lower right second mandibular molar (LR7).

Chief Complaint

The patient was pain free but complained of the presence of a 'gumboil' adjacent to the LR7 for the last few weeks.

Medical History

Unremarkable.

Dental History

His dentist had replaced a defective subgingival restoration four months previously. The patient then developed a poorly localised ache in the jaw, which resolved after a gingival swelling appeared next to the tooth. The first molar (LR6) had been extracted as a teenager and the LR7 had tilted into the first molar's position.

Pitt Ford's Problem-Based Learning in Endodontology, Second Edition. Edited by Elizabeth Shin Perry, Shanon Patel, Shalini Kanagasingam, and Samantha Hamer.

Clinical Examination

There were no remarkable extraoral findings. Intraorally, there was a buccal gingival swelling and a sinus tract adjacent to the LR7. There was a localised mid-buccal periodontal probing defect deeper than 10 mm (Figure 4.6.1), with periodontal probing depths of 1–3 mm elsewhere in the mouth. The LR7 was restored with a disto-occlusal (DO) composite restoration with poor marginal adaptation and was unresponsive to thermal sensibility tests. The rest of his dentition was moderately restored.

Radiographic Examination

- Alveolar bone heights within normal limits.
- LR7 had a DO restoration with subgingival distal caries, a calcified pulp chamber with long mesial and distal roots with severe curvatures in the apical third. Both apices were associated with an apical radiolucency that extended into the furcation area (Figure 4.6.2a).

Diagnosis and Treatment Planning

A diagnosis of pulp necrosis and asymptomatic apical periodontitis with suppuration associated with the LR7 was reached.

The treatment options for the LR7 were:

- No treatment.
- Non-surgical root canal treatment and cuspal coverage restoration.
- Extraction (and replacement).

The patient was keen to have root canal treatment to prevent further worsening of his symptoms and retain the tooth.

Treatment

The restorability of the tooth was investigated by removal of the existing composite restoration and distal caries. A gingivectomy with electrosurgery was carried out to expose the distal subgingival cavity margin. The DO cavity was restored with a resin-modified glass ionomer cement.

Which root canal preparation strategy was followed?

A multitude of instrumentation techniques and instruments are available and the clinician should always consider the biological and mechanical aims of the instrumentation process when choosing which one to use (Table 4.6.1). In this case, a crown-down approach was used to negotiate

Table 4.6.1 Aims of root canal preparation.

Biological

- Obtain access to the apical terminus
- Remove bacterial biofilm from the canal walls
- Remove debris and pulp tissue
- Create access and space for disinfection and medication
- Facilitate root canal obturation

Mechanical

- Respect the original shape of the canal
- Avoid obstruction of the root canal
- Avoid excessive root dentine removal

Table 4.6.2 Advantages of crown-down preparation strategies.

- Eradicate the bulk of the infection from the coronal third and prevent pushing bacteria into the apical third and beyond the apex
- Reduce canal blockages by permitting early penetration of irrigants and lubrication
- Remove coronal interferences to avoid file binding coronally ('taper lock')
- Minimise changes in working length during preparation
- Improve tactile feedback
- Reduce extrusion of debris

and instrument the root canals. With this approach, the coronal half of the root canals is prepared first, followed by the use of sequentially smaller instruments in an apical direction. Preparing the canal in a corono-apical direction has both biological and mechanical advantages over a step-back approach (Table 4.6.2).

The cusps were reduced to provide stable coronal reference points and shorten the working length (WL) of the canals. Three root canals were located on access. The coronal half of the root canals was explored with small (no. 08–15) stainless steel (SS) hand files and enlarged with reciprocating nickel titanium (NiTi) instruments sizes 25, 7% taper and 20, 7% taper in a crown-down fashion. Reciprocating instruments use unequal back-and-forth rotations that facilitate apical advancement of the file and reduce mechanical stress on the file (Table 4.6.3). The apical half of the canals was then scouted with SS files until resistance was met and a mechanical glide path was created to that point with a rotary file with an apical size 15 and increasing taper over its active portion. SS instruments were again used to

Table 4.6.3 Advantages of reciprocating instrumentation.

- Fewer instruments required for shaping
- Reduction of cyclic fatigue
- Decreased torsional stress
- Maintenance of original root canal anatomy
- Faster root canal preparation
- More effective gutta percha removal

electronically determine the WL (28 mm in this case). The canal preparation was completed with the rotary glide-path file and a reciprocating shaping file size 20 7% (Figure 4.6.2b).

What clinical situations benefit from the use of hand files?

Small (sizes 08–15) SS instruments possess adequate stiffness while maintaining considerable flexibility, allowing initial negotiation of curved and calcified root canals. The process of scouting with small SS files is essential to gain knowledge about the degree and location of curvatures and create a glide path for automated instruments. The tip of small hand files can be pre-curved to scout abrupt curvatures and renegotiate ledged canals.

SS hand files are made to match ISO standards that require them to have a 2% taper (0.02). The minimal taper facilitates better tactile feedback from the tip of the instrument and allows the clinician to differentiate whether the instrument is cutting dentine, has encountered a blockage caused by dentine chips or pulp remnants, or is engaged in gutta percha. Hand files are also very useful to gauge the canal diameter.

The successful use of SS hand files in these complex scenarios requires clinical skills that are developed through training and practice.

What are the properties and clinical advantages of nickel titanium instruments?

NiTi files have super-elastic properties, giving them the ability to recover their original shape after strain is removed (shape memory) even beyond the plastic deformation point. Clinically, this means they are more flexible than SS instruments and when used correctly can rotate within a curved canal before fracturing. The superior flexibility and lower restoring force allow them to shape curved canals while preserving the original root canal anatomy and minimising instrumentation mishaps. NiTi instruments can be manufactured with tapers greater than SS files and can shape canals more rapidly with fewer instruments (Table 4.6.4). They also have a high resistance to torsional stresses.

Table 4.6.4 Stainless steel vs. nickel titanium (NiTi) files.

	Stainless steel hand files	NiTi rotary files
Vision of tooth under treatment	Poor	Good
Number of instruments required	Multiple	Few
Speed of root canal preparation	Slow	Fast
Tactile feedback	Good	Poor
Selective instrumentation of irregularities	Yes	No
Evenly tapered preparation	No	Yes
Risk of preparation mishaps	High	Low
Warning signs (unwinding) of deformation	Yes	Sometimes
Pre-curve for negotiation of canal aberrations	Yes	Some
Operator fatigue	Yes	No
Expensive	No	Yes

Recent variations in the structure and thermal treatment of NiTi alloys have improved the cyclic fatigue resistance and flexibility of the instruments even further. New-generation heat-treated files can also be pre-curved (controlled memory) for easier introduction into the canals of posterior teeth. These improved properties make more conservative access preparations possible. When choosing this approach, the clinician should be aware of the risks, which may include missed anatomy and compromised disinfection (refer to Case 4.1).

What factors determine the difficulty in managing curved canals?

With the exception of some anterior teeth, most canals have curvatures in multiple planes throughout their length. The position of the tooth in the arch and the degree of mouth opening determine ease of access and influence the complexity of the treatment. Teeth restored with crowns or having moderate or severe inclination and rotation are also more difficult to access and treat. The degree of curvature is only one of the parameters that has to be taken into consideration. The abruptness and coronal position of the curvature have a major impact on the complexity of preparation and the increased risk of file fracture. The difficulty in negotiation and instrumentation is further complicated if the canals are long or calcified. Most curved canals can be successfully managed if basic principles are followed (Table 4.6.5).

Table 4.6.5 Preparation of curved root canals.

- Assess the location, degree, abruptness and number of curvatures radiographically (ideally with cone beam computed tomography)
- Determine the estimated working length (WL) from pre-operative imaging
- Use a crown-down preparation technique
- Keep the canal flooded with sodium hypochlorite throughout root canal negotiation and preparation
- Examine the root canal anatomy with small (08–15) pre-curved hand files following preparation of the coronal third
- Advance with glide path and shaping instruments to the apical third (or to an estimated length coronal to the second curvature or abrupt apical curve)
- Establish WL with an apex locator
- Create a manual (up to size 15) or rotary glide path to the full WL. Use intermediate size files to reduce stress on hand files if required
- If an obstruction is encountered, use a sharp curve near the tip of the hand file to negotiate apical curvatures and bypass ledges
- Use size 08/10 files to recapitulate frequently and avoid blockages
- Complete root canal instrumentation. Use instruments with small taper and diameter, especially in canals with coronal, acute or double curvatures

In this case, the canals were dressed with calcium hydroxide for four weeks. At the obturation appointment the swelling and sinus tract had resolved and the mid-buccal probing defect had decreased to 4 mm. Disinfection throughout the treatment was carried out with sodium hypochlorite and ethylenediaminetetraacetic acid (EDTA), which were manually activated with a matched gutta percha cone. The root canals were obturated with warm vertical compaction of gutta percha and the access was restored with a modified glass ionomer cement (Figure 4.6.3a). The patient was followed up 12 months later, with an absence of symptoms, resolution of the periodontal probing defect and radiographic healing evident (Figure 4.6.3b). A four-year review showed that the tooth had been restored with a ceramic onlay, there were no remarkable soft tissue and periodontal findings (Figure 4.6.4a) and there was an absence of apical changes radiographically (Figure 4.6.4b).

Discussion

Modern preparation techniques and instruments facilitate the negotiation and shaping of even the most complex root canal systems, as long as the clinician is aware of their characteristics and potential for use in different scenarios. Likewise, a thorough knowledge of the basic principles of root canal instrumentation and root canal anatomy is essential to achieve a successful outcome.

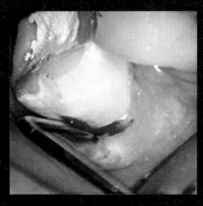

Figure 4.6.1 Buccal swelling, sinus tract and periodontal probing defect.

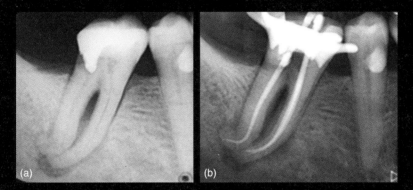

Figure 4.6.2 (a) Pre-operative radiograph. (b) Cone fit radiograph.

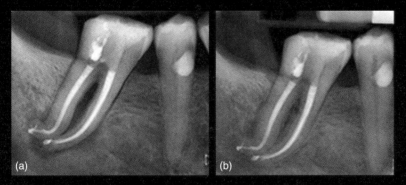

Figure 4.6.3 (a) Final radiograph. (b) 12-month recall.

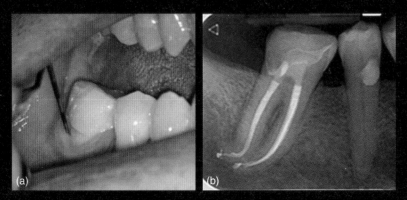

Figure 4.6.4 Four-year review. Note (a) the absence of periodontal probing and (b) resolution of the apical radiolucency.

Further Reading

Hülsmann, M., Peters, O.A., and Dummer, P.M.H. (2005). Mechanical preparation of root canals: shaping goals, techniques and means. *Endodontic Topics* 10: 30–76.

Peters, O.A., de Azevedo Bahia, M.G., and Pereira, E.S. (2017). Contemporary root canal preparation: innovations in biomechanics. *Dental Clinics of North America* 1: 37–58.

Yared, G. (2008). Canal preparation using only one Ni-Ti rotary instrument: preliminary observations. *International Endodontic Journal* 4: 339–344.

Zupanc, J., Vahdat-Pajouh, N., and Schäfer, E. (2018). New thermomechanically treated NiTi alloys – a review. *International Endodontic Journal* 10: 1088–1103.

4.7 Accessory Canals and Complexities of the Root Canal System

Frédéric Bukiet, Thomas Giraud, and Benoit Ballester

Objectives

At the end of this case, the reader should appreciate the anatomical variations and the complexities of the root canal system and how it could impact the management and prognosis of treatment.

Introduction

A 28-year-old female had continued pain despite treatment with a course of antibiotics from her general dentist. After consulting a dental emergency department, she was finally referred to an endodontist for the management of the symptomatic tooth.

Chief Complaint

The patient complained of spontaneous throbbing symptoms from the lower right second premolar (LR5) that had resolved since she presented to a dental emergency department.

Medical History

Unremarkable.

Dental History

The patient attended her general dental practitioner regularly and had a minimally restored dentition. She presented to her dentist with spontaneous pain and biting sensitivity from the LR5. Antibiotics were prescribed.

Pitt Ford's Problem-Based Learning in Endodontology, Second Edition. Edited by Elizabeth Shin Perry, Shanon Patel, Shalini Kanagasingam, and Samantha Hamer.
© 2025 John Wiley & Sons Ltd. Published 2025 by John Wiley & Sons Ltd.

However, the symptoms became worse one month later and the patient presented to an emergency dental department for pain relief. Root canal treatment was initiated, but technical difficulties were encountered by the practitioner. A temporary dressing was placed and antibiotics were prescribed. The patient was referred to a specialist endodontist.

Clinical Examination

Extraoral examination was unremarkable. Intraoral examination revealed a provisional restoration on the tooth LR5. The oral hygiene was good and the periodontal probing depths were all less than 2 mm. The adjacent teeth were unrestored. The LR5 was tender to percussion; the LR4 and LR6 were both responsive to sensibility tests while the LR5 was not.

What did the periapical radiograph of tooth LR5 reveal (Figure 4.7.1)?

- Distal perforation at the alveolar crest of LR5.
- LR5 restoration extending into pulp chamber with bifurcation of root canal at mid-root level, two roots with canal only visible in the mesial root.
- LR5 periapical radiolucency surrounding the mesial and distal apices and the bifurcation area.

A cone beam computed tomography (CBCT) scan was taken to fully assess the complexity of the root canal anatomy.

What did the cone beam computed tomography reveal (Figure 4.7.2)?

- A C-shaped cross-sectional morphology with multiple root canal irregularities indicating possible fins, cul-de-sacs and most likely internal resorption defects (moth-eaten appearance). The presence of accessory canals was also suspected.
- A large bone destruction including the buccal cortex from the middle third to the periapical area.
- A suspected subgingival perforation on the distal aspect of LR5.

Diagnosis and Treatment Planning

The diagnosis of the LR5 was pulpal necrosis with symptomatic apical periodontitis and internal inflammatory root resorption.

What were the treatment options for the patient?

- No treatment (not suitable considering the history and the diagnosis).
- Non-surgical root canal treatment.
- Extraction.

After discussion with the patient, it was decided to attempt non-surgical root canal treatment on tooth LR5 with management of the distal subgingival perforation. The purpose of the treatment was to maintain the tooth but also to regenerate the bone support.

Treatment

Under local anaesthesia and after dental dam placement, the provisional restoration was removed. The distal perforation was temporarily restored to prevent saliva leaking into the root canal and to prevent irrigant leaking out into the soft tissues. Two canals were located and shaped and thoroughly cleaned and disinfected with 3% sodium hypochlorite. Then 17% EDTA was used to remove the smear layer after root canal preparation, followed by a final sodium hypochlorite agitation/rinse. After gutta percha cone adjustment (Figure 4.7.3), the canals were dried with sterile paper points, obturated, and a provisional restoration was placed. The post-operative radiograph showed satisfactory obturation (Figure 4.7.4). An apical delta, a loop accessory canal and many root canal irregularities previously observed on the pre-operative CBCT appeared as obturated on the immediate post-operative radiographs.

The patient was scheduled to return the next week to place a cuspal coverage composite restoration to reduce the risk of fracture. The subgingival distal perforation was sealed using a resin-modified glass ionomer cement. At 12-month review, the patient was asymptomatic and the tooth was functional. The periapical radiograph revealed clear signs of bone healing (Figure 4.7.5), which was confirmed by the one-year review CBCT (Figure 4.7.6).

Discussion

This case highlights the complexity of root canal anatomy and the importance of thorough disinfection. The endodontic literature is polarised on the clinical implications of the sealing of these ramifications and irregularities of the root canal space, but also at what level this may jeopardise the outcome of the endodontic treatment.

Root canal ramifications have been termed lateral, secondary, accessory, auxiliary or furcation canals, mainly depending on their location, orientation, dimensions and length, making the terminology very complex and confusing. A simpler terminology has been suggested, using the term 'accessory' to define a branch leaving the root canal regardless of its location (coronal, middle or apical third), orientation or type (patent, blind or loop) (Figure 4.7.7).

Accessory canals are detected with the highest frequency in the apical third (Figure 4.7.8), especially in posterior teeth, and are commonly considered to be a potential cause of persistent apical periodontitis. It is well known that apical periodontitis is due to root canal infection by microorganisms. This inflammatory response is most often triggered by the release of bacterial by-products through the apical foramen or accessory foramina.

Accessory canal diameter is highly variable (between 10 and 200 μm) and remains larger than the size of most bacteria (between 0.2 and 10 μm). Accessory canals and canal irregularities can act as potential shelters for microorganisms, making thorough disinfection of the root canal space much more challenging. In addition, accessory canals, when connected to accessory foramina, provide pathways for diffusion of microorganisms and by-products from the root canal space to periodontal tissue and vice versa. This can lead to endo-perio lesions and explains why a radiolucency can be observed laterally around the root in the coronal or middle third, including the furcation region.

How can accessory canals/irregularities be detected?

In most cases, accessory canals cannot be detected by the clinician prior to root canal treatment. The small diameter of accessory canals further precludes radiographic detection even with CBCT. Accessory anatomy is also difficult to detect on a periapical radiograph when traversing the root in a bucco-lingual direction. Thus, irregularities and accessory canals are usually detected retrospectively; that is, after obturation due to the passage of radiopaque materials within these tiny spaces (Figure 4.7.9). When filling complex anatomy in the apical third, it is sometimes difficult to differentiate the sealer within the canal ramifications from the sealer surplus in the bone trabeculae (Figure 4.7.10). However, in the present case, it was possible to detect multiple root canal irregularities on CBCT slices and this was confirmed after obturation.

In case of an accessory canal, the following findings can be located anywhere on the external surface of the root:

- Localised thickening of the adjacent periodontal ligament.
- Localised discontinuity of the lamina dura.
- Lateral and/or periapical radiolucency.
- Localised external resorption.
- Sinus tract.

The pulp of an accessory canal can remain vital and inflamed. From the main canal, low molecular weight bacterial by-products can penetrate into an accessory canal and migrate towards periodontal tissue, generating inflammation of the vital pulp and causing a lateral periodontitis. Once a root canal infection is well established with a significant bacterial load, the pulp of the accessory canal can become partially or totally necrotic. The differential diagnosis with other lateral pathosis such as vertical root fracture, root perforation and periodontal disease must be considered to avoid inappropriate treatment.

Can accessory canals anatomy be predictively disinfected and obturated?

The primary goal of root canal therapy is to prevent and to treat apical periodontitis. The reduction of the bacterial load within all the ramifications/irregularities of the root canal space is essential. Obturation of accessory canals and canal irregularities is considered by some as a sign of technical success and reflects positively on the clinician's ability. A study histologically assessed root-filled teeth in which the accessory canals appeared to be filled radiographically and concluded that the accessory anatomy was not well obturated. Indeed, the accessory anatomy that was radiographically well obturated was in fact partially filled with sealer binding to pulp tissue (inflamed or necrotic) remnants. However, the antibacterial properties of root canal sealers may play a role in inactivating or entombing residual bacteria in the accessory anatomy and contribute to the healing process. A significant reduction of the bacterial load within the main canal followed by optimal obturation may be sufficient to prevent the passage of the by-products through the accessory canals.

Considering the dimensions and orientation of accessory anatomy, it is not possible to mechanically instrument them. Moreover, it has been demonstrated that root canal shaping leads to smear layer and debris impaction into these accessory canals. Advanced irrigation and activation technologies may be promising to enhance cleaning and disinfections of the irregularities of the root canal space. However, given the current state of knowledge, it is not possible to predictably disinfect, dry and obturate all accessory canals. Therefore, even with the best of efforts, the reality is that all accessory canals cannot be predictably disinfected, dried or obturated with current endodontic techniques.

Conclusion

The practitioner should be aware that accessory canals provide pathways for diffusion of microorganisms and by-products from the root canal space to periodontal tissue and vice versa. Presently, there is no clear evidence that obturation of accessory canals improves endodontic outcomes. However, the practitioner should always attempt to diligently three-dimensionally clean, disinfect and fill the complexities of root canal space as thoroughly as possible.

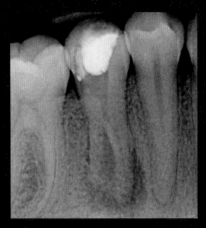

Figure 4.7.1 Pre-operative radiograph demonstrating a complex root canal anatomy, a possible subgingival perforation and a periapical radiolucency associated with the LR5.

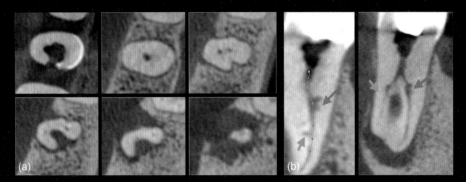

Figure 4.7.2 Cone beam computed tomography (a) axial and (b) coronal views showing the C-shaped cross-sectional morphology and a large bone destruction. Multiple root canal irregularities indicating possible fins, cul-de-sacs, ramifications (blue arrows) and most likely internal resorptions (moth-eaten appearance) (orange arrows) can also be observed.

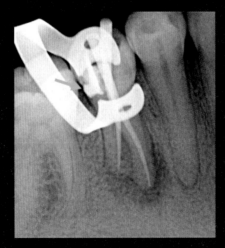

Figure 4.7.3 Intraoperative radiograph showing master gutta percha cone adjustment. The perforation was temporarily restored during root canal treatment (green arrow).

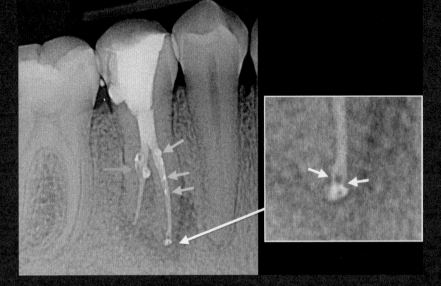

Figure 4.7.4 Post-operative radiograph showing obturation of the root canal irregularities previously detected on cone beam computed tomography (green arrows). Notice the apical delta (yellow zoom area) and a filled loop (blue arrow).

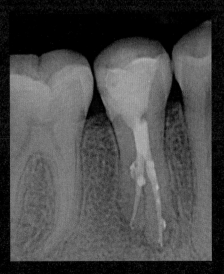

Figure 4.7.5 One-year follow-up radiograph showing the final restoration including the distal perforation management. An unexpected void between the restoration and the root canal obturation can be noted. However, it did not impact the healing of the lesion.

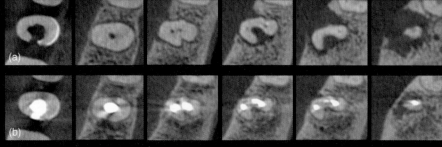

Figure 4.7.6 Comparison between (a) pre-operative and (b) one-year review cone beam computed tomography axial views illustrating the ongoing bone healing.

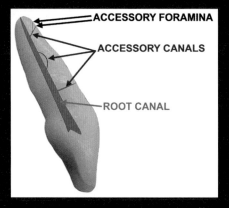

Figure 4.7.7 Simplification of the terminology used for the ramifications of the root canal space.

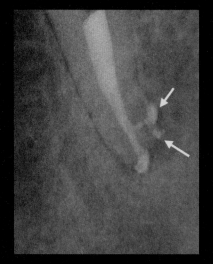

Figure 4.7.8 Radiograph showing the obturation of a wide accessory canal terminating in two accessory foramina (yellow arrows) on the external surface of the root in the

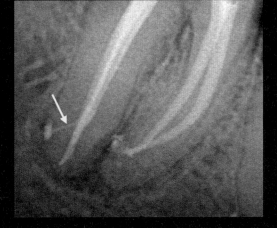

Figure 4.7.9 Radiograph showing the passage of radiopaque materials into an accessory canal after obturation of a mandibular molar (yellow arrow).

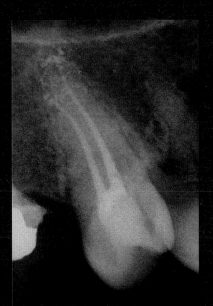

Figure 4.7.10 Radiograph showing root canal anatomy complexity in the apical third. It is difficult to distinguish between the filled accessory canals and the sealer extruded in

Further Reading

Ahmed, H.M.A., Neelakantan, P., and Dummer, P.M.H. (2018). A new system for classifying accessory canal morphology. *International Endodontic Journal* 51: 164–176.

Ricucci, D. and Siqueira, J.F. Jr. (2010). Fate of the tissue in lateral canals and apical ramifications in response to pathologic conditions and treatment procedures. *Journal of Endodontics* 36: 1–15.

Venturi, M., Prati, C., Capelli, G. et al. (2003). A preliminary analysis of the morphology of lateral canals after root canal filling using a tooth-clearing technique. *International Endodontic Journal* 36: 54–63.

4.8 Obturation of the Root Canal 1

Kreena Patel

Objectives

At the end of this case, the reader should appreciate the importance of root canal obturation and understand the different materials available and methods of obturation.

Introduction

A 45-year-old male patient presented with pain associated with the upper right first molar (UR6). The tooth had been restored with a composite restoration three years ago.

Chief Complaint

An intermittent, dull, throbbing pain was localised to the UR6. The patient was struggling to eat on the right side of his mouth.

Medical History

Unremarkable.

Dental History

The patient was a regular attender at the dentist.

Clinical Examination

Extraoral examination was unremarkable. Intraoral examination revealed a swelling on the buccal mucosa associated with the UR6 (Figure 4.8.1).

Pitt Ford's Problem-Based Learning in Endodontology, Second Edition. Edited by Elizabeth Shin Perry, Shanon Patel, Shalini Kanagasingam, and Samantha Hamer.
© 2025 John Wiley & Sons Ltd. Published 2025 by John Wiley & Sons Ltd.

The UR6 was restored with mesio-occlusal composite restoration and with recurrent caries. The tooth was tender on percussion and biting. Periodontal probing depths were 1–3 mm and the tooth did not respond to pulp tests.

What did the periapical radiograph reveal?

- Alveolar bone height within normal limits.
- Marginal defect and caries under the mesial aspect of the composite restoration.
- Calcifications in the pulp chamber.
- The distal and palatal roots have visible root canals; the mesial root has a 30° distal curvature with indistinct canal path.
- Periapical radiolucencies were associated with the apices of the mesial, distal and palatal roots.
- Mesial radiolucency on the UR7 requiring further investigation with a bitewing radiograph (Figure 4.8.2).

Diagnosis and Treatment Planning

What is the diagnosis?

Pulpal necrosis with symptomatic apical periodontitis with sinus suppuration was the diagnosis for tooth UR6.

What are the treatment options for tooth UR6?

- Non-surgical root canal treatment, subject to restorability.
- Extraction.
- No treatment.

The patient was keen to save tooth UR6 and opted to proceed with root canal treatment. The existing restoration and caries were removed. The tooth was found to be restorable and a composite pre-endodontic restoration was placed.

Dental dam isolation and access were carried out. The calcifications in the pulp chamber were removed using a piezo-electric endodontic ultrasonic tip. Four canals were located (palatal, disto-buccal, first mesio-buccal and second mesio-buccal) and prepared using hand and rotary files. Sodium hypochlorite and ethylenediaminetetraacetic acid (EDTA) were used to disinfect the root canal system.

The master cone gutta percha (GP) points were tried into the canals and checked for apical tugback. It is important to leave fluid in the canal when trying in the master cone because it mimics the lubricant effect of the sealer and aids in the seating of the cone.

A post-obturation radiograph was taken (Figure 4.8.3).

What is the purpose of obturating the root canal system?

Obturation aims to three-dimensionally seal the root canal system. The purpose is to:

- Prevent microorganisms entering the root canal system and causing reinfection *(coronal seal).*
- Prevent tissue fluids entering the root canal system and providing nutrients for any remaining microorganisms *(apical seal).*
- Entomb any remaining microorganisms and their by-products and prevent their spread through the apex.

What are the ideal properties of a root canal filling material?

- Dimensionally stable
- Non-irritant, ideally biocompatible
- Antimicrobial
- Radiopaque
- Does not discolour tooth structure
- Sterile
- Easily manipulated to conform to the shape of different canals
- Insoluble
- Good handling and working time
- Easily removed if necessary

What are the constituents of gutta percha cones?

65% zinc oxide, 20% GP, 10% radiopacifiers, 5% plasticisers.

GP exists in two crystalline forms (α and β). Processed GP cones normally exist in the β-phase, where they are a solid structure that can be compacted. When the material is heated it transitions to the α-phase, which is tackier and more pliable. Cooling of the α-phase back to the β-phase results in shrinkage.

What are the advantages and disadvantages of using gutta percha as an obturation material?

See Table 4.8.1.

How should gutta percha cones be disinfected prior to obturation?

Ideally, GP cones should be disinfected by submerging them in sodium hypochlorite solution for one minute and drying prior to use.

What is the purpose of a root canal sealer?

Sealers adhere to dentine and fill the irregularities between the core filling material and the canal walls. Sealers can also flow into lateral and accessory canals. It also acts as a lubricant during the obturation procedure.

Table 4.8.1 Advantages and disadvantages of gutta percha as an obturation material.

Advantages	Disadvantages
Plasticity: can be adapted to seal the irregular shapes of root canals	Lack of adhesion to dentine
	A sealer is required to fill the voids around the filling material
Dimensionally stable	
Not soluble	
Minimal toxicity	
Radiopacity	
Easy to remove	
Less costly	

What different types of root canal sealers are available (Table 4.8.2)?

- Zinc oxide eugenol
- Calcium hydroxide
- Resin
- Calcium Silicate Based Sealers

The canals were dried using sterile paper points prior to obturation. A warm vertical obturation technique was used. The pulp chamber space was cleaned using an ultrasonic scaler to remove traces of excess sealer (Figure 4.8.4), the tooth was restored using a composite restoration and a post-operative periapical radiograph was taken (Figure 4.8.5).

Why is it important to dry the root canal system prior to obturation?

It is important that the root canal is dry in order to increase the adhesion of sealers. Obturation of a wet canal can reduce the sealing ability and promote leakage. If there is persistent seepage of purulent or serous exudate, then an inter-appointment calcium hydroxide medicament should be placed. Prior to obturation, it is important to remove the intracanal medicament as any remaining calcium hydroxide will compromise the seal of the root filling.

Table 4.8.2 Comparing different root canal sealers.

Sealers	Properties
Zinc oxide eugenol Tubli-Seal (Kerr) Pulp Canal Sealer (Kerr) Pulpdent Root Canal Sealer (Pulpdent) CRCS (Ivoclar Vivadent)	– Long-term success rate – Antibacterial – Good handling – Some solubility
Calcium hydroxide Sealapex (Kerr) Apexit or Apexit Plus (Ivoclar Vivadent)	– Claimed to be antimicrobial and osteogenic due to sustained release of CaOH; however, lose many of these properties once set – Some solubility
Resin AH Plus (Dentsply Sirona)	– Antibacterial – Good handling and flowability – Good adhesion to dentine – Slight shrinkage on setting
Calcium silicate-based (bioceramic) sealers Endosequence BC (Brasseler USA) TotalFil BC Hiflow (FKG) Endoseal MTA (Maruchi) MTA Fillapex (Angelus) BioRoot (Septodont)	– Biocompatible – Antibacterial – Osteogenic ('bioactive') – Excellent sealing – Expensive – May be challenging to remove during retreatment – Heat can have a detrimental effect
Silicone RoekoSeal (Coltene) GuttaFlow (Coltene)	– Biocompatible – Setting time can be inconsistent/delayed when using NaOCl as a final irrigant – More evidence required to assess sealing ability

Angelus, Londrina, Brazil; Brasseler USA, Savannah, GA, USA; Coltene, Altstätten, Switzerland; Dentsply Sirona, Charlotte, NC, USA; FKG Dentaire Sarl, Switzerland; Kerr Dental, Uxbridge, UK; Maruchi, Vineland, NJ, USA; Pulpdent, Watertown, MA, USA; Septodont, Paris, France.

What different obturation techniques are available?

As there is no evidence to support one obturation technique over another, the choice of obturation technique will depend on the root canal system (Table 4.8.3).

Table 4.8.3　Comparison of different obturation techniques.

Technique	Method	Advantages/ disadvantages
Single gutta percha (GP) point and sealer	A master cone coated in sealer is placed to the working length (WL)	Advantages: Simplicity, efficiency Disadvantages: Sealer is soluble and the weakest part of a root canal filling. In this method it is used to obturate a significant part of the canal. The technique is unlikely to be able to completely fill and seal the root canal system. Calcium silicate based sealers (CSBS) have the potential to overcome this problem, however the long-term efficacy of 'hydraulic condensation' with CSBS will require further clinical research.
Cold lateral condensation	A master cone coated in sealer is placed to the WL Accessory GP points are inserted alongside it and condensed laterally using a spreader until the canal space is completely filled Spreaders: – Finger spreaders provide better tactile sensation – Nickel-titanium finger spreaders are more flexible	Advantages: Allows for good length control during compaction Disadvantages: May not fill canal irregularities as well as the warm techniques. Sealer is required to fill the spaces between the GP/ accessory cones; it does not produce a homogenous mass of GP Risk of root fracture if excessive forces are applied
Warm lateral condensation	The cold lateral technique is modified by heating the spreader prior to it being placed in the canal	Advantages: Softened GP is easier to compact, resulting in a more homogenous mass

Table 4.8.3 (Continued)

Technique	Method	Advantages/ disadvantages
Warm vertical condensation	A master cone coated in sealer is placed to the WL. A heated plugger is placed into the root canal. The coronal GP is removed with a heated plugger and the apical GP is softened and compacted using hand pluggers. Warm plasticised GP is injected above this to fill the coronal part of the canal	Advantages: Ability to fill canal irregularities and accessory canals. Softened GP is easier to compact, resulting in a homogenous mass Disadvantages: Less length control compared to cold lateral condensation. Pluggers are not able to reach the desired length (5 mm from the WL) in curved canals Excessive heat generation can damage the surrounding tissues Small risk of root fracture if excessive forces are applied
Thermo-mechanical	A slow handpiece-driven compactor file is rotated into the GP. The compactor file has flutes similar to a Hedström file but in reverse. The frictional heat produced softens the material and pushes it into the root canal	Advantages: Simplicity. Ability to fill canal irregularities Disadvantages: There is limited length control and risk that softened GP can be extruded apically. Risk of instrument fracture
Carrier-based techniques	The carrier is made of a central rigid core, which is surrounded by a layer of GP. This central core was previously made from metal or plastic, but more recently is from a more compacted GP First, a layer of sealer is placed on the canal walls. Then the carrier is placed in a heating device, and once the outer layer is softened it is placed to the WL	Advantages: Ability to fill canal irregularities. Disadvantages: There is limited length control and risk that softened GP can be extruded apically. It can be difficult to remove the central core during root canal retreatment.

What are the consequences of gutta percha and sealer extrusion?

When extruded through the apical foramen, most sealers would be dissolved or phagocytosed, whereas GP remains unchanged. This has not been shown to directly cause failure; however, the presence of GP and sealer in the periradicular tissues may prolong inflammation and delay healing. If a root is in close proximity to important anatomical structures such as the mandibular canal and the maxillary sinus, the effects of extrusion of root-filling materials may be more severe. Therefore, clinicians should avoid extrusion of root-filling materials.

What are the radiographic criteria for evaluating a root canal obturation?

The taper, density and length of a root canal filling should be assessed. In addition, the root canal filling should end below the level of the cemento-enamel junction in anterior teeth and at the level of the canal entrance in posterior teeth. There should not be a gap between the root filling and the core material. The condensation should be uniform in density with no over-extension or under-extension, terminating within 2 mm of the radiographic apex.

How should the tooth be definitively restored?

In this case, the tooth was restored with an onlay. A full-coverage crown would have been too destructive as it results in excessive removal of sound tooth structure.

There is significant evidence to show that endodontically treated premolar or molar teeth that have lost a marginal ridge have a high risk of fracture if they are not protected with a cuspal coverage restoration.

Discussion

Success of root canal treatment is primarily dependent on thorough disinfection of the root canal system. However, the obturation stage is also important. A systematic review found that four factors influenced the success rate of primary root canal treatment: the absence of a pre-operative periapical radiolucency, no voids in the root canal filling, obturation to within 2 mm of the apex and a good coronal seal.

The final coronal seal is of the utmost importance. Bacteria from the oral environment can leak through defective restorations and even a well-condensed root canal filling within a short period of time can impact the success of endodontic treatment. A good-quality coronal restoration should be placed as soon as possible after the endodontic treatment has been completed.

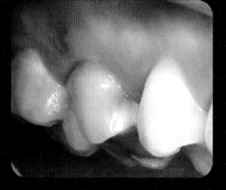

Figure 4.8.1 Pre-operative photograph showing buccal sinus.

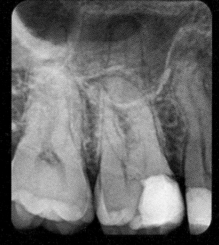

Figure 4.8.2 Pre-operative radiograph showing mesio-occlusal restoration with deficient margins, recurrent caries and restoration in proximity to pulp chamber, with curved canals and apical radiolucency.

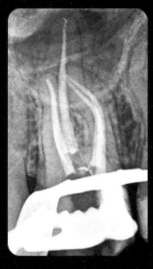

Figure 4.8.3 Obturation radiograph showing a well-condensed obturation terminating 0.5 mm from the radiographic apex.

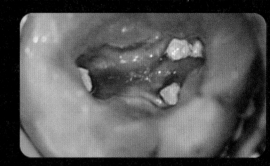

Figure 4.8.4 Magnified photograph showing a clean access cavity and obturated root canals.

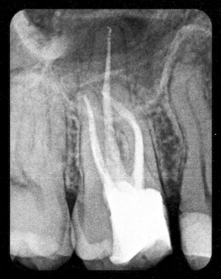

Figure 4.8.5 Post-operative radiograph showing obturated canals and a coronal restoration.

Further Reading

Allison, D.A., Weber, C.R., Walton, R.E., and Ga, A. (1979). The influence of the method of canal preparation on the quality of apical and coronal obturation. *Journal of Endodontics* 10: 229–204.

Klevant, F.J.H. and Eggink, C.O. (1983). The effect of canal preparation on periapical disease. *International Endodontic Journal* 16: 68–75.

Ørstavik D. (2005) Materials used for root canal obturation: technical, biological and clinical testing. *Endod Topics* 12: 25–38

Zavattini, A, Knight, A, Foschi, F, Mannocci, F. (2020) Outcome of root canal treatments using a new calcium silicate root canal sealer: A non-randomised clinical trial. Journal of *Clinical Medicine* 9(3): 782

4.9

Obturation of the Root Canal 2

Frédéric Bukiet, Maud Guivarc'h, and Thomas Giraud

Objectives

This case aims to discuss the use of calcium silicate–based sealers (CSBS) for root canal space obturation. The reader should be aware of their specific properties and understand why, when and how to use them.

Introduction

A 28-year-old male patient presented with spontaneous pain and biting sensitivity from the lower right first molar (LR6). He mentioned having received a root canal treatment on this tooth six months before the consultation.

Chief Complaint

Pain from a tooth on the lower right and cheek swelling.

Medical History

The day before the endodontic consultation, the patient was prescribed systemic antibiotics. The medical history was unremarkable except for elevated body temperature and asthenia during the infectious episode.

Dental History

The discomfort started one year ago. A primary root canal treatment of tooth LR6 was performed six months ago.

Clinical Examination

Extraoral examination revealed a right cheek swelling (Figure 4.9.1a). Intraoral examination highlighted a non-fluctuant swelling in the buccal

Pitt Ford's Problem-Based Learning in Endodontology, Second Edition. Edited by Elizabeth Shin Perry, Shanon Patel, Shalini Kanagasingam, and Samantha Hamer.
© 2025 John Wiley & Sons Ltd. Published 2025 by John Wiley & Sons Ltd.

sulcus adjacent to tooth LR6. Tooth LR6 was restored with an occlusal composite restoration and was tender to percussion. Pulp sensibility tests were negative on tooth LR6. Periodontal probing depths were 3 mm or less around tooth LR6. A pre-operative periapical radiograph was taken (Figure 4.9.1b).

The periapical radiograph revealed:

- Good bone levels.
- Extensive coronal restoration with a mesial void.
- An existing root canal filling sparsely condensed, with evidence of a possible unobturated second canal in the distal root.
- A large apical radiolucency associated with the mesial and distal roots.

Diagnosis and Treatment Planning

The diagnosis for tooth LR6 was an acute apical abscess associated with an existing root canal filling.

What were the treatment options for the patient?

- No treatment (not suitable considering the history and the diagnosis).
- Root canal retreatment.
- Apical microsurgery.
- Extraction.

After discussion with the patient and considering the clinical and radiograph information, it was decided to attempt a root canal retreatment on tooth LR6.

Treatment

The retreatment of the tooth LR6 was scheduled over two visits.

First visit

After local anaesthesia and dental dam placement, the occlusal restoration was removed and the access cavity was revised. After filling materials were removed, two additional canal entrances were identified in the distal root (Figure 4.9.2):

- One corresponding to the disto-lingual canal that was missed during the primary root canal treatment.
- One additional canal starting lingually from the disto-lingual canal. Scouting this canal revealed an abrupt initial curvature. A radix entomolaris was suspected.

Root canal shaping and disinfection were initiated. A cone beam computed tomography (CBCT) scan was carried out to assess the complex root canal anatomy before calcium hydroxide (Ca[OH]$_2$) intracanal dressing for one week.

Cone beam computed tomography analysis

The CBCT analysis (Figures 4.9.3–4.9.5) revealed:

- Significant bone destruction surrounding the mesial and distal root from the middle third to the periapical area.
- A narrow pathway through the buccal cortical plate connecting the periapical lesion and the soft tissues, explaining the cellulitis.
- The presence of a disto-lingual canal merging the disto-buccal in the middle third.
- A fused radix entomolaris containing a separate canal.

Second visit

Root canal shaping was completed after electronic working length determination. A 17% ethylenediaminetetraacetic acid (EDTA) solution was used to remove calcium hydroxide remnants and smear layer. Then 3% NaOCl solution agitation/rinse was performed. After gutta percha master cone adjustment, a final rinse with sterile water was implemented and the canals were slightly dried with a micro suction tip and one sterile paper point per canal.

A calcium silicate–based sealer was injected within the root canals before gutta percha cone insertion to the full working length (hydraulic condensation). They were then sectioned and gently condensed with a vertical plugger at the level of the canal entrances. A temporary restorative material was placed. The immediate post-operative periapical radiographs showed satisfactory obturation (Figure 4.9.6). The patient was scheduled the next week to place a direct composite restoration (Figure 4.9.7).

Follow-up

At eight-month review, the patient was asymptomatic and the tooth was functional. Periapical radiographs and review CBCT revealed clear signs of bone healing (Figure 4.9.8).

Discussion

CSBS have grown in popularity over time. This discussion aims to address their specificities and their clinical use.

What is a calcium silicate–based sealer?

ProRoot® mineral trioxide aggregate (MTA; Dentsply Sirona, Charlotte, NC, USA) was the first calcium silicate–based material introduced to dentistry in 1993. Since its release, several modified formulations have been progressively developed. Despite variation in compositions, in most of these formulations the main components remain calcium silicates, leading to them being categorised as 'calcium silicate–based materials'. More recently, the reduction of the particle size led to the development of CSBS for root canal obturation in association with gutta percha. Among the available CSBS, differences can be highlighted regarding their composition and handling (pre-mixed or hand-mixed formulations) The specific compositions can be found in the safety data sheet provided by the manufacturers. The composition differences between the formulations can significantly impact their clinical properties.

Unlike conventional sealers, CSBS are hydraulic and their setting process is based on a hydration reaction. In the presence of water, calcium silicates form a calcium silicate hydrate gel and subsequently $Ca(OH)_2$. The OH^- ions increase environmental pH and this alkalisation provides antimicrobial properties. Si^{4+} and Ca^{2+} induce mineralisation processes by promoting cell mineralisation activity. Moreover, in the presence of phosphate, deposition of apatite precursors and hydroxyapatite occurs on the material surface, resulting in a mineral infiltration zone into the dentine (Table 4.9.1).

Table 4.9.1 Schematic representation of the setting reaction of calcium silicate–based sealers.

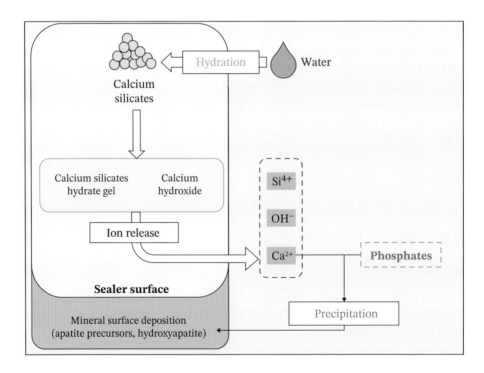

Calcium silicate–based sealers and conventional sealers are compared in Table 4.9.2.

Table 4.9.2 Comparison of the properties of calcium silicate–based sealers (CSBS) and conventional sealers. Overall, the composition of CSBS can significantly impact their properties.

Physico-chemical properties
Flowability/consistency of CSBS can be considered to be comparable to conventional sealers
Setting times appear to be quicker for CSBS, but this can be affected by the moisture content of the root canal
Radiopacity of CSBS is comparable to conventional sealers
Dimensional stability of CSBS is overall better than conventional sealers, especially zinc oxide eugenol–based sealers. A slight hygroscopic expansion is observed for some CSBS formulations
Film thickness of CSBS is globally higher compared to conventional sealers and sometimes close to the limit values of the standard recommendations
Solubility of CSBS is highly variable and shows higher values than conventional sealers. This higher solubility could at first sight be considered as negative in terms of long-outcome sealing. However, CSBS solubility is essential to trigger ion release and activation of bioactivity
Biological properties
Biological properties of CSBS rely on hydration by-products
CSBS show similar or increased antimicrobial properties in comparison to conventional sealers. These effects can last long after CSBS setting due to the extended alkalisation of the environment
CSBS exhibit better biocompatibility than conventional sealers
CSBS present a certain bioactivity. Their use promotes regeneration processes and control of inflammation steps, both involved in tissue healing

How has introduction of calcium silicate based sealers impacted root canal obturation strategies?

The single-cone technique initially used with zinc oxide eugenol–based sealers has fallen out of favour. However, since CSBS release, interest has been regained in the single-cone technique due to their excellent dimensional stability. CSBS behave like a true filling material, while the gutta percha cone functions as a carrier, helping CSBS distribution into the root canal space. It has to be noted that obturation with CSBS is not limited to the single-cone technique. Depending on the root canal anatomy, accessory gutta percha cones can also be used. This method of obturation is sometimes named hydraulic condensation.

What are the relevant indications for calcium silicate–based sealers?

- *Related to the root canal anatomy*: in narrow, long, curved canals, but also anatomy showing deep ramifications, implementing warm vertical compaction with appropriate penetration of the plugger can be difficult, and even impossible. Since the gutta percha is not melted in the apical third, the obturation behaves like a single-cone technique in the last mm. Using hydraulic condensation with CSBS in such situations makes obturation easier and faster while taking advantage of the physico-chemical and biological properties of CSBS. CSBS can also be indicated with hydraulic condensation in case of large foramen (young teeth, external inflammatory apical resorption).
- *Related to a biological purpose*: the antibacterial, alkalisation and biomineralisation abilities of CSBS might stimulate and enhance the healing process. They should be suitable in cases of apical periodontitis, external inflammatory root resorption or maxillary sinusitis of dental origin (especially in immunocompromised patients with contraindications to zinc-oxide eugenol or formaldehyde-based sealers). CSBS might also be suitable in patients presenting risk of osteonecrosis, for whom it is desirable to reduce bone aggression factors. CSBS usage with hydraulic condensation can also simplify the management of middle or apical third perforation while taking advantage of the biological properties.
- *Related to operative accessibility*: when dealing with restricted operative access (limited mouth opening, conservative access cavity), hydraulic condensation with CSBS facilitates the obturation process compared to methods based on gutta percha compaction.

Does calcium silicate–based sealer usage impact the clinical protocol?

A wide variation in clinical use of CBCS is highlighted in the literature and is based on practitioners' clinical experience due to the limited available evidence at the time of writing.

- *Do CSBS require the use of specific gutta percha cones?* To improve the adhesion between CSBS (hydrophilic) and gutta percha (hydrophobic), some manufacturers recommended the use of specific pre-impregnated gutta percha cones. So far, there have been no consistent and independent studies confirming the benefit of such a strategy.
- *Do CSBS affect the irrigation protocol and the root canal drying technique?* CSBS need water to initiate the hydration reaction that conditions their setting process. Therefore, intracanal dentine desiccation should be avoided and the recommendation is to gently dry the root canal before obturation, especially for pre-mixed formulations. Since previous studies showed that most irrigants may negatively affect the properties of CSBS, it seems advisable to perform a final rinse with sterile water. Then root canal drying is implemented with intracanal micro-suction before usage of one sterile paper point.

● *How can the quality of obturation be improved when using CSBS?* Several methods have been proposed to reduce void occurrence when applying hydraulic condensation in oval or wide canals. Before master cone insertion, using a device that helps the sealer's distribution/ penetration into the root canal space (such as a Lentulo spiral at 700 rpm, flexible injection tip or sonic or ultrasonic activation) may improve the quality of the obturation.

● *Can CSBS be used with warm gutta percha obturation techniques?* While this approach may appear consistent to combine the advantages of these techniques and CSBS use, temperature rise (especially above 100 °C) can negatively affect physical properties of most CSBS formulations. However, new formulations that can be used with warm gutta percha have been released.

● *Can CSBS impact the difficulty of non-surgical retreatments?* Most studies showed that apical patency could be properly reestablished during retreatment if the master cone was adjusted to the full working length. This may be obvious since the gutta percha cone can be easily and quickly removed from the root. A non-surgical retreatment approach is usually indicated in a case of obturation short of the working length. In such situations, some studies reported that it was impossible to achieve apical patency especially in curved canals due to the presence of the 'hard' CSBS just beyond the tip of the master cone.

Conclusion

Overall, CSBS present comparable or better properties than conventional sealers. Considering the popularity of these sealers and the ever increasing number of formulations, CSBS users should pay careful attention to the specific composition of the constituents which affect their biological properties and clinical behaviour. Clinicians should take this into consideration to ensure correct clinical usage and predictable outcomes.

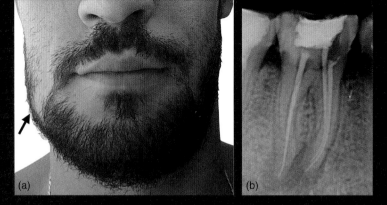

Figure 4.9.1 (a) Extraoral examination showing a right cheek swelling (arrow). (b) Pre-operative radiograph of the LR6.

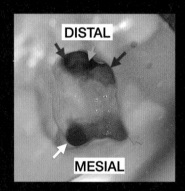

Figure 4.9.2 Clinical view of the pulp floor after filling material removal and initiation of root canal shaping. Five canals were located, including three canals in the distal: mesio-buccal: blue arrow, mesio-lingual: white arrow, disto-buccal: purple arrow, disto-lingual: green arrow and suspected radix root canal: red arrow.

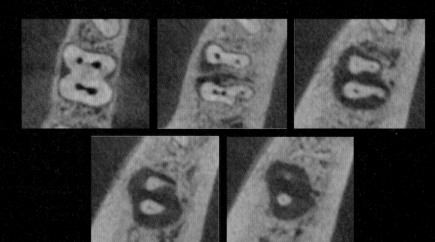

Figure 4.9.3 Cone beam computed tomography axial views from the coronal to the apical third highlighting the particular anatomy, especially the fused radix entomolaris and the bone destruction.

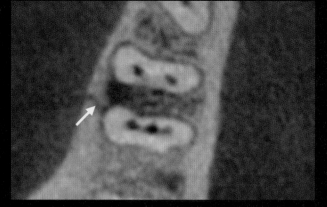

Figure 4.9.4 Cone beam computed tomography axial view showing a narrow pathway through the buccal cortical plate (yellow arrow) connecting the periapical lesion and the soft tissues and explaining the cellulitis.

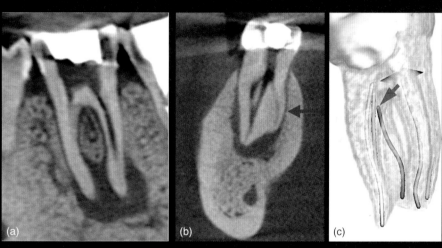

Figure 4.9.5 (a) Cone beam computed tomography (CBCT) sagittal view illustrating the extensive bone destruction. (b) CBCT coronal view showing the distal root configuration. (c) Volume rendering simulating the root canal trajectories and showing the fused radix entomolaris (red arrow).

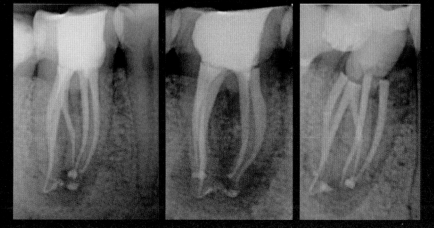

Figure 4.9.6 Immediate post-operative radiographs using three different angulations.

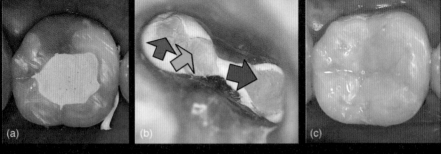

Figure 4.9.7 Restorative treatment. (a) Pre-operative clinical view. (b) Clinical view centred on the distal root. Notice the calcium silicate–based sealer volume (white material) and the gutta percha cones (radix: red arrow, disto-lingual: green arrow and disto-buccal: purple arrow). (c) Post-operative occlusal view after direct composite restoration.

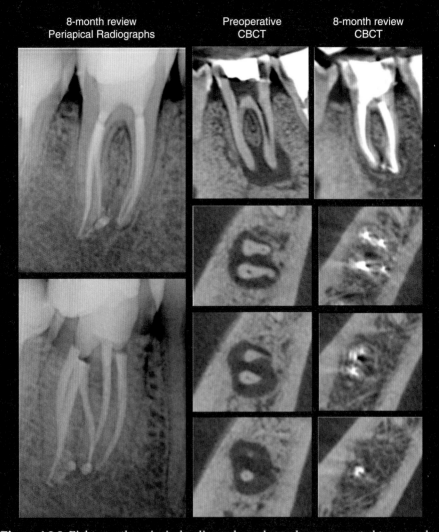

Figure 4.9.8 Eight-month periapical radiographs and cone beam computed tomography (CBCT) review showing the bone healing.

Further Reading

Camilleri, J. (2017). Will bioceramics be the future root canal filling materials? *Current Oral Health Reports* 4: 228–238.

Guivarc'h, M., Jeanneau, C., Giraud, T. et al. (2020). An international survey on the use of calcium silicate-based sealers in non-surgical endodontic treatment. *Clinical Oral Investigations* 24: 417–424.

Prati, C. and Gandolfi, M.G. (2015). Calcium silicate bioactive cements: biological perspectives and clinical applications. *Dental Materials* 31: 351–370.

Sfeir, G., Zogheib, C., Patel, S. et al. (2021). Calcium silicate-based root canal sealers: a narrative review and clinical perspectives. *Materials (Basel).* 14 (14): 3965.

Torabinejad, M., Parirokh, M., and Dummer, P.M.H. (2018). Mineral trioxide aggregate and other bioactive endodontic cements: an updated overview – Part II: Other clinical applications and complications. *International Endodontic Journal* 51: 284–317.

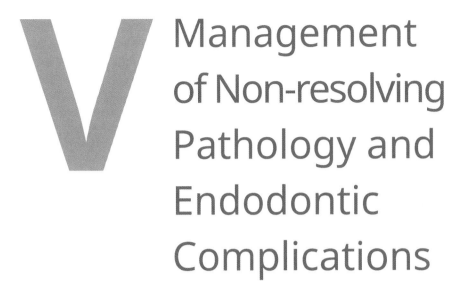

V Management of Non-resolving Pathology and Endodontic Complications

5.1 Post-Treatment Periapical Periodontitis

David Figdor

Objectives

At the end of this chapter the reader should understand the possible causes of endodontic treatment failure and have an understanding of the management of cases with signs or symptoms of post-treatment periapical periodontitis.

Introduction

A male, 60 years old, presented to his dentist regarding the lower left second molar (LL7). The tooth had been root treated over 10 years ago.

Chief Complaint

Pain on biting.

Dental History

Regular dental attendance with historical high dental treatment need.

Medical History

Tamsulosin for management of benign prostatic hyperplasia.

Clinical Examination

Extraoral examination was unremarkable.

Intraoral examination revealed an extensively restored dentition with good oral hygiene.

Pitt Ford's Problem-Based Learning in Endodontology, Second Edition. Edited by Elizabeth Shin Perry, Shanon Patel, Shalini Kanagasingam, and Samantha Hamer. © 2025 John Wiley & Sons Ltd. Published 2025 by John Wiley & Sons Ltd.

The LL7 was firm with slight tenderness on percussion and no tenderness or swelling in the buccal sulcus. There was gingival inflammation and probing of 4 mm on the disto-lingual aspect of the LL7; all other probing depths were <3 mm. The tooth was restored with an amalgam overlay, with a crack visible in the buccal enamel; however, there was no isolated deep probing depth associated with this area. The tooth was unresponsive to sensibility testing.

Radiographic Examination

Periapical radiograph

The periapical radiograph of the LL7 (Figure 5.1.1) revealed:

- Good bone levels.
- Large amalgam restoration with the core build-up extending into the mesial and distal canals and satisfactory margins.
- Both roots have a slightly curved morphology.
- Existing root filling in both roots, terminating short of the radiographic apices.
- A uniform and intact periodontal ligament.

Conventional two-dimensional (2D) radiographs have limitations and are affected by superimposition, geometrical distortion and anatomical noise. If the periapical lesion is confined to the cancellous bone it may not be detected with conventional radiographs. Cone beam computed tomography (CBCT) scans are three-dimensional (3D) and have a higher sensitivity and specificity for the detection of periapical pathology when compared to conventional radiographs. The ionising radiation associated with CBCT needs to be justified such that the additional information from the scan provides beneficial information for the management of the case. A high-resolution, small field-of-view CBCT (Morita 3De) was warranted in this case to check for pathology (Figure 5.1.2).

Findings from cone beam computed tomography for the LL7

- The mesial root has an S-shape morphology. There is radiolucent bone in the furcation, but essentially a normal lamina dura.
- In the sagittal plane, there is a slightly widened apical lamina dura around the distal root.

Diagnosis and Treatment Planning

What is the diagnosis?

The symptoms (specifically, tenderness to chewing) are consistent with periradicular inflammation, possibly due to infection. The differential diagnosis could include (i) post-treatment endodontic infection, (ii) a crack, or

(iii) occlusal trauma. However, there were no corroborating findings seen clinically or radiographically, so the precise aetiology was uncertain.

As clinicians, we are accustomed to operative intervention; indeed, many patients expect it. Yet when there is an uncertain aetiology due to a mismatch in history, symptoms and clinical findings, or when the findings are inconclusive, it is certainly acceptable to wait, monitor and review.

Depending on the diagnosis, the potential treatment options might include monitor and review, endodontic retreatment or extraction. In this case, as the symptoms were settling and the diagnosis was uncertain, in discussion with the patient the decision was to recall in one year but review at any time if there were recurrent symptoms or signs.

Review

One year later, the patient returned for review. Over the year, there had been intermittent mild symptoms with occasional tenderness to chewing.

A new periapical radiograph revealed a developing periapical radiolucency (Figure 5.1.3). Therefore, with this new radiographic finding it was then possible to clarify the diagnosis as symptomatic apical periodontitis associated with the previously root-filled lower left second molar.

What is the most likely aetiology?

The possible reasons for the recurrent periapical infection could be renewed endodontic infection via coronal microleakage, or a crack, or infection that persisted after the previous root canal treatment and some ecological disturbance that allowed the infection to reach a clinical level. Special properties are required by microorganisms for long-term survival in the inhospitable environment of the filled root canal (Table 5.1.1).

Table 5.1.1 Properties required by microorganisms to survive in the root-filled canal and cause post-treatment apical periodontitis.

- Survive antimicrobial treatment
- Survive root filling
- Survive starvation
- Find substrates for growth
- Endure host defence
- Induce and maintain periapical inflammatory response

What are the treatment options?

The potential treatment options discussed with the patient were:

- No treatment
- Extraction
- Endodontic retreatment

Leaving the tooth alone was not a feasible option as the tooth was occasionally symptomatic. The ideal approach was to save this tooth as a functional unit of the dentition, and tooth retention was the patient's clear preference.

Before attempting retreatment, the patient should be advised that the prognosis of retreatment depends on removal of the existing root filling material and control of the root canal infection. The structural integrity of the tooth also has a significant impact on prognosis. The presence of a crack or insufficient sound remaining coronal tooth structure could adversely impact on the prognosis.

It is important that the patient has a realistic understanding of the complexity of both the problem and the treatment. Expecting a certain successful outcome is unrealistic and there is a risk that the disease may not resolve, or the tooth structure may fail, necessitating extraction. Nevertheless, if the retreatment is well done, it is reasonable to expect around a 75% chance of favourable healing. Cuspal coverage with a crown is the ideal restoration after endodontic retreatment.

The patient was fully informed about the details, difficulties, risks and prognosis and decided to proceed with endodontic retreatment.

Treatment

Endodontic retreatment

The tooth was carefully isolated with dental dam in a leak-free manner to allow work in a clean and sterile field. The tooth and surrounding dental dam were cleaned with hydrogen peroxide and disinfected with a chlorhexidine-alcohol tincture.

An access cavity was prepared in the occlusal surface through the amalgam restoration to reach the pulp chamber. Working with the operating microscope, amalgam was carefully removed over the orifice of each canal using ultrasonic tips. Gutta percha was removed in the coronal section of the canals with Gates-Glidden burs, followed by chloroform and hand instruments in the apical half to complete the removal of gutta percha. The canals were further negotiated using small-sized (10–20) stainless steel hand files to the apex. Canal measurements were confirmed on radiographs and the canals were cleaned and shaped using alternating 15% ethylenediamine-tetraacetic acid (EDTA) and 4% sodium hypochlorite (NaOCl) irrigation solutions. The canals were dressed with calcium hydroxide paste and the access cavity sealed with a temporary restorative material. Insertion of the temporary filling deep into the pulp chamber and over the orifice of the canals helps ensure a reliable inter-appointment seal.

One week later, the patient returned for the second completion of the root canal treatment (Figure 5.1.4). The patient was advised to return to the referring dentist for permanent restoration with a crown.

Post Treatment

The healing response was monitored over time. Fourteen months post-retreatment, a follow-up conventional radiograph showed resolution of the original periapical lesion (Figure 5.1.5), which was confirmed with a high-resolution CBCT scan (Figure 5.1.6).

Discussion

Post-treatment apical periodontitis is primarily associated with persisting infection of the root canal system. Experience has shown that most cases are associated with shortcomings in the quality of the previous treatment that are linked to failure to control the root canal infection. Common examples include inadequate access, missed canals, errors in instrumentation and leakage of the coronal restoration. Thus, it makes good sense to focus treatment measures on infection control. Attention to the fine details can make a significant difference to treatment outcome.

In this case, endodontic retreatment taking care with aseptic control resulted in a favourable healing outcome, shown by resolution of the periapical radiolucency. The post-treatment review CT scan revealed filling material in the isthmus between the mesio-buccal and mesio-lingual canals at the mid-root level. Whether or not this site was a nidus for persisting infection is uncertain, but it is known that small numbers of microbes may persist at these sites following endodontic treatment.

Because the success rate for retreatment is generally favourable (around 75%), in most cases it is well worth attempting to retain teeth by endodontic retreatment, as a first choice for management. In this case, the favourable outcome with periapical bone repair means that it should be feasible to get many more years of service life from this previously extensively treated tooth.

The microbial flora in a poorly treated root canal is similar to that seen in a previously untreated case, so it is a reasonable expectation that thorough application of the antimicrobial techniques of isolation, asepsis, instrumentation, irrigation and dressing should be effective in control of the root canal infection.

The microbial flora in the untreated root canal differs considerably from that seen in a well-treated case. In the former, there is typically a polymicrobial flora dominated by obligate anaerobes. In the previously filled canal the flora consists mostly of a mono-infection dominated by Gram-positive facultative and obligate anaerobes. Common isolates are *Enterococci*, *Candida* and *Streptococci*, which share characteristics of resistance to antimicrobial measures and an ability to survive in the low nutrient environment of the filled root canal.

While most post-treatment disease is associated with persistent intraradicular infection, a small proportion of well-treated cases are related to extraradicular infection and non-microbial factors, such as cysts or a foreign body reaction. A few lesions can heal by scar tissue, which on follow-up radiographs may be confused with persistent apical periodontitis (Table 5.1.2).

Diagnosis should be based on assembling all available information (history, examination, tests and radiography) and integrating it to reach a conclusion consistent with the facts. If the findings are ambiguous or inconsistent, it is reasonable to wait and review, consider or discuss with a colleague, keeping the final diagnosis open until an appropriate time.

In summary, most cases of post-treatment disease are associated with persisting infection of the root canal system. The treatment of first choice is root canal retreatment to a high standard with a particular focus on infection control. A comprehensive history including details of previous treatment is helpful for establishing the diagnosis and planning the optimal approach to treatment. Informed discussion allows the patient to compare treatment options, and balance benefits and risks to make an appropriate decision. Retreatment is generally a more complex process than primary endodontic treatment and the practitioner should include referral to a specialist endodontist as a sensible and prudent management option.

Table 5.1.2 Causes of post-treatment persistent periapical radiolucency.

- Intraradicular infection
- Extraradicular infection (mostly periapical actinomycosis)
- True cysts
- Foreign body reaction (e.g. to filling materials, paper points and cholesterol crystals)
- Healing by scar tissue[a]

[a] Not a true failure of treatment.

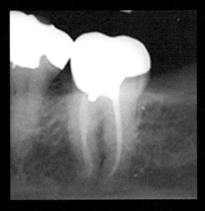

Figure 5.1.1 Periapical radiograph taken at the time of initial consultation reveals a uniform and intact periodontal ligament.

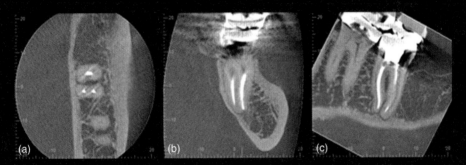

(a)　　　　　　　(b)　　　　　　　(c)

Figure 5.1.2 Cone beam computed tomography reveals slightly widened apical lamina dura around the distal root.

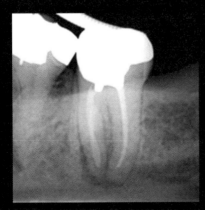

Figure 5.1.3 One year after the initial consultation, the periapical radiograph revealed a developing periapical radiolucency.

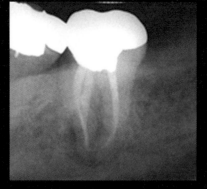

Figure 5.1.4 Periapical radiograph of retreatment of the root canal.

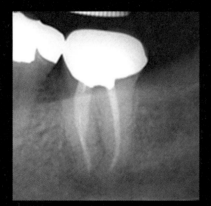

Figure 5.1.5 Fourteen months post retreatment, periapical radiograph shows resolution of the original periapical lesion.

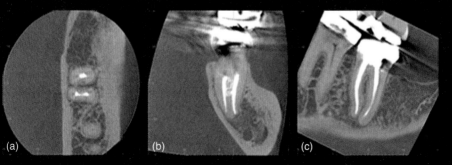

Figure 5.1.6 Cone beam computed tomography confirms resolution of the original

Further Reading

Al-Nuaimi, N., Patel, S., Austin, R.S., and Mannocci, F. (2017). A prospective study assessing the effect of coronal tooth structure loss on the outcome of root canal retreatment. *International Endodontic Journal* 50: 1143–1157.

Davies, A., Patel, S., Foschi, F. et al. (2016). The detection of periapical pathoses using digital periapical radiography and cone beam computed tomography in endodontically retreated teeth - part 2 : a one year post-treatment follow-up. *International Endodontic Journal* 49: 623–635.

Figdor, D. and Gulabivala, K. (2011). Survival against the odds: microbiology of root canals associated with post-treatment disease. *Endodontic Topics* 18: 62–77.

Molander, A., Reit, C., Dahlén, G., and Kvist, T. (1998). Microbiological status of root-filled teeth with apical periodontitis. *International Endodontic Journal* 31: 1–7.

Nair, P.N.R. (2004). Pathogenesis of apical periodontitis and the causes of endodontic failures. *Critical Reviews in Oral Biology & Medicine* 15: 348–381.

Nair, P.N.R., Henry, S., Cano, V., and Vera, J. (2005). Microbial status of apical root canal system of human mandibular first molars with primary apical periodontitis after "one-visit" endodontic treatment. *Oral Surgery, Oral Medicine, Oral Pathology, Oral Radiology and Endodontology* 99: 231–252.

Sjögren, U., Hagglund, G., Sundqvist, G., and Wing, K. (1990). Factors affecting the long-term results of endodontic treatment. *Journal of Endodontics* 16: 498–504.

Sundqvist, G. and Figdor, D. (2003). Life as an endodontic pathogen. Ecological differences between the untreated and root-filled root canals. *Endodontic Topics* 6: 3–28.

Sundqvist, G., Figdor, D., Persson, S., and Sjögren, U. (1998). Microbiologic analysis of teeth with failed endodontic treatment and the outcome of conservative re-treatment. *Oral Surgery, Oral Medicine, Oral Pathology, Oral Radiology and Endodontology* 85: 86–93.

5.2 Non-surgical Retreatment and Disassembly

John Rhodes

Objectives

At the end of the case the reader should be aware of the assessment, treatment options and technical aspects of disassembling a tooth that has been restored with a post crown.

Introduction

A 54-year-old man was referred with occasional pain and tenderness over the apex of his root-filled maxillary right lateral incisor (UR2). The tooth had been restored with a post crown for over 15 years.

Chief Complaint

A tender spot on the gum above the tooth and the tooth occasionally ached.

Medical History

Unremarkable.

Dental History

A regular attender at the dentist with a well-maintained dentition.

Clinical Examination

There were no extraoral signs or swelling. Intraoral examination revealed a well-cared-for dentition with various restorations, no caries and healthy periodontium.

The crown on UR2 was reasonable and there was staining on the UR1 and UR3

(Figure 5.2.1). The gingiva was tender when palpated over the apex of UR2.

Pitt Ford's Problem-Based Learning in Endodontology, Second Edition. Edited by Elizabeth Shin Perry, Shanon Patel, Shalini Kanagasingam, and Samantha Hamer. © 2025 John Wiley & Sons Ltd. Published 2025 by John Wiley & Sons Ltd.

What does the periapical radiograph reveal?

- Alveolar bone height within normal limits.
- The UR2 had been restored with a post crown and large metal parallel serrated or screw post that extended 2–3 mm below crestal bone level.
- A laterally condensed gutta percha root filling was in place; the filling could be slightly short.
- There was a periapical radiolucency associated with the UR2.
- The UR1 had also been root filled more recently and there may be periapical radiolucency associated with this tooth (Figure 5.2.2).

A small-volume cone beam computed tomography (CBCT) scan of the anterior maxilla was exposed to confirm the presence or absence of periapical pathology on the UR1 and to prepare for the possibility of a microsurgical treatment approach on the UR2 (Figure 5.2.3).

The CBCT showed:

- There was no periapical radiolucency associated with the UR1.
- A periapical radiolucency was evident on the UR2. The cortical plate was intact.
- There were no other problems identified.

Diagnosis and Treatment Planning

The diagnosis for the UR2 was symptomatic apical periodontitis associated with an existing root canal treatment.

Treatment options for tooth UR2

- Non-surgical root canal retreatment
- Microsurgical root end surgery
- Extraction and replacement
- No treatment

Technical challenges

What technical challenges could be faced during treatment?

Non-surgical retreatment will require the removal of the large metal post. Using force there is a risk that the root could fracture while this is being done. The tooth would definitely require a new coronal restoration for which the patient would incur additional cost.

Microsurgical treatment avoids the need to replace the crown and has a similar success rate in the short term to a non-surgical approach. However, there is more risk of postoperative pain and swelling.

The general consensus is that if the previous root filling is technically poor and can be improved using a non-surgical approach, this will improve the long-term prognosis. However, in anterior teeth with post crowns, if the post crown restoration is good it is often possible to disinfect the apical portion of the root beyond the post using a modern microsurgical approach and bespoke ultrasonic instruments.

The tooth is restorable and functional and it would be difficult to justify extraction and replacement. Equally, doing nothing risks the chance of an acute flare-up.

Treatment plan

After discussing all of the options the patient elected to have non-surgical root canal retreatment.

Single- or multiple-visit treatment?

Due to the concern that a temporary post crown could allow microleakage between visits, there was no clinical justification for completing treatment over two visits. In this case, due to the possibility of contamination with multiple-visit treatment, single-visit treatment may be associated with a higher chance of success.

Treatment

After application of local anaesthetic, the crown on the UR2 was removed by sectioning and elevated with an Ash crown remover (Dentsply Sirona, Charlotte, NC, USA).

The root was isolated with dental dam and a wingless EW clamp (Ash, Denstply Sirona) (Figure 5.2.4).

Disassembly

Core material was removed from around the metal post using a Start-X no. 3 ultrasonic tip (Dentsply Sirona) on a medium power setting. Cement was removed from around the post using the same ultrasonic tip (Figure 5.2.5).

Post removal – what is the most efficient means?

- Cement should be removed conservatively to preserve valuable coronal tooth substance. This can be achieved with ultrasonic tips and when the post is cylindrical with a Masserann trephine.
- Ultrasonic tips can be used to vibrate and loosen metal and cast restorations. Heat is created when using ultrasound and it is important to use water coolant to prevent damage to the periodontium.

- Do not try to remove the post with forceps or apply lateral force, as this will increase the likelihood of root fracture.
- If after a few minutes nothing seems to be happening, consider using a different technique such as a post-puller.

The post was removed using a combination of a Masserann trephine and a Start-X no. 4 ultrasonic tip. The tip was used with water coolant to prevent heating. The Masserann trephine was used to remove cement conservatively from around the circumference of the post. It can also be used to grip the post and help unscrew it (Figure 5.2.6).

Gutta percha root filling material was removed using a Gates-Glidden no. 2 and Hedström file no. 30.

The root length was estimated with an electronic apex locator and size 30 FlexoFile and confirmed with a radiograph. This was also a good opportunity to confirm that all the gutta percha had been removed (Figures 5.2.7 and 5.2.8).

Preparation and Disinfection

A single, large reciprocating nickel titanium (NiTi) instrument was used to prepare the canal to the full working length.

Irrigation was carried out with 3% sodium hypochlorite agitated with an ultrasonic tip and final rinsing with 17% ethylenediaminetetraacetic acid (EDTA).

Sealing the Canal

The apical part of the root canal was obturated using vertically compacted gutta percha and AH Plus Sealer (Dentsply Sirona).

Restoration

What are the optimum requirements for a post crown using a fibre post and composite core?

- You should allow an apical seal with gutta percha of 3–5 mm.
- The post should be as long as practicably possible, extend below crestal bone level and be tapered.
- Post width in this case was dictated by the previous restoration, but never enlarge the post hole excessively as this will weaken the tooth. Approximately one-third of the root width is sufficient.
- Aim to provide 1.5–2.0 mm of ferrule. This acts as a bracing element for lateral forces, which would otherwise be exerted through the post itself and could result in failure of the restoration.

A fibre post (Dentsply Sirona) was selected that fitted snugly into the post hole. It was not necessary to enlarge the post hole as this would remove valuable tooth substance and weaken the tooth unnecessarily.

After etching with phosphoric acid and rinsing, a dual-cure bonding agent was applied to the walls of the post hole. The fibre post was cemented with a dual cure composite (Core-X Flow, Dentsply Sirona) and a core built up. (It is important to use a dual-cure system when cementing fibre posts as light penetration is reduced at the base of the post hole.)

The core material was prepared and a temporary acrylic crown was fabricated (Figure 5.2.9).

A final periapical radiograph showed the completed root filling. A good homogenous seal had been created from coronal to apical (Figure 5.2.10).

Reviews

Reviews were carried out at one year and four years.

The tooth had been restored with a permanent crown at one year and was sign and symptom free. There was some reduction in the size of the apical radiolucency on radiograph. At a four-year review there was good evidence of apical healing (Figures 5.2.11 and 5.2.12).

Discussion

In this case the tooth could have been extracted and replaced with an implant-supported crown; however, this was not considered to be a justifiable treatment option. Indeed, endodontically treated teeth can survive as well as single-unit implant restorations with fewer post-operative problems.

Studies report that no significant difference was found between restored single-unit implants (95%) and endodontically treated teeth (94%) over six years. In a study at the University of Minnesota, matched pairs of endodontically treated teeth and single-unit implants were compared; after seven to nine years, the positive outcome was 74% for implants and 84% for endodontically treated teeth. The rate of complications and necessary interventions was significantly higher in the implant group, and it took longer for patients to adjust to the implant restoration. It has also been found that the survival of restored endodontically treated teeth (83.34%) and implants (80.8%) in the same arch showed no significant difference after eight years.

It would also have been possible to treat the tooth using a microsurgical endodontic approach, disinfecting the apical part of the root canal with specialised ultrasonic tips. Surgical treatment of such cases compared with a non-surgical approach has a highly favourable outcome. When non-surgical and surgical treatment were compared in 95 randomly assigned cases, there was a higher healing rate with surgery at 12 months, no difference in healing at 48 months and no systematic difference in outcome long term. More favourable early success was noted in the surgical group, but a more favourable outcome was shown for non-surgical treatment in the long term.

There are many factors for the clinician to consider when deciding between a non-surgical or surgical approach and these are outlined in Table 5.2.1.

Metal cast posts and cores have historically been used to restore root-filled teeth, with success rates of 84–94% at 10 years. Two disadvantages of metal posts include greater removal of pericervical root canal dentine and the potential risk of coronal leakage during temporisation. Flexible post systems such as fibre posts have been developed to facilitate more uniform stress distribution compared to metal posts. To date, however, there is no reported evidence that fibre posts reduce the occurrence of root fractures in vivo. A meta-analysis of the literature showed that no evidence was identified

Table 5.2.1 Comparison of non-surgical and microsurgical endodontic techniques.

Non-surgical	Microsurgical
Patient factors	
More destructive/expensive for patient	More invasive, longer recovery
Greater surgery time	Less surgery time
Late healing	Early healing
Minor post-operative discomfort	Greater risk of discomfort, swelling and bruising
	Requires greater operator skill and specialised equipment
Decision-making factors	
Restoration defective/technically poor endodontic treatment	Optimal restoration
Marginal bone loss	Good periodontal condition and buccal cortical bone present
Anatomical features, e.g. mental nerve, maxillary antrum, palatal neurovascular bundle	Disassembly likely to render tooth unrestorable
Some medical conditions	Multiple teeth

for a difference in failure rates between fibre posts and metal posts. These findings were independent of the type of metal post and position within the dental arch. Fibre posts are therefore considered a reliable means of providing additional retention, certainly in anterior teeth.

Conclusion

In this case non-surgical retreatment of a failed root filling in a tooth restored with a metal post and crown was completed. The tooth was restored with a fibre post, composite core and crown. There was good evidence of osseous healing at four years.

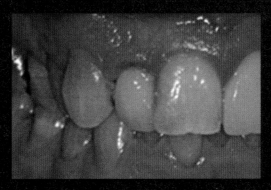

Figure 5.2.1 An intraoral photograph showing the crown on tooth UR2.

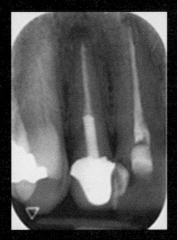

Figure 5.2.2 The paralleling pre-operative radiograph shows a technically good root filling and post crown restoration. The post is metal and has a serrated or crew thread.

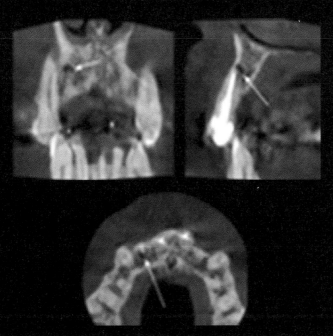

Figure 5.2.3 A small-volume cone beam computed tomography scan confirming a periapical lesion on the UR2. There was no radiolucency around the apex of the UR1.

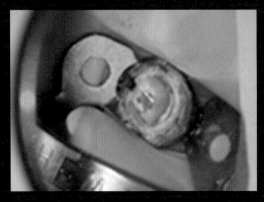

Figure 5.2.4 Isolated with dental dam. Core material can be removed using ultrasonics.

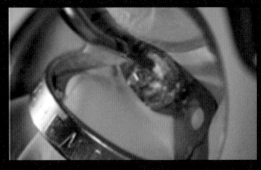

Figure 5.2.5 A Start-X no. 3 ultrasonic tip being used to remove cement.

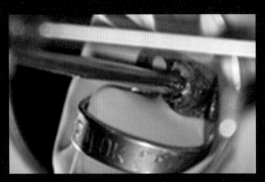

Figure 5.2.6 The Masserann trephine can be used to remove material conservatively from around the post. It will also help with retrieval.

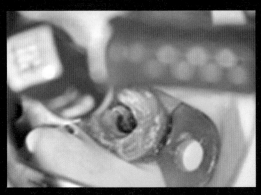

Figure 5.2.7 A FlexoFile was used for working length estimation and removal of gutta percha tags.

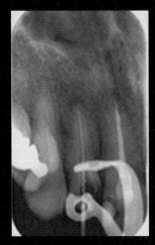

Figure 5.2.8 A diagnostic working length radiograph showed that the file was at good length and the gutta percha had been completely removed.

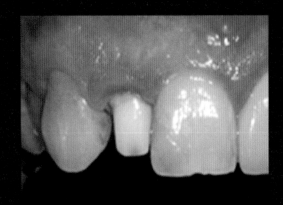

Figure 5.2.9 The dual-cure composite core has been prepared prior to fabrication of a temporary acrylic crown.

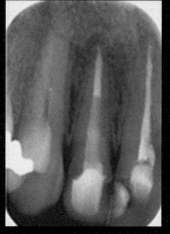

Figure 5.2.10 Post-operative radiograph shows a good coronal-apical homogenous seal

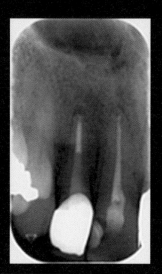

Figure 5.2.11 Review at one year; the tooth is symptom and sign free and has been permanently restored, with apical radiolucency decreasing in size.

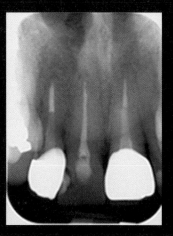

Figure 5.2.12 Review at four years; the tooth is symptom and sign free, with good evidence of osseous healing.

Further Reading

Cloet, E., Debels, E., and Naert, I. (2017). Controlled clinical trial on the outcome of glass fiber composite cores versus wrought posts and cast cores for the restoration of endodontically treated teeth: a 5-year follow-up study. *International Journal of Prosthodontics* 30: 71–79.

Davies, H., Ahmed, S., and Edwards, D. (2021). Metal vs fibre posts – which is clinically superior for the restoration of endodontically treated teeth? *Evidence-Based Dentistry* 22: 162–163.

Del Fabbro M, Taschieri S, Testori T, Francetti L, Weinstein RL. (2007) Surgical versus non-surgical endodontic re-treatment for periradicular lesions. Cochrane Database of Systematic Reviews 18(3): CD005511.

Doyle, S.L., Hodges, J.S., Pesun, I.J. et al. (2006). Retrospective cross sectional comparison of initial nonsurgical endodontic treatment and single-tooth implants. *Journal of Endodontics* 32: 822–827.

Ferrari, M., Mannocci, F., Vichi, A. et al. (2000). Bonding to root canal: structural characteristics of the substrate. *American Journal of Dentistry* 13: 255–260.

Iqbal, M.K. and Kim, S. (2007). For teeth requiring endodontic treatment, what are the differences in outcomes of restored endodontically treated teeth compared to implant-supported restorations? *International Journal of Oral & Maxillofacial Implants* 22 (Suppl): 96–116.

Kvist, T. and Reit, C. (1999). Results of endodontic retreatment: a randomized clinical study comparing surgical and nonsurgical procedures. *Journal of Endodontics* 25: 814–817.

Mannocci, F., Bhuva, B., Roig, M. et al. (2021). European Society of Endodontology position statement: the restoration of root filled teeth. *International Endodontic Journal* 54: 1974–1981.

Ng, C.C., Dumbrigue, H.B., Al-Bayat, M.I. et al. (2006). Influence of remaining coronal tooth structure location on the fracture resistance of restored endodontically treated anterior teeth. *Journal of Prosthetic Dentistry* 95: 290–296.

Sathorn, C., Parashos, P., and Messer, H.H. (2005). Effectiveness of single versus multiple-visit endodontic treatment of teeth with apical periodontitis: a systematic review and meta-analysis. *International Endodontic Journal* 38: 347–355.

Torabinejad, M., Corr, R., Handysides, R., and Shabahang, S. (2009). Outcomes of nonsurgical retreatment and endodontic surgery: a systematic review. *Journal of Endodontics* 35: 930–937.

Vozza, I., Barone, A., Quaranta, M. et al. (2011). A comparison between endodontics and implantology: an 8-year retrospective study. *Clinical Implant Dentistry and Related Research* 15: 29–36.

5.3 *Endodontic Microsurgery*

Elizabeth Shin Perry

Objectives

Endodontic microsurgery describes minimally invasive surgical procedures that address non-resolving endodontic pathology when non-surgical root canal therapy has been adequately performed.

Modern endodontic microsurgical techniques involve the use of a surgical operating microscope and specialised microsurgical instruments, together with contemporary root end filling materials, to result in a more precise and predictable outcome than traditional surgical techniques.

At the end of this case, the reader should understand the principles of endodontic microsurgical procedures and identify clinical situations in which these procedures would be appropriate.

Introduction

A 52-year-old male presents with a history of swelling and pain to pressure above his upper left central incisor.

Chief Complaint

The patient presented with the chief complaint '15 years ago I fell and hit my front teeth and they were messed up since then'. He reports that one month previously, he had swelling and pain above the upper left central incisor. His dentist prescribed a course of antibiotics, and he has been comfortable ever since.

The Medical History

The patient had a history of controlled hypertension, diabetes and joint prostheses of both hips.

Pitt Ford's Problem-Based Learning in Endodontology, Second Edition. Edited by Elizabeth Shin Perry, Shanon Patel, Shalini Kanagasingam, and Samantha Hamer.
© 2025 John Wiley & Sons Ltd. Published 2025 by John Wiley & Sons Ltd.

Dental History

The patient received routine dental care from his general dentist and no significant issues were reported.

Clinical Examination

Extraoral examination was unremarkable. Intraoral examination revealed tenderness to palpation in the anterior buccal sulcus over tooth UL1. The tooth was tender to percussion, but exhibited no mobility and was non-responsive to pulp sensibility testing. No evidence of caries, prior restorations or fractures was seen. Periodontal probing depths were within normal limits. All adjacent teeth exhibited no tenderness to percussion or palpation and tested within normal limits to pulp sensibility testing.

What do the periapical radiographs reveal?

A periapical radiographs of tooth UL1 revealed an 8.5 × 10.5 mm well-defined, periapical radiolucency. The apical lesion was seen to extend towards, but did not encompass, the apex of tooth UL2 (Figure 5.3.1a, b).

Diagnosis and Treatment Planning

Diagnosis of tooth UL1 was pulpal necrosis with symptomatic apical periodontitis.

Treatment options discussed with the patient were:

- Non-surgical root canal therapy
- Extraction
- No treatment (not advisable)

The patient was interested in saving the tooth and consented to non-surgical root canal treatment.

Treatment

Non-surgical root canal therapy of tooth UL1 was initiated. Local anaesthetic was delivered and the tooth was isolated with a dental dam. The canal was accessed and the pulp chamber and access opening were examined with the surgical operating microscope for any evidence of cracks, fractures or other compromise. As no compromise of the tooth structure was seen, the canal was debrided and disinfected. The canal was dried and calcium hydroxide was placed. The access opening was sealed with a temporary restoration.

The patient returned in two weeks and reported that his symptoms had subsided. The calcium hydroxide was removed and root canal treatment was completed (Figure 5.3.1c).

One year later, the patient returned to report that his symptoms had returned. Radiographic examination with periapical radiographs revealed that a 6.9×8.2 mm apical radiolucency persisted (Figure 5.3.2a).

Further imaging with cone beam computed tomography (CBCT) revealed a $8 \times 9 \times 7$ mm apical radiolucency with perforation of the buccal cortical plate associated with tooth UL1 (Figure 5.3.2b).

Why is cone beam computed tomography imaging important to assess a tooth that has continued symptoms after non-surgical root canal therapy has been completed?

The use of CBCT has allowed the practitioner to identify factors that directly influence treatment planning decisions. These factors include but are not limited to inadequate obturation of the root canal, untreated root canal anatomy, root fractures, perforations, separated endodontic instruments, over-extended root canal filling, resorption and periodontal compromise. As further treatment options include non-surgical or surgical endodontic treatment versus extraction, CBCT is an important addition for accurate diagnosis and treatment planning. If additional therapy includes a surgical approach, CBCT is indispensable for pre-surgical treatment planning. The three-dimensional imaging allows the practitioner to visualise root anatomy as it relates to the surrounding anatomical structures and landmarks. In addition, CBCT allows for localisation of the extent of the periapical pathology, which is important to plan for the surgical incision and access during the surgery.

What are the reasons for persistent endodontic pathology after non-surgical endodontic treatment?

- Intraradicular infection.
- Extraradicular infection.
  - Bacterial plaque on the apical root surface.
  - Bacteria within the apical lesion such as *Actinomyces*.
- Extruded root canal filling or other exogenous materials causing a foreign body reaction.
- Accumulation of endogenous materials such as cholesterol crystals that cause irritation of periapical tissues.
- True cystic lesions.

Table 5.3.1 Reasons for persistent endodontic pathology.

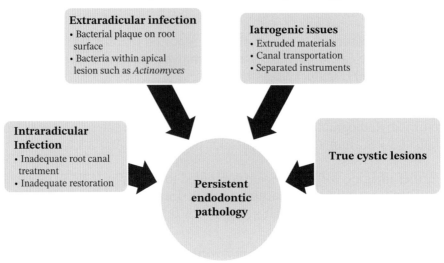

It is clear from the endodontic literature that the main cause of non-resolution of endodontic pathology after non-surgical endodontic treatment is persistent intraradicular infection. Clinical or radiographic examination does not allow the practitioner to differentiate the reason for the non-resolution of the pathology.

What are the treatment options for a tooth with persistent endodontic pathology after root canal therapy has been completed?

- Non-surgical retreatment of the root canal
- Endodontic microsurgery
- No treatment
- Extraction

Retreatment of the root canal should be considered as the first treatment of choice when possible. However, there are situations in which retreatment is not possible or advisable due to the presence of large posts or obstructions within the root canal, suspected longitudinal root fractures or individual patient concerns.

Additionally, if the non-surgical treatment has been carried out using a strict aseptic technique and to a high standard, the CBCT reveals no other reasons for compromise and apical pathology persists, orthograde retreatment does not guarantee elimination of the residual infection. In such cases, surgical intervention may be considered. Surgical management of these cases allows for the removal of any extraradicular elements preventing resolution of the pathology. In addition, a surgical approach allows for resection of the root apex and retrograde access to eliminate any potential infection in the apical portion of the root canal system.

Table 5.3.2 Indications and contraindications for microsurgery.

Endodontic Microsurgery	
Indications	**Contraindications**
• Continued symptoms of swelling or sinus tract after quality endodontic treatment and restoration done with strict asepsis • Complications from unsuccessful endodontic treatment such as blocked or transported canals • Large post or restoration in root canal that will compromise the structural integrity of the root if removal is attempted	• Poor-quality endodontic treatment that can be improved • Poor-quality restoration or caries causing contamination of the root canal system • Anatomical location in the arch making surgical approach difficult • Significant periodontal compromise or unfavorable crown to root ratio • Patient on IV Bisphosphonates or IV Antiangiogenics

Indications and contraindications for endodontic microsurgery are outlined in Table 5.3.2.

Endodontic microsurgery was recommended to the patient. The procedure was discussed in detail, risks and benefits were reviewed and he consented to treatment.

Endodontic microsurgery was performed with the aid of a surgical operating microscope. A submarginal (Ochsenbein-Luebke) flap was raised to expose the defect (Figure 5.3.3a). The entire apical lesion was curetted out in toto and sent for biopsy. Then 3 mm of the root end was resected with a surgical high-speed handpiece (Figure 5.3.3b, c) and retrograde preparation was performed using ultrasonic instrumentation to a depth of 3 mm (Figure 5.3.4a, b). A retrograde bioceramic paste and putty were placed using microsurgical pluggers (Figure 5.3.4c, d). A periapical radiograph was taken to confirm the quality of the retrograde fill (Figure 5.3.5a). The flap was repositioned and 6×0 monofilament sutures were placed. Saline-moistened gauze was placed directly on the repositioned flap and gentle pressure was applied for several minutes to aid in healing and stabilisation of the flap.

The patient returned two days later for removal of the sutures. At that time, the soft tissue healing was progressing well and the patient was comfortable. The pathology report identified the area of pathology to be a periapical cyst. The patient returned at four weeks and the soft tissues were seen to have healed completely with no residual scar visible (Figure 5.3.5b).

Follow-up visit at nine months revealed the apical lesion to have significantly decreased in size (Figure 5.3.6a). Two year follow-up with periapical radiograph and CBCT revealed complete resolution of the apical lesion (Figure 5.3.6b, c)

Would a bone graft have been beneficial in this case?

In cases that involve endodontic pathology limited to the periapex, as in this case, evidence confirms that placement of bone graft and membrane materials provides little or no benefit to the elimination of disease and healing of the apical pathology. In addition, placement of radiopaque bone grafting materials makes radiographic interpretation of the periapical lesions difficult. However, endodontic lesions that erode both the buccal and lingual cortical plates ('through and through') or apico-marginal lesions that involve lateral periodontal loss of bone have been shown to benefit from the adjunctive treatment with bone graft and membrane materials. Also, in situations where the preservation of thickness of bone in the cortical plate is desired, for instance for possible implant placement in the future, placement of a bone graft and membrane may be warranted.

What medications are recommended after endodontic microsurgery?

Endodontic microsurgery is a minimally invasive procedure that, when done correctly, requires minimal post-operative medications. A non-steroidal anti-inflammatory is generally adequate for post-operative discomfort and inflammation. A chlorhexidine mouth rinse beginning the day after surgery has been shown to be effective in reducing biofilm formation and gingival inflammation when the patient's oral hygiene ability is compromised.

Studies have shown that supplemental antibiotics following adequate drainage and debridement in cases of localised endodontic infections are ineffective. Thus, the use of antibiotics is typically not indicated after endodontic microsurgery and should be avoided. Additional medications such as narcotic pain medications and corticosteroids are generally not necessary and should be avoided as well.

Discussion

Endodontic microsurgery is a valuable option for treatment of persistent endodontic pathology. Consideration of each individual case, along with accurate diagnosis, careful treatment planning and follow-up, is important to determine the best course of treatment for the patient (Table 5.3.3). It is important to prepare the patient for all possibilities, including the need for surgical intervention if an area of pathology does not respond to non-surgical treatment. In this case, endodontic microsurgery was recommended for the persistent pathology due to the large size of the lesion, history of trauma 15 years previously, known details of the initial endodontic treatment and the patient's medical history.

Table 5.3.3 Considerations prior to undertaking endodontic microsurgery.

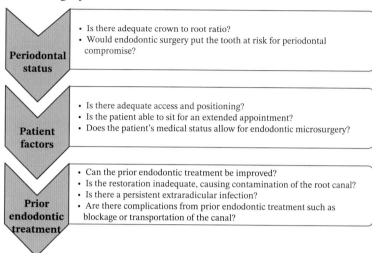

Periodontal status	• Is there adequate crown to root ratio? • Would endodontic surgery put the tooth at risk for periodontal compromise?
Patient factors	• Is there adequate access and positioning? • Is the patient able to sit for an extended appointment? • Does the patient's medical status allow for endodontic microsurgery?
Prior endodontic treatment	• Can the prior endodontic treatment be improved? • Is the restoration inadequate, causing contamination of the root canal? • Is there a persistent extraradicular infection? • Are there complications from prior endodontic treatment such as blockage or transportation of the canal?

In endodontics, microsurgical techniques have revolutionised the procedures used to treat persistent apical pathology after non-surgical treatment of the root canal has been performed. A microsurgical approach to endodontic surgery involves the magnification and illumination of a surgical operating microscope combined with microsurgical instruments and contemporary biocompatible root end filling materials to allow for a more predictable outcome (Table 5.3.4).

Table 5.3.4 Comparison of microsurgery and conventional endodontic surgery techniques.

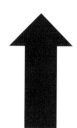

Microsurgery
• Minimal to no bevel
• Small osteotomy
• Minimal compromise of buccal cortex
• Decreased risk of periodontal compromise
• Increased accuracy of canal identification

Conventional endodontic surgery
• Acute bevel (45–60 degrees)
• Large osteotomy
• Greater compromise of buccal cortex
• Increased risk of periodontal communication
• Inability to visualize and locate canals

Microsurgical techniques are specifically tailored to the precise nature of the procedure and allow for an atraumatic and conservative approach to access and treatment of the root end, thus allowing for a more comfortable patient experience and enhanced healing. Endodontic literature has shown that microsurgical techniques result in more predictable and successful outcomes and have been shown to be more successful than traditional root end surgical techniques. Endodontic microsurgery is a valuable adjunct to the practitioner's skillset to enhance the long-term success of modern-day endodontic procedures.

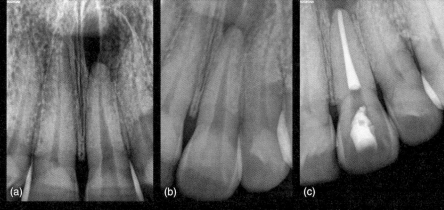

Figure 5.3.1 (a, b) Pre-operative radiographs. (c) Post-operative radiograph following root canal therapy.

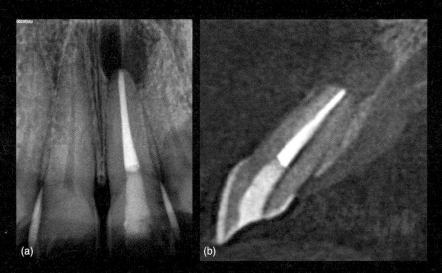

Figure 5.3.2 (a) One-year follow-up with persistent apical pathology. (b) One-year follow-up cone beam computed tomography shows an apical radiolucency with perforation of the buccal cortical plate.

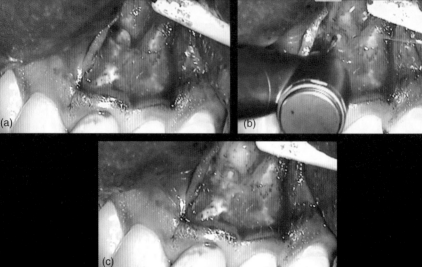

Figure 5.3.3 (a) Root end exposure after apical curettage. (b) Apical resection. (c) Resected root end.

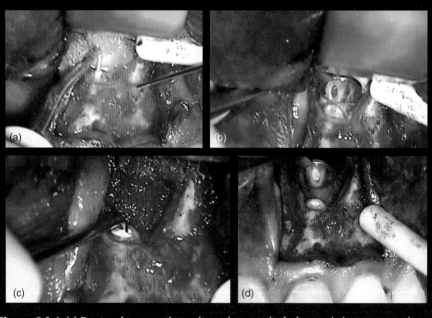

Figure 5.3.4 (a) Root end preparation using microsurgical ultrasonic instrumentation. (b) Inspection of root end preparation with microsurgical mirror. (c) Placement of bioceramic root end filling with microsurgical plugger. (d) Inspection of final root end filling with microsurgical mirror.

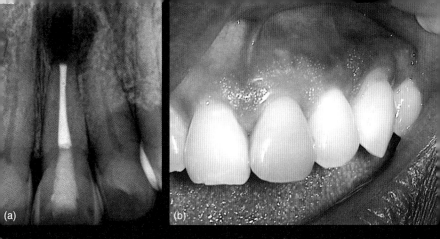

Figure 5.3.5 (a) Post-surgery radiograph. (b) Four-week follow-up; note the minimal scarring of the soft tissue.

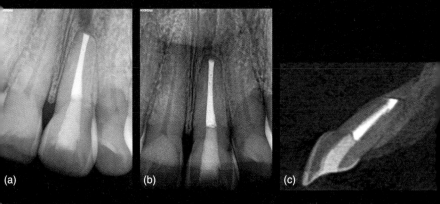

Figure 5.3.6 (a) Nine-month follow-up radiograph, showing significant resolution of the apical lesion. (b) One year follow-up radiograph shows complete resolution of the apical lesion. (c) Two-year follow-up cone beam computed tomography shows complete resolution of the apical lesion and the reestablishment of the buccal cortical plate over the apex of the tooth.

Further Reading

American Association of Endodontists (2017). AAE guidance on the use of systemic antibiotics in endodontics. Chicago, IL: AAE. https://www.aae.org/specialty/wp-content/uploads/sites/2/2017/06/aae_systemic-antibiotics.pdf.

Kim, S., Kratchman, S., Karabucak, B., and Kohli, M. (2017). Microsurgery in Endodontics. Wiley-Blackwell.

Kim, S., Pecora, G., and Rubinstein, R. (2000). *Color Atlas of Microsurgery in Endodontics*. St. Louis, MO: W.B. Saunders.

Royal College of Surgeons of England, Faculty of Dental Surgery (2023). Clinical Guidelines. London: FDS. https://www.rcseng.ac.uk/dental-faculties/fds/publications-guidelines/clinical-guidelines.

Setzer, F.C., Shah, S.B., Kohli, R.K. et al. (2010). Outcome of endodontic surgery: a meta-analysis of the literature – Part 1: Comparison of traditional root-end surgery and endodontic microsurgery. *Journal of Endodontics* 36: 1757–1765.

Torabinejad, M., Corr, R., Handysides, R., and Shabahang, S. (2009). Outcomes of nonsurgical retreatment and endodontic surgery: a systematic review. *Journal of Endodontics* 35 (7): 930–937.

5.4 Non-surgical Management of Perforation

Taranpreet Puri

Objectives

At the end of this case, the reader should understand the causes and management of an iatrogenic perforation. The reader should also appreciate the factors that influence prognosis of perforations, as well as knowledge of current materials used in perforation repairs.

Introduction

A female, 26 years old, was referred by her general dental practitioner regarding the lower right first molar (LR6). Root canal treatment had been initiated on this tooth three months previously.

Chief Complaint

The patient was asymptomatic on presentation.

Medical History

Unremarkable.

Dental History

Regular dental attendance, historical high caries risk status. The LR6 had been severely painful, with spontaneous throbbing pain. The symptoms resolved following emergency dental treatment three months before.

Clinical Examination

Extraoral examination was unremarkable.

Pitt Ford's Problem-Based Learning in Endodontology, Second Edition. Edited by Elizabeth Shin Perry, Shanon Patel, Shalini Kanagasingam, and Samantha Hamer.
© 2025 John Wiley & Sons Ltd. Published 2025 by John Wiley & Sons Ltd.

Intraoral examination revealed a moderately restored dentition with satisfactory oral hygiene.

The LR6 was firm with slight tenderness on percussion and no swelling or tenderness in the buccal sulcus. The tooth had an existing glass ionomer restoration, with signs of secondary caries and marginal defects. There were no periodontal probing depths greater than 2 mm and the tooth was unresponsive to sensibility testing (Figure 5.4.1).

What were the radiological findings?

A periapical radiograph of the LR6 revealed (Figure 5.4.2):

- Good bone levels.
- The LR5 had a disto-occlusal restoration with good marginal adaptation and existing root canal filling, terminating short of the radiographic apex, with an intact and uniform periodontal ligament.
- The LR6 had a disto-occlusal restoration extending into the pulp chamber, with straight mesial and distal roots with visible root canals. There was a perforation in the furcation of the pulp chamber floor with furcal radiolucency. Apical radiolucency was associated with the mesial and distal roots.
- The LR7 had mesial caries.

In order to aid in investigation and treatment planning, cone beam computed tomography (CBCT) imaging (Figure 5.4.3) was performed, which highlighted the precise location, extent and size of the perforation, as well as the presence of an additional distal canal.

Diagnosis and Treatment Planning

Diagnosis

The diagnosis for the LR6 was symptomatic apical periodontitis associated with a necrotic pulp and iatrogenic furcal perforation.

What were the treatment options?

LR6 chronic apical periodontitis associated with a necrotic pulp and perforation:

- Non-surgical perforation repair and root canal treatment with cuspal coverage restoration.
- Extraction with or without prosthetic replacement.
- Leave alone.

LR5 technical deficiencies in root canal filling with no associated apical pathology:

- Monitor with annual periapical radiograph.
- Review need for root canal retreatment if cuspal coverage restoration required.

LR7 mesial enamel lesion:

- Advise patient on diet, fluoride and oral hygiene. Regular monitoring with bitewing radiographs.
- Restoration.

Treatment Plan

Following discussion with the patient, she was keen to save the tooth in question. It was decided to perform non-surgical root canal treatment of the LR6 with internal repair of the perforation followed by cuspal coverage restoration.

What are the general considerations prior to commencing treatment in cases of preexisting perforations?

- Knowledge of prognosis of perforation repairs, to manage the patient's expectations and predict likelihood of success.
- Staged and logical planning of treatment in order to minimise the potential risk of accidental irrigant extrusion.
- Appreciation of materials available and their handling properties.
- Planning and designing the definitive restoration of the endodontically treated tooth in the short and long term.

Treatment was performed over two visits. In the first visit, the tooth was isolated with dental dam and the existing restoration was removed to assess restorability and the perforation site. A pre-endodontic composite build-up was performed. Careful irrigation was initially carried out with saline, to reduce the risk of extrusion. A cotton pledget soaked in hypochlorite was then used to disinfect the perforation site and allow haemostasis (Figure 5.4.4a). The canals were located and protected with paper points. The perforation was repaired with a calcium silicate cement and protected with a cover of glass ionomer restoration (Figure 5.4.4b). This was to enable the preparation of the canals and further use of irrigation solutions without compromising the perforation seal. Once canals were fully prepared and disinfected with hypochlorite, the tooth was stabilised with a composite restoration, and occlusal access was preserved with glass ionomer for subsequent visits.

At a subsequent visit the root canal treatment was completed (Figure 5.4.5a). A composite core was placed in preparation for a full cuspal coverage restoration (Figure 5.4.5b).

The tooth was later restored with a full-coverage crown. The patient was reviewed 12 months following treatment (Figure 5.4.6). The tooth was asymptomatic and fully retained in function. Clinical examination showed that the tooth was not tender to percussion or palpation, and there were no probing depths greater than 2 mm.

How are perforations diagnosed? What are the clinical and radiographic signs?

Clinical signs:

- Patient may feel pain during treatment.
- Bleeding (may or may not be uncontrollable) from perforation site.
- Erroneous and conflicted readings on electronic apex locator, zero reading when file is clearly not at the estimated working length.
- Periodontal pocket at perforation site, more than 4 mm isolated probing depth.

Radiographic signs:

- Radiolucency at the site of perforation (chronic and delayed presentation).
- Clear deviation from the original path of the canal.
- Diagnostic radiograph with file at the length and site of suspected perforation.

What materials are used to repair perforations?

Current literature supports the use of calcium silicate cements as the ideal materials of choice for internal perforation repairs.

Calcium silicate cements such as Biodentine® (Septodont, New Castle, DE, USA), BC putty (Brasseler USA, Savannah, GA, USA) or Well-Root™ putty (Vericom, Knoxville, TN, USA) have been advocated over mineral trioxide aggregate (MTA) due to the faster setting time compared with MTA. This allows for obturation ideally in the same visit as the repair, which can reduce risk of bacterial contamination. Another advantage of is the reduced risk of discoloration, which is particularly relevant in management of crestal and coronal perforations in anterior teeth.

One disadvantage of Biodentine is that the radiopacity is similar to dentine, therefore it is harder to see evidence of repair radiographically. Also, limited evidence and a lack of long-term studies exist in the literature in relation to the use of Biodentine and other calcium silicate cements specifically for perforation repairs in comparison to MTA.

Alternative materials available are intermediate restorative material (IRM), glass ionomer cement or composite, depending on the clinical situation and approach for the repair (surgical exposure). Glass ionomer–based materials are prone to leakage and therefore are least desirable for use in perforation repairs due to suboptimal sealing ability and lack of long-term stability.

Discussion

Perforations are severe complications in endodontic treatment and can reduce the odds of success of root canal treatment by 56%. The site of perforation can impact prognosis, with crestal and coronal perforations having the highest risk of failure due to pocket formation, which serves as a point of communication from the oral environment. Immediate repair and single-visit root canal treatment are ideal in the management of perforations. Delayed presentation of perforations, along with radiographic signs of associated pathology, and perforations larger than 3mm have poorer success rates.

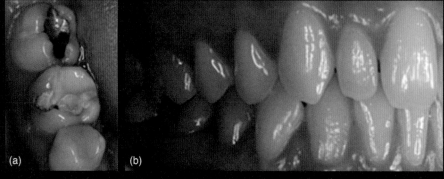

Figure 5.4.1 (a) Occlusal view of the LR6. (b) Buccal view of the LR6.

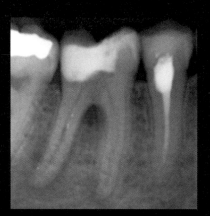

Figure 5.4.2 Pre-operative radiograph of the LR6.

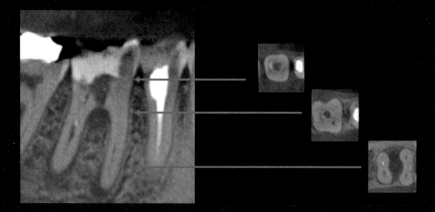

Figure 5.4.3 Cone beam computed tomography: sagittal view of the LR6 and corresponding axial views, showing furcal perforation and two canals in the distal root.

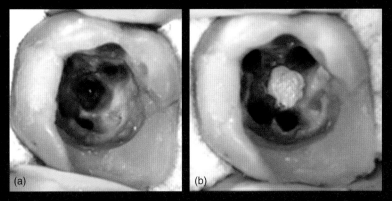

Figure 5.4.4 (a) Furcation perforation site exposed following identification and mild flaring of canals, as well as the pre-endodontic composite build-up. (b) Perforation repair with calcium silicate cement (Biodentine) and glass ionomer cement covering the site is shown. Subsequently the canals were fully prepared.

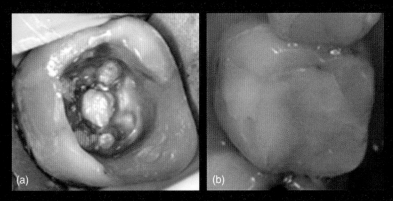

Figure 5.4.5 (a) Obturation of canals. (b) Postoperative composite core.

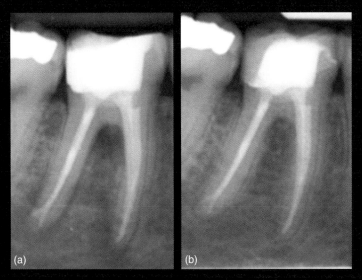

Figure 5.4.6 Periapical radiographs: (a) post treatment; (b) 12 months following treatment.

Further Reading

Clauder, T. (2022). Present status and future directions – managing perforations. *International Endodontic Journal* 55 (S4): 872–891.

Gorni, F., Andreano, A., Ambrogi, F. et al. (2016). Patient and clinical characteristics associated with primary healing of iatrogenic perforations after root canal treatment: results of a long-term Italian study. *Journal of Endodontics* 42 (2): 211–215.

Krupp, C., Bargholz, C., Brusehaber, M., and Hulsmann, M. (2013). Treatment outcome after repair of root perforations with mineral trioxide aggregate: a retrospective evaluation of 90 teeth. *Journal of Endodontics* 39 (11): 1364–1368.

Ng, Y.L., Mann, V., and Gulabivala, K. (2011). A prospective study of the factors affecting outcomes of nonsurgical root canal treatment: part 1: periapical health. *International Endodontic Journal* 44 (7): 583–609.

Pontius, V., Pontius, O., Braun, A. et al. (2013). Retrospective evaluation of perforation repairs in 6 private practices. *Journal of Endodontics* 39 (11): 1346–1358.

5.5 *Inadvertent Extrusion*

Samantha Hamer and Shalini Kanagasingam

Objectives

At the end of this case, the reader should be able to identify the signs and symptoms associated with inadvertent extrusion of endodontic materials beyond the confines of the root canal. The reader should be aware of the management strategies and appreciate the measures that can be taken to prevent the occurrence of extrusion accidents.

Introduction

A 53-year-old female patient presented complaining of acute pain, facial swelling and mucosal ulceration. The patient had been referred by her general practitioner, who had seen her the previous day for root canal treatment of the upper right canine (UR3). During the irrigation procedure, the patient experienced sudden severe pain. The referring dentist provided additional local anaesthetic, provisionally restored the tooth and prescribed analgesics.

Chief Complaint

The patient complained of a constant dull ache associated with the upper right quadrant since the endodontic procedure. She was also very distressed by the facial swelling and bruising she experienced, which was still present after 24 hours.

Medical History

Unremarkable.

Dental History

Regular attender and has had restorations replaced recently.

Pitt Ford's Problem-Based Learning in Endodontology, Second Edition. Edited by Elizabeth Shin Perry, Shanon Patel, Shalini Kanagasingam, and Samantha Hamer. © 2025 John Wiley & Sons Ltd. Published 2025 by John Wiley & Sons Ltd.

Clinical Examination

Extraoral examination revealed moderate swelling and bruising over the right cheek with loss of the right nasolabial fold (Figure 5.5.1a). This area was found to be slightly tender to palpation. Intraoral examination revealed a moderately restored dentition. An access cavity on the palatal aspect of the UR3 had been restored with glass ionomer cement. A 12 mm × 3 mm ulcer was noted on the labial mucosa, apical to the UR3 (Figure 5.5.1b).

Tooth UR3 was tender to percussion. There was no loss of motor or sensory function of the surrounding tissues in the upper right quadrant. A periapical radiograph revealed a UR3 with a single canal and a periapical lesion. There were no signs of perforation of the root or root resorption. The tooth had a closed root apex and there was no sign of excessive apical preparation.

Diagnosis and Treatment Planning

A diagnosis of previously initiated therapy and symptomatic apical periodontitis was reached for the UR3. A sodium hypochlorite extrusion incident occurred during the previous canal instrumentation procedure.

The anticipated short-term and long-term sequelae of the sodium hypochlorite extrusion (including further swelling, bruising, paraesthesia and scarring) were explained to the patient. She received advice on pain management, use of warm compress, warm saline rinses and reassurance that her symptoms would be expected to subside after a week and may take up to a month to completely resolve. Rarely, some patients may have sensory or motor impairment after one year. Due to the presence of the ulceration, the patient was referred to an Oral and Maxillofacial (OMFS) unit.

The treatment options for tooth UR3 were discussed with the patient:

- No treatment
- Continuation of root canal treatment followed by definitive restoration
- Extraction

What are the consequences of sodium hypochlorite (NaOCl) extrusion?

The antibacterial properties and organic tissue-dissolving capacity of sodium hypochlorite make it a highly effective root canal irrigant. However, it is also cytotoxic and caustic. If it is extruded into the periapical vital tissues, it will cause oxidation of the surrounding tissues, leading to haemolysis, ulceration and damage to endothelial and fibroblast cells and inhibition of neutrophil migration.

Patients' initial symptoms include:

- Sudden onset of severe pain (despite presence of local anaesthetic).
- Profuse haemorrhage in the root canal.
- Swelling.
- Burning pain in the throat or sinus (if extrusion involves the maxillary sinus). The accessed tooth will present with little or no bleeding from the canal and there are usually no signs of immediate swelling. The patient may experience sinus congestion and nasal bleeding.

Subsequent symptoms may include the following:

- Haemolysis leading to interstitial bleeding (haematoma).
- Mucosal necrosis.
- Neurological signs (paraesthesia).
- Trismus.
- Swallowing difficulties/airway distress.

How can the severity of the injury be assessed and what is the optimal management?

The management of NaOCl extrusion is based on the severity of the tissue injuries. Figure 5.5.2 highlights the relevant management strategies. Reassuring the patient and daily contact are important to monitor changes in the patient's condition and provide reassurance.

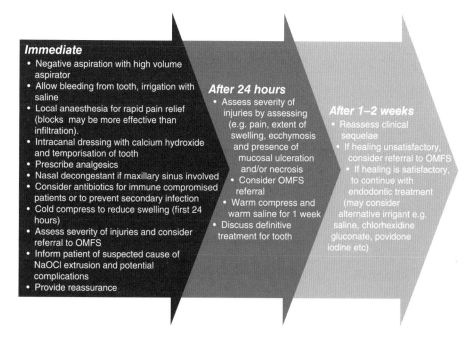

Immediate
- Negative aspiration with high volume aspirator
- Allow bleeding from tooth, irrigation with saline
- Local anaesthesia for rapid pain relief (blocks may be more effective than infiltration).
- Intracanal dressing with calcium hydroxide and temporisation of tooth
- Prescribe analgesics
- Nasal decongestant if maxillary sinus involved
- Consider antibiotics for immune compromised patients or to prevent secondary infection
- Cold compress to reduce swelling (first 24 hours)
- Assess severity of injuries and consider referral to OMFS
- Inform patient of suspected cause of NaOCl extrusion and potential complications
- Provide reassurance

After 24 hours
- Assess severity of injuries by assessing (e.g. pain, extent of swelling, ecchymosis and presence of mucosal ulceration and/or necrosis
- Consider OMFS referral
- Warm compress and warm saline for 1 week
- Discuss definitive treatment for tooth

After 1–2 weeks
- Reassess clinical sequelae
- If healing unsatisfactory, consider referral to OMFS
- If healing is satisfactory, to continue with endodontic treatment (may consider alternative irrigant e.g. saline, chlorhexidine gluconate, povidone iodine etc)

Figure 5.5.2 Guidance on the important management strategies for NaOCl extrusion.

Mild injuries are indicated by the patient complaining of a relatively low degree of pain localised to the tooth undergoing endodontic treatment. The presence of swelling would be less than 30% compared to the contralateral side with localised ecchymosis. These injuries will be suitable to be managed by a general dentist or endodontist.

Moderate to severe injuries will involve a more intense inflammatory reaction, resulting in diffuse ecchymosis and larger swelling. Mucosal ulceration may occur adjacent to the tooth being treated. Neurovascular deficits may be noted and oedema can compromise the patient's airway. More severe injuries will require referral to hospital (Oral Maxillofacial Deparment).

Treatment

The patient was reviewed after two days; the swelling and bruising were still present. Ecchymosis was noted on the patient's right infraorbital region. The patient mentioned that the tooth was not as tender on biting. Intraorally, tissue sloughing was observed at the site of the ulceration. At the one-week review, the patient had a reduced right cheek swelling. The intraoral ulceration had healed. Facial symmetry was noted after three weeks (Figure 5.5.1c–f). The patient decided to complete the root canal treatment of the UR3. This was carried out, followed by the definitive restoration.

Disussion

What are the consequences of extrusion of other endodontic materials?

There have been case reports of the damaging effects of other endodontic materials such as medicaments and sealers on the tissues surrounding the root apex, including extrusion into nerves, arteries and the sinus. Root apices can be in close proximity to the mental foramen or inferior dental canal. Pathways of spread to the periapical region include drainage through lymphatic vessels, systemic dispersion via the periapical vein and spreading towards soft tissues between bone and mucosal membrane. Extruded irrigants, endodontic files and materials affecting the neurovascular bundle could result in permanent paraesthesia.

Paraesthesia can be caused by several mechanisms:

- *Mechanical*: damage caused by over-instrumentation or severing a nerve during surgery, or compression from extruded materials.
- *Pathological*: compression of a nerve from periapical swelling or microbes diffusing through the marrow space.
- *Physical*: excess heat from insufficient cooling of drills, ultrasonics or prolonged use of thermoplastic obturation techniques.

- *Chemical*: from local anaesthetics, endodontic sealers or irrigants.
- *Microbiological*: from extraradicular infections or aspergillosis.

Endodontic Sealer Extrusion

Aspergillosis is a fungal infection associated with over-extension of root fillings in antral teeth, which can trigger unilateral chronic sinusitis, especially in immunocompromised patients. It is frequently seen in with zinc oxide eugenol–based sealers, which have a characteristic appearance of radiopaque foreign body material in a homogenously clouded maxillary sinus, as seen in panoramic radiographs and cone beam computed tomography (CBCT) scans. Patients may have a history of nasal obstruction post endodontic treatment.

Despite the known biocompatibility of bioceramic sealer, its extrusion has been reported to cause persistent prolonged paraesthesia, affecting temperature sensation. Patients have reported the detriment to their quality of life as the paraesthesia was affecting drinking, eating, kissing, brushing teeth and applying makeup.

Calcium Hydroxide Extrusion

Calcium hydroxide is a widely used and effective antibacterial intracanal medicament, due to its high pH and destructive effects on bacterial cell walls and protein structures. It has been noted that calcium hydroxide creates a favourable environment for periapical healing and osseous repair. However, if it is extruded there have been case reports of deleterious effects:

- Extrusion into surrounding soft tissues leading to localised mucosal necrosis.
- Extrusion into the external carotid artery leading to necrosis of the ear lobe and skin over the cheek.
- Extrusion into the inferior alveolar nerve leading to paraesthesia.

Extrusion is more likely with pre-mixed injectable calcium hydroxide. Nonetheless, accurate placement can be achieved with the use of a rubber stopper and pre-measuring the needle at least 2mm short of working length. Calcium hydroxide can also be placed using Lentulo spiral fillers or hand files.

Management of Extrusion of Endodontic Material and Sealers

In a systematic review of 84 cases of altered sensation following extrusion of root canal filling materials, 53% made a full recovery, 38% a partial recovery and 9% had persistent altered sensation. These varied in severity, with some having permanent disability with a significant effect on their quality of life. Mandibular second molars (72%) was the most common tooth, followed by mandibular second premolars (19%). In cases involving mandibular premolars, 83% of patients fully recovered, whereas in cases involving mandibular molars only 33% of patients fully recovered. In one study, eight patients had extrusion of sealer into the inferior alveolar canal but suffered no alteration in sensation.

There is limited evidence on how to manage these cases. In the review, 77% of cases were managed with surgical or combined surgical and non-surgical treatment, with 46% making a full recovery; 24% of the cases were managed with a non-surgical treatment, with 63% making a full recovery. This is based on low-level evidence, but early intervention was advised to prevent or minimise long-term damage.

Non-surgical treatment

There is no consensus on the management of extrusion and proposed treatment varies from conservative monitoring (Figure 5.5.3) to invasive sagittal split osteotomy surgical intervention. Non-surgical options include:

- Monitoring and follow-up.
- Anti-inflammatory medication (e.g. ibuprofen, diclofenac).
- Steroids (e.g. prednisolone).
- Anticonvulsants (e.g. pregabalin).
- B vitamin supplements and adenosine triphosphate.

Surgical treatment

Nine patients were observed with pre-mixed injectable non-setting calcium hydroxide extruded into the inferior alveolar nerve. The mean time from nerve injury to surgery was 61.6 days (9–152 days). The surgical procedures performed included foreign removal and microsurgical external and internal decompression via decortication of small bony window or sagittal split osteotomy. Recovery was observed in the early and late surgical intervention cases; however, it was noted that recovery was less likely with extensive nerve injury. Surgical intervention cannot resolve all nerve injuries and the procedure also carries the risk of causing secondary nerve injury.

What measures can be taken to minimise the risk of extrusion of endodontic materials?

- Pre-operative assessment:
  - Anticipate potential risk factors, open apices, existing perforations, root fractures or root resorption.
  - Check proximity to adjacent structures, such as the maxillary sinus, mental foramen or inferior dental canal. Pre-operative CBCT should be used when possible.
- Accurate depth of insertion of syringe (keeping at least 2 mm from working length when dispensing irrigant, medicament and sealer).

- Safe irrigation technique including preventing wedging of the irrigation syringe in the canal, keeping the syringe constantly moving during irrigation, use of a side-venting irrigation needle and avoiding forceful injecting of irrigant by using the index finger instead of the thumb.
- Accurate working length determination and instrumentation.

Conclusion

Meticulous pre-assessment and maintenance of working length in all root canals are essential for the prevention of extrusion of endodontic materials. Should inadvertent extrusion occur, prompt recognition and diagnosis are essential to facilitate effective management. This chapter has highlighted more severe forms of extrusion of materials and consequences. Most cases of slight extrusion of obturation materials such as endodontic sealers are well tolerated and would be resorbed over time. Studies have reported lower healing rates in cases with extruded gutta percha material compared to those which were obturated within 2mm of the radiographic apex. However, slight extrusion of gutta percha may not cause significant symptoms. It may be prudent to monitor these cases more closely. From a medico-legal point of view, the clinician must clearly communicate the risks and potential complications to the patient. Accurate contemporaneous records of all patient safety incidents are essential, with subsequent reporting to the relevant national authority.

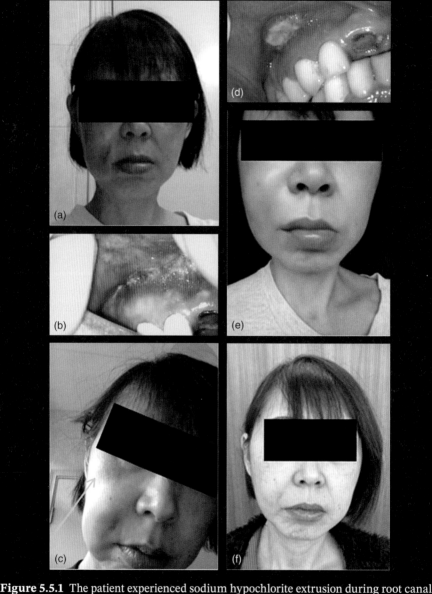

Figure 5.5.1 The patient experienced sodium hypochlorite extrusion during root canal treatment of the UR3. (a) Within 24 hours of the incident diffuse swelling and bruising on her right cheek had developed with loss of the nasolabial fold. (b) An ulcer was noted on the labial mucosa apical to the UR3. The patient was reviewed at 48 hours. (c) The swelling and bruising on her right cheek persisted and ecchymosis was also noted at the right infraorbital region (blue arrow). (d) Intraorally, tissue sloughing was observed at the site of the ulceration. (e) At one week post extrusion, the right cheek swelling had decreased. (f) At the three-week review, facial symmetry was noted. Source: Courtesy of Dr. J Rajan.

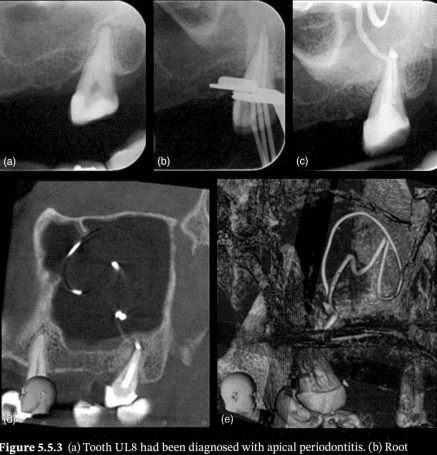

Figure 5.5.3 (a) Tooth UL8 had been diagnosed with apical periodontitis. (b) Root canal treatment was completed in a single visit. (c) Post-obturation radiograph revealed a significant amount of extruded thermo-plasticised gutta percha. (d, e) Cone beam computed tomography scan of the palatal root tip, which extended into the maxillary sinus and had been over-instrumented, which resulted in the overfill of gutta percha extending into the sinus cavity. The patient had no symptoms and was managed with conservative monitoring.

Further Reading

Alves, F.R.F., Dias, M.C.C., Mansa, M.G.C.B., and Machado, M.D. (2020). Permanent labiomandibular paraesthesia after bioceramic sealer extrusion: a case report. *Journal of Endodontics* 46: 301–306.

Bosch-Aranda, M.L., Canalda-Sahli, C., Figeiredo, R., and Gay-Escoda, C. (2012). Complications following an accidental sodium hypochlorite extrusion: a report of two cases. *Journal of Clinical and Experimental Dentistry* 4: 194–198.

Byun, S.H., Kim, S.S., Chung, H.J. et al. (2016). Surgical management of damaged inferior alveolar nerve caused by endodontic overfilling of calcium hydroxide paste. *International Endodontic Journal* 49: 1020–1029.

Farook, S.A., Shah, V., Lenouvel, D. et al. (2014). Guidelines for management of sodium hypochlorite extrusion injuries. *British Dental Journal* 217: 679–684.

Guivarc'h, M., Ordioni, U., Ahmed, H.M.A. et al. (2017). Sodium hypochlorite accident: a systematic review. *Journal of Endodontics* 43: 16–24.

Guivarc'h, M., Ordioni, U., Catherine, J.H. et al. (2015). Implications of endodontic-related sinus aspergillosis in a patient treated by infliximab: a case report. *Journal of Endodontics* 41: 125–129.

Kanagasingam, S. and Blum (2020). Sodium hypochlorite extrusion accidents: management and medico-legal considerations. *Primary Dental Journal* 9 (4): 59–63.

Lopez-Lopez, J., Estrugo-Devesa, A., Jane-Salas, E., and Segura-Egea, J.J. (2012). Inferior alveolar nerve injury resulting from overextension of an endodontic sealer: non-surgical management using the GABA analogue pregabalin. *International Endodontic Journal* 45: 98–104.

Rosen, E., Goldberger, T., Taschieri, S. et al. (2016). The prognosis of altered sensation after extrusion of root canal filing materials: a systematic review of the literature. *Journal of Endodontics* 42: 873–879.

5.6 *Intentional Reimplantation*

Rahul Bose and Bhavin Bhuva

Objectives

At the end of this case, the reader should appreciate when intentional reimplantation can be used as a valid treatment option and appreciate the procedural factors that will facilitate a favourable outcome.

Introduction

A 27-year-old male was referred by his general dental practitioner (GDP) for endodontic assessment and management of his upper right central incisor (UR1).

Chief Complaint

The patient complained of a severe, constant, dull throbbing ache localised to the UR1. A swelling subsequently developed in the region, which was managed with analgesics and antibiotics prescribed by the patient's GDP.

Medical History

Unremarkable.

Dental History

There was a history of dento-alveolar injury at the age of 12. The patient attended annually for dental check-up appointments and hygienist maintenance.

Pitt Ford's Problem-Based Learning in Endodontology, Second Edition. Edited by Elizabeth Shin Perry, Shanon Patel, Shalini Kanagasingam, and Samantha Hamer.
© 2025 John Wiley & Sons Ltd. Published 2025 by John Wiley & Sons Ltd.

Clinical Examination

Extraoral examination was unremarkable. The patient had an unrestored dentition and oral hygiene was good.

The UR1 was discoloured (Figure 5.6.1), tender to labial palpation and did not respond to electric or thermal sensibility testing. Both neighbouring teeth (UR2 and UL1) responded to sensibility testing. Periodontal probing depths were within normal limits and there was no associated mobility.

What did the radiographic examination reveal?

A periapical radiograph of the UR1 and UR2 (Figure 5.6.2) showed:

- Alveolar bone height within normal limits.
- UR1 had an intact crown with a subcrestal radiolucency on the mesial cervical aspect of the root; there was incomplete root development with an open apex and evidence of root blunting. A large periapical radiolucency extended from the mesial aspect of the UR1 to the mesial aspect of the UR3.
- UR2 had an intact crown with visible root canal, complete root development, and mature apex; there was an apical radiolucency extending from the mesial aspect of the UR1 to the mesial aspect of the UR3, encompassing the periapex of the UR2.

Cone beam computed tomography (CBCT) of the UR1 and UR2 (Figure 5.6.3) showed the following:

- The coronal view revealed that the UR1 had a subcrestal radiolucency on the mesial cervical margin of the root, with no pulpal communication, a visible root canal, open apex and large periapical radiolucency.
- The axial view demonstrated that the UR1 mesial radiolucency in the root did not extend into the root canal, and the buccal and palatal cortical plates were intact. There was partial loss of the outline of the incisive canal associated with the periapical radiolucency.
- The sagittal view showed that the UR1 had a wide-open apex, external root resorption at the apex and a large periapical radiolucency with an intact palatal cortical plate.

Diagnosis and Treatment Planning

What was the diagnosis?

Diagnosis for the UR1 was symptomatic apical periodontitis associated with an infected necrotic pulp and external cervical resorption (ECR).

ECR develops in the cervical region of a tooth, as a result of damage to, and/ or deficiency of, the subepithelial cementum. The aetiology is unknown, but some predisposing factors include trauma, parafunction, orthodontic treatment, periodontal treatment, dentoalveolar surgery, intracoronal bleaching, playing woodwind instruments, bisphosphonate therapy, varicella zoster virus infection and idiopathic causes. Early lesions can be asymptomatic and can sometimes appear clinically as a pink spot on the cervical margin. Early lesions are more often a chance radiographic finding. To assess the true extent of an ECR lesion, a CBCT scan is required. Lesions can then be classified using the Patel classification for ECR lesions (Table 5.6.1). The classification will help to formulate a treatment plan. This ECR lesion was classified as Patel 2Ap.

What were the treatment options?

- Orthograde root canal treatment followed by external repair and intentional reimplantation (IR).
- Surgical repair of ECR and orthograde root canal treatment.
- Root canal treatment and periodic review (no treatment of ECR).
- Extraction and replacement with single-tooth implant, resin-bonded bridge or removable partial denture.
- No treatment.

What are the possible consequences of not treating the tooth?

- Endodontic flare-up.
- Progression of the ECR lesion with possible perforation into the root canal.
- Fracture (decoronation) of the tooth due to the weakening effect of progressive resorption.

Table 5.6.1 Patel classification of external cervical resorption.

Height	Circumferential spread	Proximity to the root canal
1: At cemento-enamel junction level or coronal to the bone crest (supracrestal) **2:** Extends into coronal third of the root and apical to the bone crest (subcrestal) **3:** Extends into mid-third of the root **4:** Extends into apical third of the root	**A:** ≤90° **B:** >90° to ≤180° **C:** >180° to ≤270° **D:** >270°	**d:** Lesion confined to dentine **p:** Probable pulpal involvement

Why was intentional reimplantation indicated?

The ECR lesion was located interproximally, encased within the buccal and palatal cortices, meaning that surgical access would have required significant buccal crestal bone removal. This would have resulted in a poor aesthetic result and/or compromised future replacement with a dental implant.

Root treatment without repairing the resorptive defect would have resolved the patient's presenting symptoms; however, untreated, progressive ECR would ultimately result in decoronation.

After discussing the treatment options, the patient decided to proceed with root canal treatment of the UR1 followed by intentional reimplantation to permit repair of the ECR lesion.

Treatment

Root canal treatment of the UR1 was carried out under local anaesthetic and dental dam in a single visit. No communication was observed between the root canal and the ECR lesion. Chemo-mechanical debridement was completed using stainless steel hand files and activated irrigation with sodium hypochlorite and ethylenediaminetetraacetic acid (EDTA) solution. The root canal was obturated with calcium silicate cement (CSC) due to the open apex. Using a CSC for the orthograde obturation would also help to minimise extraoral dry time during the IR, as the root apex will only require resection rather than both resection and retrograde preparation and filling. The access cavity was restored with composite (Figure 5.6.4).

The IR of the UR1 was planned for three months after the endodontic treatment was completed. This was to ensure that the root canal infection had resolved prior to IR. As part of the contingency planning, a resin-bonded bridge was constructed in case the UR1 crown fractured during the extraction procedure.

A putty index was taken to facilitate accurate repositioning of the replanted tooth. Following local anaesthesia, the UR1 was atraumatically extracted using periotomes and forceps. Pressure was applied coronal to the cemento-enamel junction to reduce damage to the periodontal ligament (PDL) and surrounding alveolar bone. Two clinicians were required to ensure that the procedure was performed efficiently, thus ensuring extraoral time of less than 15 minutes.

The first clinician managed the extracted tooth. The UR1 was first placed in Hanks' balanced salt solution (HBSS; Save-a-Tooth™, SmartPractice, Phoenix, AZ, USA) and then transferred to a gauze soaked in HBSS.

The lesion was identified under an operating microscope and the granulation tissue within the defect was gently debrided using excavators and a sterile diamond bur. The ECR defect was restored with resin-modified glass ionomer cement (GC Fuji IX GP™, GC Corporation, Tokyo, Japan). Composite resin was not used in this circumstance, as the etch/bond could cause additional damage to the PDL cells. The root apex was resected by 3 mm. During this time, the second clinician gently curetted the extraction socket to remove granulation tissue. Sterile gauze soaked in saline was used to cover the socket and prevent contamination with saliva (Figure 5.6.5).

The tooth was replanted into the socket within 10 minutes, initially being held with finger pressure before being stabilised with a flexible (composite and wire) splint for two weeks (International Association of Dental Traumatology 2020 guidelines for avulsed teeth). The patient was seen at two weeks for the removal of the splint, and thereafter, reviewed at four weeks, three months, six months and annually. At the one-year review, the patient was asymptomatic and the periapical radiograph showed good evidence of healing (Figure 5.6.6).

What are the main prognostic factors for the success of intentional reimplantation?

Key prognostic factors for the success of IR include:

- Atraumatic extraction using periotomes, and if forceps are necessary, they should only engage the crown of the tooth, therefore minimising damage to the PDL cells. Additionally, orthodontic extrusion can facilitate atraumatic extraction.
- Minimise extraoral dry time (EDT) to less than 15 minutes. The shorter the EDT, the higher the chance of maintaining PDL fibre and cementum viability, thus limiting the subsequent inflammatory response.

What are the benefits of using Hanks' balanced salt solution?

The key benefit of using HBSS is to maintain the PDL cell viability, differentiation and proliferation capacities. Periodic submersion of the tooth in HBSS can help avoid desiccation.

What are the contraindications to intentional replantation?

Contraindications include advanced, unstable periodontal disease, existing vertical root fracture and increased risk of crown and/or root fracture during extraction (e.g. divergent or curved roots, extensive root resorption). Patients who are contraindicated for dento-alveolar surgery (due to being immunocompromised, having haematological disorders and/or those who are at risk of medication-related osteonecrosis of the jaw) will not be suitable for IR.

Does the tooth have a favourable outcome?

The outcome of IR is supported by recent outcome studies: taking into account the key prognostic factors, reported survival rates of 95% with a mean follow-up period of 25 months have been reported. Longer-term outcome studies have revealed a retention rate of 93% after 12 years.

Discussion

IR is a pragmatic treatment option in specific situations; that is, when teeth are not amenable to conventional endodontic (surgical) treatment.

IR is defined as the intentional 'extraction and reinsertion of an endodontically treated tooth into its socket'. It is a viable alternative for the management of endodontic disease that is not easily accessible via non-surgical or surgical approaches. These include roots in close proximity to anatomical structures (e.g. inferior alveolar nerve, mental nerve, extensive palate-gingival grooves).

Case selection is imperative and clear communication of the risk of failure and complications must be included in the shared decision-making and consent process. Clinicians should be aware that the majority of complications, in particular external replacement resorption, occur within the first year after treatment. However, long-term follow-up is desirable as late failures have been reported.

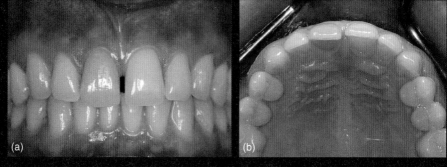

Figure 5.6.1 (a) Labial view of the anterior maxillary and mandibular teeth, showing discoloration of the UR1. (b) Occlusal view of the maxillary anterior teeth, showing the slightly palatal position of the UR1.

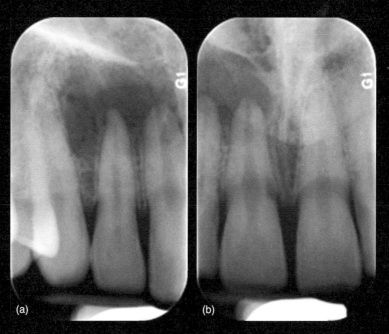

Figure 5.6.2 (a, b) Periapical radiographs showing the UR1 and UR2, with subcrestal radiolucency in the mesial cervical region of the UR1. A large periapical radiolucency extended from the midline suture to the mesial aspect of the UR3.

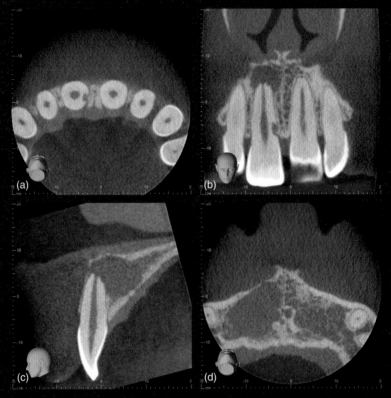

Figure 5.6.3 Cone beam computed tomography. (a) Axial view showing UR1 mesial radiolucency with thick buccal and palatal bone overlying the lesion. (b) Coronal view showing subcrestal mesial radiolucency not communicating with the root canal, and periapical radiolucency. (c) Sagittal view showing apical external inflammatory root resorption, an open apex and extensive periapical radiolucency, with intact cortical plates. (d) Axial view showing the extensive radiolucency with partial loss of the outline of the incisive canal.

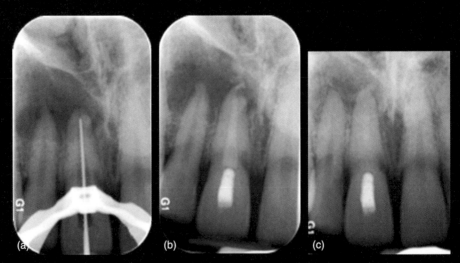

Figure 5.6.4 (a) UR1 orthograde root canal treatment working length radiograph. (b) UR1 post-operative radiograph with calcium silicate cement obturation. (c) UR1 three-month review radiograph prior to intentional reimplantation, showing early periapical healing.

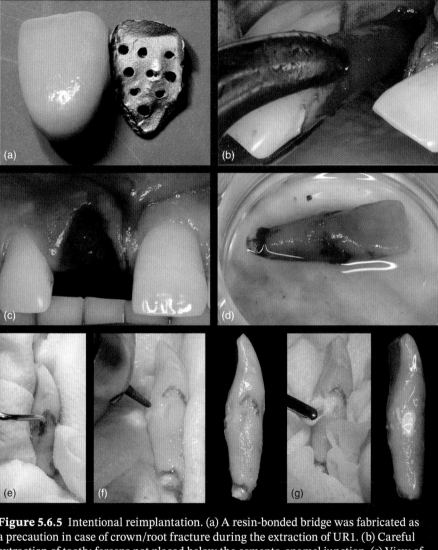

Figure 5.6.5 Intentional reimplantation. (a) A resin-bonded bridge was fabricated as a precaution in case of crown/root fracture during the extraction of UR1. (b) Careful extraction of tooth; forceps not placed below the cemento-enamel junction. (c) View of socket following extraction; buccal and palatal cortices intact. (d) The tooth is immersed in Hanks' balanced salt solution (HBSS) in a sterile well plate to maintain vitality of the periodontal ligament cells. (e) The tooth is then carefully held with gauze soaked in HBSS. (f) Excavation of the resorptive lesion with a sterile bur. (g) Glass-ionomer cement restoration.

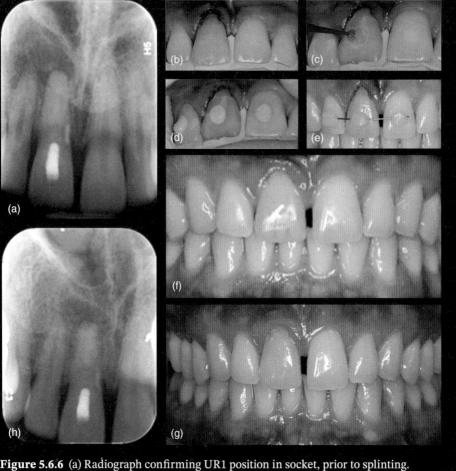

Figure 5.6.6 (a) Radiograph confirming UR1 position in socket, prior to splinting. (b) Putty index used to aid in accurate repositioning of UR1. (c) Etching and bonding of UR2, UR1 and UL1. (d) Composite resin placement prior to splinting. (e) Flexible composite/wire splint on UR1, UR2 and UL1. (f) Photograph following splint removal at two weeks. (g) Photograph at one-year follow-up. (h) Periapical radiograph at one-year follow-up, showing good periapical healing.

Further Reading

Bender, I.B. and Rossman, L.E. (1993). Intentional replantation of endodontically treated teeth. *Oral Surgery, Oral Medicine, and Oral Pathology* 76: 623–630.

Cho, S.Y., Lee, Y., Shin, S.J. et al. (2016). Retention and healing outcomes after intentional replantation. *Journal of Endodontics* 42: 909–915.

Choi, Y.H., Bae, J.H., Kim, Y.K. et al. (2014). Clinical outcome of intentional replantation with pre-operative orthodontic extrusion: a retrospective study. *International Endodontic Journal* 47: 1168–1176.

Cunliffe, J., Ayub, K., Darcey, J. et al. (2020). Intentional replantation – a clinical review of cases undertaken at a major UK dental school. *British Dental Journal* 229: 230–238.

Fouad AF, Abbott PV, Tsilingaridis G, et al. International Association of Dental Traumatology guidelines for the management of traumatic dental injuries: 2. Avulsion of permanent teeth. Dental Traumatology 2020; 36(4): 331–342.

Patel, S., Foschi, F., Condon, R. et al. (2018). External cervical resorption: part 2 – Management. *International Endodontic Journal* 51: 1224–1238.

Plotino, G., Abella Sans, F., Duggal, M.S., Grande, N.M., Krastl, G., Nagendrababu, V., and Gambarini, G. (2021). European Society of Endodontology position statement: Surgical extrusion, intentional replantation and tooth autotransplantation: European Society of Endodontology developed by. *International Endodontic Journal* 54: 655–659.

Plotino, G., Abella Sans, F., Duggal, M.S., Grande, N.M., Krastl, G., Nagendrababu, V., and Gambarini, G. (2022). Present status and future directions; Surgical extrusion, intentional reimplantation, tooth autotransplantation 55(Suppl. 3): 827–842.

Torabinejad, M., Dinsbach, N.A., Turman, M. et al. (2015). Survival of intentionally replanted teeth and implant-supported single crowns: a systematic review. *Journal of Endodontics* 41: 992–998.

5.7 Fractured Endodontic Instruments

Luis Ferrandez

Objectives

At the end of the chapter, the reader should appreciate the reasons for file fracture, understand how to avoid it and identify the most appropriate management option.

Introduction

A 50-year-old male was referred by his general dentist to a specialist endodontic practice for management of a root canal–treated tooth with a separated instrument in the apical third. The tooth had recently caused symptoms.

Chief complaint

The patient complained of swelling under his jaw and a loose and broken filling in the mandibular left second molar (LL7).

Medical history

Unremarkable.

Dental history

Root canal treatment of the LL7 had been completed over five years previously and had not caused problems until recently. The mandibular left third molar (LL8) had been extracted within the last year and the lower left first molar (LL6) had recently had distal caries, which had been restored with a composite resin restoration.

Clinical Examination

Extraorally, the left submandibular lymph nodes were swollen and tender to palpation. Intraorally, the soft tissues adjacent to the LL7 were within normal limits and there were no periodontal defects. The LL7 was

Pitt Ford's Problem-Based Learning in Endodontology, Second Edition. Edited by Elizabeth Shin Perry, Shanon Patel, Shalini Kanagasingam, and Samantha Hamer.
© 2025 John Wiley & Sons Ltd. Published 2025 by John Wiley & Sons Ltd.

restored with multiple composite restorations with secondary caries. The LL6 and LL5 were minimally restored with well-adapted composite restorations.

Radiographic Examination

- Alveolar bone height within normal limits.
- The LL7 had a subgingival mesio-occlusal restoration with marginal defect and a void between the coronal restoration and the root canal filling. The existing root canal filling was sparsely condensed and terminated short of the radiographic apex in the mesial canal, with a 3 mm instrument fragment in the apical third. Apical radiolucency was associated with the mesial and distal apices (Figure 5.7.1).

Diagnosis and Treatment Planning

A diagnosis of symptomatic apical periodontitis associated with an existing root canal filling for tooth LL7 was reached.

What other diagnostic tests could be carried out to assist with treatment planning in teeth with broken files?

Pre-operative cone beam computed tomography (CBCT) imaging is strongly recommended and can provide valuable information about the location and length of the file fragment, multiplanar canal curvatures and root canal anatomy, such as the size and shape of the canal and whether the canal is confluent with another or independent (Figure 5.7.2).

How do endodontic files break and what can be done to minimise occurrence of this?

Endodontic files fracture through one or a combination of two mechanisms:

- Torsional fatigue
- Cyclic fatigue

Torsional failure occurs when the tip of the instrument is engaged in the root canal but the file continues rotating to the point that the elastic limit of the instrument is surpassed. Both hand files and rotary instruments can fracture in this manner. The clinician should avoid excessive apical pressure, especially when the instrument is not advancing to prevent it. Flexural (cyclic) failure occurs when the instrument is rotating in the area of the canal curvature, subjecting it to repeated tensile and compressive stresses. This causes cracks in the material, eventually leading to file fracture. This mode of failure is characteristic of rotary endodontic instruments. Careful pre-operative radiographic assessment of the root canal anatomy and initial canal negotiation with hand files are key to providing the clinician with knowledge of the degree and abruptness of the canal curvature in the different planes (Table 5.7.1).

Table 5.7.1 Recommendations to reduce incidence of instrument fracture.

Enhancement of operator skills
● Cone beam computed tomography assessment of the degree and radius of canal curvature in all planes
● Recognition of the importance of file size and design
● Use of heat-treated nickel titanium instruments
● Single instrument use
● Canal orifice relocation if necessary
● Clinical assessment of canal size and curvature with small hand files
● Establishment of a glide path
● Use of recapitulating and patency hand filing
● Avoidance of apical pressure
● Use of rotary instruments within a soaked or lubricated canal
● Regular visual examination of unwinding of the file
● Use of a crown-down shaping strategy
● Use of a short pecking motion

What are the options for management of a tooth with a fractured instrument?

- Root canal retreatment leaving the file in situ.
- Root canal retreatment attempting instrument bypass.
- Root canal retreatment attempting instrument removal.
- Periapical microsurgery.
- Intentional replantation.
- Extraction.

The factors influencing the decision on how to treat a root-treated tooth with a broken instrument are:

- The position of the tooth in the arch.
- The restorative status of the tooth.
- The location of the instrument within the canal (straight or curved canal/coronal, middle or apical third).
- The length of the fractured instrument and the type of instrument (rotary files are much harder to remove, as they tend to screw into

the dentine and due to their greater taper they tend to fully occlude the canal, making bypass more difficult).

- The pulpal and periapical diagnosis.
- The root canal anatomy and the expected effect (destruction) of the procedure on radicular dentine (how much dentine will remain following removal to gain access to the instrument) (Table 5.7.2).

Table 5.7.2 Decision-making tree for management of instrument fracture.

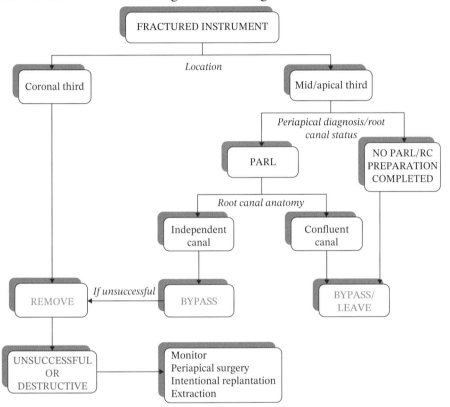

What are the objectives of the treatment when a fractured file is present?

The fractured file itself does not constitute a problem. However, it can hinder root canal disinfection by blocking the passage of shaping instruments that allow access of disinfectant solutions to the apical third of the canal. Instrument removal techniques invariably need additional root canal preparation coronal to and around the head of the file. The chosen treatment option should ensure disinfection of the apical canal while avoiding excessive removal of radicular dentine, thus aiming to achieve periapical health without challenging the ultimate objective of tooth retention (Table 5.7.3).

Table 5.7.3 Bypass vs removal of a fractured instrument.

	Bypass	**Removal**
Use of specialised systems	No	Yes
Magnification required	Occasionally	Yes
Technically challenging	Yes	Yes
Root dentine removal around the file head needed	No	Yes
Possibility of mishaps (e.g. perforations)	Yes	Yes
Time-consuming	Yes	Yes
Contraindications	No	Apical third/fragment not visible

What was the treatment decision in this case?

The patient was keen to retain the tooth because he had recently lost the adjacent molar (LL8). The position and restorative status of the tooth precluded surgical options as first-line treatment. Removal of the file fragment would have been very challenging and probably destructive given its apical position. A decision was made to attempt file bypass, as the CBCT scan showed that the canals merged at the level of the instrument.

What Technique is Used to Bypass a Broken Instrument?

- Dry the canal, try to visualise the instrument and insert a small (size 8 or 10) 21 mm hand file between the fragment and the wall, preferably along the isthmus or inner curve.
- Once a 'stick' is felt, advance gently with a stem-winding motion.
- Flood the canal with sodium hypochlorite and keep using the same movement.
- Once the file loosely passes along the segment, use a short push–pull motion.
- Repeat the process with larger hand files and recapitulate as necessary.
- A rotary instrument may be used with caution after a glide path has been created with hand files (at least size 20).
- On occasion the fragment comes out of the canal while irrigating (Figure 5.7.3).

The existing restoration and caries were removed. The gutta percha was retrieved with ultrasonics and Hedström files. The instrument was bypassed and chemo-mechanical preparation of the canals completed with hand and rotary instruments. Disinfection was carried out with sodium hypochlorite and citric acid, which were ultrasonically activated. Treatment was completed in two visits with calcium hydroxide as an intracanal medicament. The root canals were obturated with warm vertical compaction of gutta percha (Figure 5.7.4). The tooth was restored with a dual-cure composite core ready for the referring dentist to provide a full-coverage restoration.

The patient returned a year later for a clinical and radiographic review. The tooth was restored with a well-fitting metal ceramic crown. There was an absence of clinical signs or symptoms and radiographically there was resolution of the pre-operative apical radiolucency (Figure 5.7.5).

What are the risks of bypassing a broken instrument?

The use of large hand or rotary instruments along the fragment can cause canal transportation and strip perforation, especially in the mid-third of thin roots. The clinician should consider abandoning the attempt to bypass the file if progress is not made relatively early, as this may lead to canal ledging and perforation.

What are the main instrument removal techniques and their mechanism of action?

- *Ultrasonics*: exposure of the file head and application of low-energy vibration.
- *Braiding technique*: bypassing the instrument on both sides with hand files, braid and pull.
- *Tube and glue*: file head exposure by ultrasonics and engagement with a tube and adhesive (e.g. Cancellier kit, SybronEndo, Orange, CA, USA).
- *Tube and file devices*: exposure of the head and engagement with a tube and internal file or shaft (e.g. instrument removal system).
- *Lasso-type devices*: exposure of the shank end of the file and loosening with ultrasonic tips followed by retrieval with a micro-lasso (e.g. Terauchi file retrieval kit TRFK, Plan B Dental, Goleta, CA, USA).

Discussion

The incidence of endodontic instrument fracture is low and frequently the result of poor operator technique. Therefore, the importance of training and practice cannot be over-emphasised.

For the clinician it can be a stressful and even embarrassing event. However, there are a myriad of treatment options and techniques to deal with the problem and, in most cases, if the appropriate decisions are taken, the prognosis of treatment is unaffected and the tooth can be retained.

Removal of the instrument should not be the main objective, although this is tempting, especially if it is the result of one's own error. The clinician should always attempt to fulfil the biological goals of the treatment without compromising the structural integrity and long-term survival of the tooth.

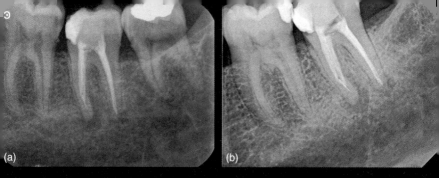

Figure 5.7.1 (a, b) Pre-operative radiographs.

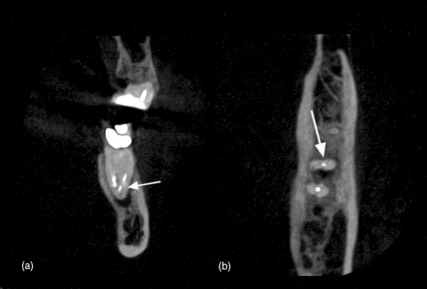

Figure 5.7.2 (a) Coronal and (b) axial slices showing the mesial canals merging and the segment centred within the root canal apically. The fragment broke in the mesio-buccal canal at the intersection with the mesio-lingual canal.

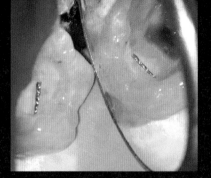

Figure 5.7.3 The broken file segment came out during irrigation after completing root canal preparation.

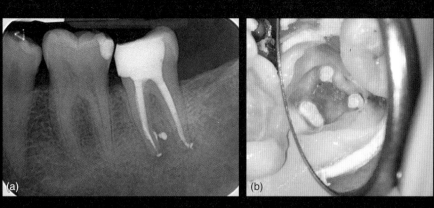

Figure 5.7.4 (a) Final radiograph. Note the inadvertent sealer extrusion through a lateral canal in the apical third of the mesial root. (b) Clinical image of the pulp chamber post obturation.

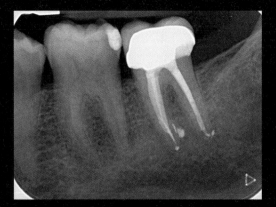

Figure 5.7.5 One-year review radiograph. Note the absence of apical findings.

Further Reading

Cheung, G.S.P. (2009). Instrument fracture: mechanisms, removal of fragments, and clinical outcomes. *Endodontic Topics* 16: 1–26.

McGuigan, M.B., Louca, C., and Duncan, H.F. (2013). Endodontic instrument fracture: causes and prevention. *British Dental Journal* 7: 341–348.

Panitvisai, P., Parunnit, P., Sathorn, C., and Messer, H.H. (2010). Impact of a retained instrument on treatment outcome: a systematic review and meta-analysis. *Journal of Endodontics* 5: 775–780.

Parashos, P. and Messer, H.H. (2006). Rotary NiTi instrument fracture and its consequences. *Journal of Endodontics* 11: 1031–1043.

Souter, N.J. and Messer, H.H. (2005). Complications associated with fractured file removal using an ultrasonic technique. *Journal of Endodontics* 6: 450–452.

VI Restoration of the Endodontically Treated Tooth

6.1 Restoration of a Root-Filled Tooth with a Fibre Post-Retained Crown

Bhavin Bhuva, Francesco Mannocci, and Massimo Giovarruscio

Objectives

At the end of this case, the reader should know when a post may be used to restore a root-filled tooth and appreciate the factors that influence the survival of compromised teeth restored with posts.

Introduction

A 37-year-old male patient presented, complaining of cold sensitivity and occasional throbbing pain associated with the upper left first premolar tooth.

Chief Complaint

The patient complained of pronounced and prolonged pain with cold foods and drinks. There was also spontaneous, poorly localised, lingering throbbing pain in the upper left premolar region.

Medical History

Unremarkable.

Dental History

The patient was an infrequent attender. He had seen an emergency dentist approximately one year previously, who had advised restoration of a carious tooth that had fractured. A temporary restoration had been placed but the patient failed to return for treatment.

Pitt Ford's Problem-Based Learning in Endodontology, Second Edition. Edited by Elizabeth Shin Perry, Shanon Patel, Shalini Kanagasingam, and Samantha Hamer.
© 2025 John Wiley & Sons Ltd. Published 2025 by John Wiley & Sons Ltd.

Clinical Examination

Tooth UL4 was restored with a disto-occlusal temporary dressing (Figure 6.1.1). The tooth was not tender to percussion, but gave a painful response to cold sensibility testing that lingered for several seconds. There were no periodontal probing depths greater than 3 mm associated with the tooth.

What does the radiograph reveal (Figure 6.1.2)?

- Extensive caries in the UL4 that appears to extend close to the pulp.
- Periodontal ligament space widening associated with the UL4.
- Tooth UL6 is root treated to a good standard and the associated peri-apical tissues appear healthy.

Diagnosis and Treatment Planning

A diagnosis of symptomatic irreversible pulpitis was made for tooth UL4.

The patient's symptoms were due to inflammation of the pulp as a result of the deep caries. Although the caries had not breached the pulp proper, the bacterial insult associated with the carious lesion had caused the pulp to become irreversibly inflamed.

What are the treatment options for this tooth?

- No treatment.
- Root canal treatment (subject to restorability assessment) followed by cuspal coverage restoration.
- Extraction followed by replacement with (i) implant-retained crown, (ii) conventional or resin-bonded bridge, or (iii) removable partial denture.

Following discussion of the various treatment options, the patient decided to proceed with root canal treatment of tooth UL4. The patient was advised that, in the first instance, the residual sound tooth structure would need to be assessed following caries removal. Only following restorability assessment can it be established whether the tooth is restorable, and whether a post may be required to retain a core, prior to cuspal coverage restoration.

When and how should we assess restorability?

- Restorability assessment is a fundamental step of endodontic treatment that should be carried out at an early stage, in order to determine the feasibility of the treatment, as well as the restorative prognosis of the tooth.

- All existing restorations and caries should be removed so that the *quality* and *quantity* of the residual tooth structure can be assessed.
- Without removing the entire existing restoration, it is not possible to detect caries, marginal leakage or cracks, even when the restoration appears clinically and radiographically acceptable.
- Complete coronal disassembly will facilitate more conservative and appropriately directed access cavity preparation. Where feasible, the operator may also be able to use the existing cavity to direct the endodontic access to prevent further removal of tooth structure. This has been described as 'restoratively driven' or 'caries-driven' access.
- The quantity and location of residual tooth structure will allow the operator to decide on the most appropriate method for restoring the tooth. It is at this stage, that the operator should plan the final restoration, so that all of the treatment steps can be carried out accordingly. The decision as to whether a post-retained restoration is required cannot be made without assessment of the remaining tooth structure following coronal disassembly.

Treatment

Following local anaesthesia, dental dam isolation of tooth UL4 was performed. The disto-occlusal caries was removed initially with a diamond bur under copious water spray. Caries removal was completed with a stainless steel rose-head bur. The tooth was deemed to be restorable following assessment of the residual sound tooth structure. The buccal and palatal cusps were undermined by the caries, such that their residual thickness was considered insufficient to avoid fracture during function, particularly as the patient had group function on lateral excursive movements.

Endodontic access revealed a hyperaemic pulp, confirming the diagnosis of irreversible pulpitis. Two canals were located and root canal instrumentation was initiated. Copious irrigation with 3% sodium hypochlorite solution was performed throughout the procedure. The working lengths of the root canals were determined using an electronic apex locator.

Root canal preparation was carried out using stainless steel hand files to obtain a glide path, followed by preparation with nickel titanium rotary instruments. After completion of the preparation, the canals were rinsed with 17% ethylenediaminetetraacetic acid (EDTA) solution, in order to remove the smear layer created during root canal preparation. A master cone periapical radiograph was taken to verify the preparation of the canals (Figure 6.1.3). Final irrigation of the canals was completed with sodium hypochlorite, which was dynamically activated using a sonic device.

The canals were dried with paper points and obturated with gutta percha and sealer, using a warm vertical condensation technique. Post spaces were left in both canals for subsequent core placement.

When is post retention necessary?

Posts are necessary when there is insufficient tooth structure to support the coronal restoration. In almost all cases where a post is required, the definitive restoration will involve the provision of an onlay or crown. The purpose of post placement in this case was to facilitate the retention of the core, as there was a large class II cavity and the residual axial walls were of insufficient thickness, and therefore strength, to prevent subsequent cusp fracture. The use of posts has been shown to be beneficial to restoration and tooth longevity in root-filled premolar teeth with class II or greater defects. Further indications for a post may be when retreatment is performed and a post was used following the initial treatment, or where there is an anatomically wide canal and the residual dentine walls are thin (for example, an immature tooth).

What is meant by the ferrule effect?

The ferrule effect refers to a circumferential collar of cast metal or ceramic (provided by the cuspal coverage restoration), which encircles the near parallel walls of dentine, coronal to the margins of the cuspal coverage preparation (Figure 6.1.4).

The presence of an adequate ferrule effect is a critical factor for the retention of a cuspal coverage restoration. Posts do not reinforce root-filled teeth and cannot retain the cuspal coverage restoration in the absence of a sufficient ferrule effect.

An adequate ferrule effect is also a significant factor in preventing root fracture of teeth restored with rigid posts and post decementation with fibre posts. In addition to the presence of an adequate ferrule effect, the longevity of root-filled teeth has been increasingly shown to be determined by the overall volume of sound tooth structure, number of residual walls, tooth location and number or proximal contacts.

What are the advantages of placing the post immediately after endodontic treatment has been completed?

- Risks of iatrogenic accidents during post preparation are minimised, as the orientation of the root and anatomy of the canal are familiar to the operator.
- Reduced risk of microleakage, as a good coronal seal is obtained immediately. Temporary post-retained onlays and crowns are

particularly poor at providing a bacteria-tight seal and are prone to debonding between appointments.

- Reduction of overall treatment time and number of appointments, potentially allowing preparation for the cuspal coverage restoration to be carried out at the same visit as the endodontic treatment.

Dental dam isolation is necessary when carrying out post placement, as it prevents bacterial contamination of the root canal space and provides a moisture-free working field, which is particularly important when the post is to be adhesively bonded. However, caution must be exercised when using a dental dam during post preparation, as it may be difficult to orientate the tooth correctly; this may lead to the misdirected use of rotary instruments within the root canal. This is of particular relevance when the post preparation is carried out at a separate appointment from the endodontic treatment and/or when treating severely proclined/retroclined teeth.

When placing a post, preparation of the root canal space should be as conservative as possible or, better still, avoided altogether. Unnecessary thinning of the root dentine, particularly in the pericervical region to facilitate post placement, will weaken the root unduly and increase the risk of subsequent root fracture. For optimal passive post placement, a well-fitting post should be chosen to minimise the thickness of the luting cement; increasing cement thickness compromises post retention. This may be a challenge in oval canals, where post adaptation will be poor in the bucco-lingual plane. Customisable glass fibres can be used to fabricate anatomically specific fibre posts at the chairside; however, these do not appear to perform as well as prefabricated designs.

A variety of passive post systems exist, which include prefabricated metal and fibre posts. The post drills of the chosen post system should be used to 'manually' gauge the correct size to be used. The selected post can then be inserted into the root canal, to ensure it reaches the coronal level of the root canal filling. To ensure optimal adaptation and bonding of materials to the root canal dentine, it is essential to ensure that there are no remnants of root filling material or sealer on the walls of the post space. Rotary reaming instruments (for example Gates-Glidden burs or Largo drills) may be useful for removing gutta percha, whilst ultrasonic instruments and/or air abrasion with concomitant magnification may also be used to ensure that all material remnants have been removed from the root canal walls.

The post spaces in both buccal and palatal canals were first cleaned using ultrasonic instruments to ensure there were no remnants of gutta percha or root canal sealer on the root canal walls (Figure 6.1.5). Well-fitting fibre posts were chosen and their adaptation within the canals was verified (Figure 6.1.6a). The posts and post space were rinsed with isopropyl alcohol, after which the dentine was etched, washed and dried, to obtain a clean bonding surface. The post was prepared for bonding by applying a silane coupling agent. A non-rinse conditioner and bonding agent were applied to the dentine surface (Figure 6.1.6b, c), after which the posts were cemented with a dual-cure resin cement (Figure 6.1.6d, e, f), which was light-cured to accelerate the polymerisation. A composite core was then built up incrementally. Once the core was complete, the posts were sectioned, using copious water spray and a diamond disc. Onlay preparation was then carried out immediately after completion of the core (Figure 6.1.7). An impression of the completed onlay preparation was taken, and a bisacryl temporary onlay was constructed using the pre-operative putty matrix. The definitive onlay was constructed (Figure 6.1.8) and then cemented two weeks later (Figure 6.1.9). The patient was reviewed one year after the completion of treatment and no symptoms were reported. A follow-up radiograph demonstrated healthy periapical tissues (Figure 6.1.10).

If a eugenol-based sealer has been used during the root canal treatment, the root canal can be rinsed with alcohol to sequester any free eugenol, thereby preventing the inhibition of polymerisation of any composite resin materials that are to be used.

What are the advantages of using a fibre post over a cast metal post?

A common mode of failure for teeth restored with cast metal posts is root fracture, which will usually result in extraction of the tooth. Conversely, teeth restored with fibre posts appear to fail due to debonding and therefore this is a more retrievable, tooth-friendly approach than those restored with cast metal posts. This is due to the more favourable modulus of elasticity of fibre posts when compared to cast posts. The main modes of failure for fibre post systems are post decementation, chipping of the composite restoration and secondary caries. Of these, post decementation would appear to be the most frequent cause of failure. Finally, superior aesthetic outcomes are achievable with translucent and/or tooth-coloured post and core materials.

There is evidence to suggest that the failure rate of fibre posts is between 7% and 11% after 7–11 years of clinical service. The incidence of secondary caries in teeth restored with fibre posts appears to be greater in teeth that have not been crowned. In addition to reducing the risk of secondary caries, a crown will reduce moisture absorption into the composite–post complex, thereby reducing the risk of post decementation. Definitive restoration with a crown or onlay also protects the remaining tooth structure, reducing the risk of terminal fractures. Therefore, in most cases, the placement of a cuspal coverage restoration should be considered as an integral final stage in the restoration process of the compromised root-filled tooth.

How wide should a post be?

Post adaptation is far more important than post diameter, as it is the luting cement that is the weakest link in the tooth–restoration complex. Although the post must be wide enough to resist fracture (most commonly at the post–core interface), it should not be so wide as to cause unnecessary stress on the root. Various suggestions on post diameter have been made; one such recommendation, which is frequently cited, is that the post should be one-third of the root diameter. In reality, the ratio of post diameter to the remaining thickness of the dentine wall is of far more importance. The preservation of a minimum dentine thickness of 1 mm has been recommended. However, one must bear in mind that the bucco-lingual width of anterior and premolar teeth is invariably less than their mesio-distal dimensions.

The dentine in the pericervical region should be preserved as much as possible to minimise the risk of dentine fracture. There are a variety of types and sizes of prefabricated post systems, and therefore it will usually be possible to match a post fairly accurately to the post space. In this way, excessive 'thinning' of the root canal dentine is minimised, and the placement of the post does not cause any additional weakening of the tooth. The advantage of newer fibre post systems is that the post has a more tapered, wider shape coronally, thereby preventing unnecessary enlargement of the root canal, but giving greater strength to the post at the critical post–core junction.

How long should a post be, and what are the factors that should be considered when deciding on post length?

The length of a post will affect its retention, but will also influence the distribution of forces imparted on the root. Longer posts will allow better stress distribution than shorter ones, and therefore are less likely to cause root fractures. However, the relationship between post length and root fracture relates to cast posts. Root fracture is not a significant mode of failure for fibre post systems, which tend to fail primarily by decementation.

Post length has been shown to be a more important variable than post width. However, as mentioned previously, it must be remembered that obtaining an adequate ferrule effect is the most critical factor in the predictable restoration of compromised teeth.

Whilst optimising post length is desirable when restoring root-filled teeth, it is also important to preserve an adequate length of root-filling material to prevent the persistence or development of apical periodontitis. Therefore, a sufficient length of well-condensed gutta percha must be maintained when preparing the post space. At least 5 mm of apical root-filling material should be preserved in order to maintain an adequate seal. It may be difficult to achieve optimal post length and preserve an adequate length of root-filling material in teeth that have relatively short root lengths. In these instances, adequate root-filling material should be preserved and an adhesive technique employed to bond the post into the root canal space. The use of a fibre post system is particularly useful in cases such as these.

Discussion

The decision to use a post is dependent on careful assessment of the residual sound coronal tooth structure, subsequent to the removal of the entire restoration and any associated caries. The purpose of a post is to retain the core, which would not otherwise be possible if the remaining tooth structure alone was used.

When a post is placed, it is important not to carry out any preparation that will remove unnecessary dentine and weaken the root in the critical pericervical region. The root canal dentine should be adequately cleaned and prepared when an adhesive post system is to be used.

Under dynamic functional loading, posts will exert stresses along the root, which may potentially lead to root fracture. When there is at least a 2 mm circumferential ring (ferrule) of dentine coronal to the margins of the crown preparation, the effect of these forces being transmitted to the root is minimised. The modulus of elasticity of fibre posts is three to four times that of dentine. This is more favourable than that of metal posts and so reduces the risk of root fracture significantly. In summary, the use of a fibre post, in conjunction with an adequate ferrule effect, will allow the predictable restoration of the compromised root-filled tooth.

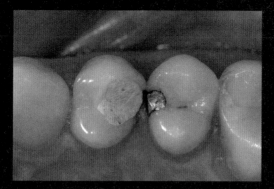

Figure 6.1.1 Occlusal view of the UL4, which has a disto-occlusal cavity that has been temporarily dressed.

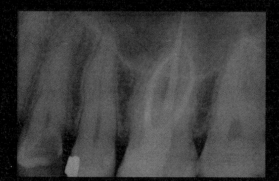

Figure 6.1.2 Periapical radiograph showing gross caries in the UL4. Radiographically, the caries appears intimate with the pulp; however, the clinical findings may be different. There is slight widening of the periodontal ligament space associated with the tooth. The UL6 has been root canal treated to a good standard and the associated periapical tissues are normal.

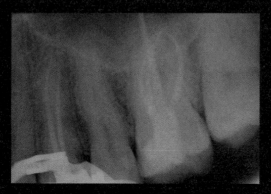

Figure 6.1.3 Master cone periapical radiograph showing adequate preparation and extension of gutta percha cones prior to obturation. The radiograph is taken with a dedicated endodontic film holder so that the clamp can be accommodated without affecting the image.

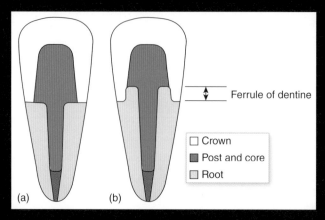

Figure 6.1.4 The 'ferrule effect' refers to the circumferential band of a crown that encircles the remaining coronal tooth structure. Ideally, there should be at least 2 mm of sound dentine (height) that is encased by the crown margins. The ferrule effect reduces the incidence of root fracture and also provides an optimal seal. (a) A post crowned tooth with no ferrule effect. The fulcrum axis is such that occlusal forces are transmitted entirely into the root with no protection from the remaining tooth structure, (b) A post crowned tooth with an adequate ferrule effect. The presence of an adequate ferrule of dentine moves the axis of rotation and dissipates forces more favourably, reducing the risk of root fracture.

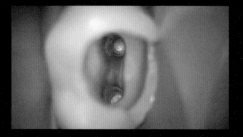

Figure 6.1.5 Occlusal view of the obturated buccal and palatal canals.

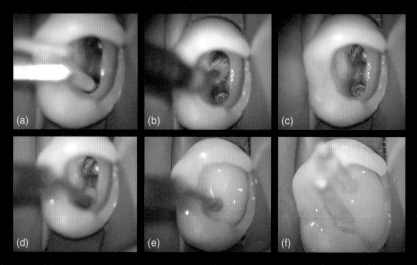

Figure 6.1.6 (a) Fibre post adaptation is verified in each canal. No preparation was carried out and the post size that was best adapted was selected. (b, c) The use of dual-cure bonding agent is advantageous when cementing posts adhesively. Light-cured materials should be avoided to prevent incomplete polymerisation and failure of optimal bonding. (d, e) A dual-cure composite resin cement is applied with a dedicated delivery tip so that it can be placed to the full depth of the post space. (f) The two posts are cemented using the resin cement. The post should not be agitated, as this may allow the inclusion of air and subsequent void formation.

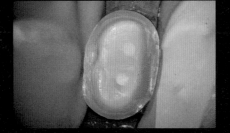

Figure 6.1.7 Following completion of the core, the preparation for a full-coverage ceramic onlay is completed.

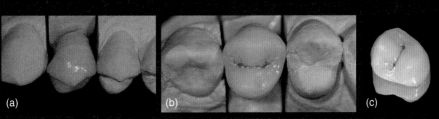

(a) (b) (c)

Figure 6.1.8 (a–c) A lithium disilicate ceramic onlay is manufactured; note the supragingival margins that facilitate preservation of residual sound tooth structure, particularly in the pericervical region of the tooth. This will distribute non-axial forces more favourably, reducing the risk of root fracture.

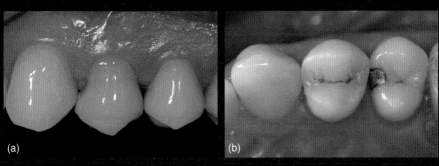

(a) (b)

Figure 6.1.9 (a, b) The final restoration has been adhesively cemented under dental dam isolation.

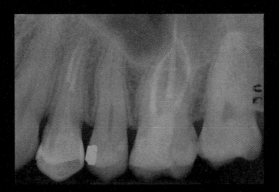

Figure 6.1.10 A follow-up radiograph taken one year after the treatment demonstrates healthy periapical tissues. The marginal fit of the restoration appears satisfactory.

Further Reading

Bhuva, B., Giovarruscio, M., Rahim, N. et al. (2021). The restoration of root filled teeth: a review of the clinical literature. *International Endodontic Journal* 54: 509–535.

Creugers, N.H., Mentink, A.G., Fokkinga, W.A., and Kreulen, C.M. (2005). 5-year follow-up of a prospective clinical study on various types of core restorations. *International Journal of Prosthodontics* 18: 34–39.

Ferrari, M., Cagidiaco, M.C., Goracci, C. et al. (2007). Long-term retrospective study of the clinical performance of fiber posts. *American Journal of Dentistry* 20: 287–291.

Fokkinga, W.A., Kreulen, C.M., Bronkhorst, E.M., and Creugers, N.H. (2007). Up to 17-year controlled clinical study on post-and-cores and covering crowns. *Journal of Dentistry* 35: 778–786.

Giok, K.C., Veettil, S.K. and Menon, R.K. (2023) Comparative effectiveness of fiber and metal posts in the restoration of endodontically treated teeth: A systematic review with network meta-analysis. *Journal of Prosthetic Dentistry*. Oct 10:S0022-3913(23)00569-3.

Mannocci, F., Bertelli, E., Sherriff, M. et al. (2002). Three-year clinical comparison of survival of endodontically treated teeth restored with either full cast coverage or with direct composite restoration. *Journal of Prosthetic Dentistry* 88: 297–301.

Mannocci, F., Bhuva, B., Roig, M., Zarow, M., and Bitter, K. (2021). European Society of Endodontology position statement: The restoration of root filled teeth. *International Endodontic Journal*, 54: 1974–1981.

Naumann, M., Schmitter, M., and Krastl, G. (2018). Postendodontic restoration: endodontic post-and-core or no post at all? *Journal of Adhesive Dentistry* 20: 19–24.

Sorenson, J.A. and Engelman, J.T. (1990). Ferrule design and fracture resistance of endodontically treated teeth. *Journal of Prosthetic Dentistry* 53: 496–500.

Standlee, J.P., Caputo, A.A., Collard, E.W., and Pollack, M.H. (1972). Analysis of stress distribution by endodontic posts. *Oral Surgery, Oral Medicine, Oral Pathology* 33: 952–960.

6.2 Restoration of an Endodontically Treated Posterior Tooth

Shanon Patel, Massimo Giovarruscio, and Bhavin Bhuva

Objectives

At the end of this case the reader should understand the biomechanical differences between endodontically treated teeth and vital teeth, and the principles of restoring endodontically treated posterior teeth.

Introduction

A 45-year-old patient presented with symptoms of a throbbing pain localised to a heavily restored upper left first premolar tooth (UL4).

Chief Complaint

The patient complained of a spontaneous throbbing ache that lasted minutes to hours. Hot and cold liquids also resulted in similar symptoms. The pain had been getting progressively worse over the last four days.

Medical History

Unremarkable.

Dental History

The patient regularly attended her dentist for annual routine examinations and saw the hygienist every six months.

Clinical Examination

The UL4 was restored with a class 2 amalgam restoration (Figure 6.2.1). The tooth was slightly tender to percussion. The patient's presenting symptoms

Pitt Ford's Problem-Based Learning in Endodontology, Second Edition. Edited by Elizabeth Shin Perry, Shanon Patel, Shalini Kanagasingam, and Samantha Hamer.

were reproduced with cold sensibility testing on the UL4. A periapical radiograph revealed a calcified pulp chamber and root canal system (Figure 6.2.2).

Diagnosis and Treatment Planning

A diagnosis of symptomatic irreversible pulpitis with symptomatic apical periodontitis was reached for the UL4. The patient was advised that endodontic treatment was necessary if she wished to retain her tooth, after which a cuspal coverage restoration (for example, crown or onlay) would be required to provide the best long-term treatment outcome.

Before embarking on endodontic treatment, how would you assess the restorability of the tooth?

The overall restorability of the tooth *must* be established before carrying out endodontic treatment (Table 6.2.1). The following factors should be assessed:

- *Periodontal status*: The periodontal probing profile should be determined by 'walking' a periodontal probe around the circumference of the tooth. Localised increased probing depths may be of significance (for example, vertical fractures, furcation defects or perforation) and generalised increased probing depths indicating periodontal disease may adversely influence the long-term prognosis of the tooth.

Table 6.2.1 Factors affecting the prognosis of a tooth requiring endodontic intervention.

General	➤ Patient's motivation to preserve tooth
	➤ Financial and time restraints
Prosthodontic	➤ Ability to remove existing restoration
	➤ Remaining sound coronal tooth structure
	➤ Ability to obtain ferrule
	➤ Occlusal factors
	➤ Ability to obtain satisfactory aesthetics
Periodontal	➤ Oral hygiene
	➤ Gingival health and periodontal probing depths
	➤ Furcation involvement
	➤ Root length and anatomy
Endodontic	➤ Development status of root
	➤ Existing root canal treatment
	➤ Presence of a periapical radiolucent lesion
	➤ Access to tooth
	➤ Ability to isolate the tooth with dental dam
	➤ Ability to identify all root canals
	➤ Ability to negotiate, shape, clean and fill all canals to length

- *Prosthodontic status*: The residual sound tooth structure should be assessed following the removal of existing restorations and/or caries, after which the restorability of the tooth may be determined. The volume and location of residual sound dentine will determine the 'survival' of the endodontically treated tooth, as the majority of teeth will fail through 'structural' (biomechanical) failure, rather than due to complications associated with the root canal treatment itself. For endodontically treated posterior teeth, in addition to the overall loss in sound tooth structure, a minimum 2 mm of supramarginal circumferential sound coronal dentine is desirable to provide a ferrule effect for the subsequent cuspal coverage restoration (for example, crown or onlay). The final restoration therefore needs to be considered and planned following coronal disassembly.

- *Endodontic status*: Is it possible to identify and negotiate all the root canals to their full working length for subsequent preparation, cleaning and obturation? If these objectives can be met, then the endodontic prognosis of the tooth in question is excellent, regardless of whether the tooth is being root treated for the first time or being retreated.

These factors will determine the overall prognosis of the tooth. It is essential to advise patients that the tooth will need to be investigated in the first instance to establish the feasibility and prognosis of treatment. Prior to embarking on the treatment, it should be discussed that if there is insufficient tooth structure and/or a deep crack is found, then extraction may be indicated. Furthermore, the patient should be advised of the importance of the final cuspal coverage restoration as an integral part of the treatment.

How do endodontically treated teeth differ from vital teeth?

Endodontically treated teeth appear to be more susceptible to fracture compared with teeth with vital pulps. This is due to a cumulative effect of the following:

- *Loss of tooth structure*: Teeth requiring endodontic treatment have usually undergone significant tooth structure loss due to caries or previous restorative procedures. This often results in loss of the marginal ridge(s). This loss of the marginal ridges, in combination with the effects of access cavity preparation, results in posterior teeth being more susceptible to fracture under functional loads. Access cavity preparation should therefore be carried out conservatively (with respect to dentine removal), but without compromising the technical objectives of the root canal treatment.

- *Root canal and/or post preparation*: Over-zealous instrumentation and post preparations may result in unnecessary and excessive removal of dentine, which may result in thinner root walls that predispose the tooth to fracture. This is particularly important in the pericervical region (the region extending approximately 4 mm coronal and apical to the crestal bone level) of the tooth, where excessive coronal preparation of the root canal will weaken the root most adversely. Larger-sized and tapered root canal instruments should therefore be avoided. For the same reasons, large post-space preparations should not be created, and when necessary posts should be placed 'passively' to be accommodated within the existing root canal anatomy.

- *Disinfection*: Excessive use of irrigants such as sodium hypochlorite and ethylenediaminetetraacetic acid (EDTA) may change the biomechanical properties of dentine. Long-term calcium hydroxide intracanal dressings may also have a similar effect, resulting in reduced fracture resistance and increased brittleness.

- *Obturation*: Excessive compaction pressure (vertical or lateral) of gutta percha may also result in root fracture of an already compromised root. Care must be taken when cementing posts for the same reason.

- *Loss of proprioception*: The loss of proprioception in pulpless teeth results in a higher loading threshold. This may result in increased stresses in a tooth that already has compromised residual sound dentine. Furthermore, endodontically treated teeth commonly present for initial treatment with cracks, and these will be subjected to higher stresses, predisposing them to propagation and, at worst, a vertical root fracture.

When there is sufficient time available, it is best to place the definitive plastic (core/foundation) restoration immediately after the endodontic treatment has been completed. The access cavity will be adequately disinfected and still isolated with dental dam; these are the ideal conditions for restoring the tooth. In these circumstances, the tooth can be restored with a definitive plastic restoration (for example, composite resin). If a cuspal coverage restoration is planned, as is the case for most posterior teeth, then the tooth may be restored with a plastic core, in advance of the subsequent onlay or crown preparation.

It has been shown that the survival of endodontically treated posterior teeth is significantly improved with cuspal coverage restoration. The last tooth in the arch (terminal tooth) is the most susceptible to fracture. Similarly, teeth without proximal contacts are more at risk of structural failure.

When should the tooth be restored with a cuspal coverage restoration?

The survival rate for well-executed endodontic treatment is over 90%. Therefore, providing the objectives of endodontic treatment have been met (i.e. identification, negotiation, preparation and obturation of all root canals to the full working length), the tooth may be restored by a cuspal coverage restoration immediately or temporized and restored within a few weeks. If the endodontic prognosis of the tooth is uncertain (for example, persistent symptoms, inability to negotiate up to the ideal working length), the provision of a cuspal coverage restoration may need to be delayed until there are definite signs of healing (for example, significant improvement in the patient's symptoms). In the interim period the tooth can be restored with a direct plastic onlay or an acrylic temporary crown.

What are the aims of restoring an endodontically treated tooth?

- Provide a coronal seal to prevent microbial leakage, and therefore contamination of the disinfected root canal system.
- Protect the remaining tooth tissue from fracture.
- Minimise undesirable stress distribution to the residual tooth structure.
- Allow the tooth to be a functional unit within the dental arch.
- Maintain or improve aesthetics.

Are there any situations when a cuspal coverage restoration is not indicated for restoring an endodontically treated posterior tooth?

An occlusal access cavity may be restored with a direct composite resin restoration when the marginal ridges of the tooth remain intact. The decision as to the most appropriate restoration must take into consideration a number of factors, which include the presence of cracks, occlusion (guidance in lateral excursive and protrusive movements), position of tooth in the arch, number of proximal contacts and whether there are any signs of heavy occlusal loading. In addition, parafunctional habits such as clenching or grinding may indicate that a cuspal coverage restoration is necessary even if the tooth has intact marginal ridges.

Treatment

In this case the existing amalgam restoration was removed to confirm that the tooth was restorable. A superficial stained crack line was noted, which did not extend into the internal walls of the pulp chamber (Figure 6.2.3a). Endodontic treatment was carried out in a single visit (Figure 6.2.3b) and temporised with a well-adapted intermediate restorative material (IRM) temporary restoration, as there was insufficient time to place a permanent restoration. At a subsequent visit, the tooth was restored with a composite resin core and prepared for a lithium disilicate ceramic onlay (Figure 6.2.4a), impressions were taken and the tooth was temporarily restored with an acrylic onlay. Two weeks later the onlay was adhesively cemented with a composite resin luting cement (Figure 6.2.4b–d). The amalgam restoration on the UL5 was replaced with a ceramic onlay based on the patient's wishes. At the review appointment the patient was asymptomatic and clinical examination was unremarkable (Figures 6.2.5 and 6.2.6).

Discussion

The restorability and type of post-endodontic restoration should always be considered *before* embarking on endodontic treatment. Failure to do so may result in treatment complications or, worse still, the inability to adequately restore the tooth once endodontic treatment has been completed.

Occlusal loading of posterior teeth during mastication, but more so with parafunction, can be considerable. Loss of the marginal ridge(s) and/or preexisting fracture lines in otherwise intact marginal ridge(s) will result in increased cuspal flexure and reduce the fracture resistance of the endodontically treated teeth. Therefore, cuspal coverage restorations (i.e. crowns and onlays) are usually indicated for endodontically treated posterior teeth when opposed by natural teeth or implant-retained crowns. The design of the cuspal coverage restoration is determined by the residual tooth structure (volume and location), tooth location in the arch and proximal contacts, occlusal considerations and thereafter material choice (for example, type and thickness of material). Given that residual tooth volume is such an important factor in determining survival, it is essential to conserve remaining tooth tissue when planning and executing the preparation of the cuspal coverage restoration. Therefore, when possible, an onlay preparation is more desirable than a full-coverage crown preparation.

Endo-crowns may be considered for posterior teeth with extensively damaged clinical crowns, decreased interocclusal clearance, as well as teeth with short, divergent roots. These are full-coverage monolithic composite or ceramic crowns that incorporate a dowel extension into the pulp chamber for retention. The margins are circular equigingival or supragingival butt margins to preserve enamel to improve retention. Clinical studies have shown good success rates for endo-crowns in root-treated premolars and molars.

Each tooth should be assessed and treated according to its unique requirements. For example, it may be possible to avoid a cuspal coverage restoration on an endodontically treated posterior tooth with a class II cavity, which does not have to withstand high occlusal loads. For example, if the treated tooth was opposed by a denture, a direct plastic restoration (for example, composite resin) may be sufficient.

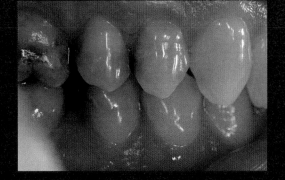

Figure 6.2.1 Photograph of the buccal view of the UL4.

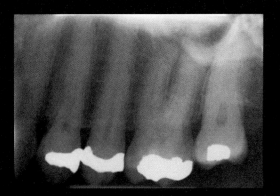

Figure 6.2.2 Pre-operative periapical radiograph of the UL4.

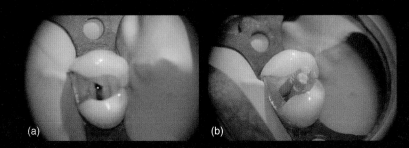

Figure 6.2.3 (a) The existing restoration was removed, along with removal of caries A superficial stained crack line that did not extend to the internal walls of the pulp chamber was noted on the UL4. The tooth was deemed restorable with three walls remaining and sufficient supragingival tooth structure in the distal-proximal box. (b) Two root canals were located, prepared and filled to good length.

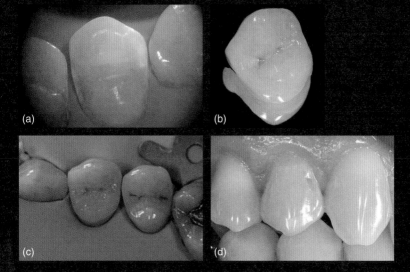

Figure 6.2.4 (a) A composite resin core is placed, after which the tooth is prepared for a conservative cuspal coverage ceramic onlay. Note how the residual walls (which have good thickness) are minimally prepared to preserve as much sound tooth structure as possible. (b) A lithium disilicate onlay has been fabricated, (c) tried in and then (d) adhesively cemented with composite luting cement. The patient requested that the amalgam restoration on the UL5 be replaced with a ceramic onlay, which was carried out at the same time as restoration of the UL4.

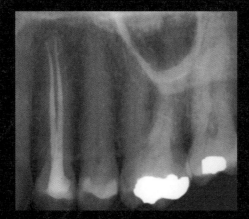

Figure 6.2.5 Post-operative periapical radiograph of the UL4 showing a good result with the endodontic treatment, well-adapted composite core and conservative cuspal protection of the tooth.

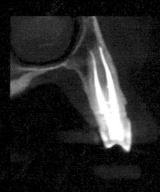

Figure 6.2.6 Cone beam computed tomography scan, eight years post treatment.

Further Reading

Bhuva, B., Giovarruscio, M., Rahim, N. et al. (2021). The restoration of root filled teeth: a review of the clinical literature. *International Endodontic Journal* 54: 509–535.

Mannocci, F., Bitter, K., Sauro, S., Ferrari, P., Austin, R., and Bhuva, B. (2022). Present status and future directions: The restoration of root filled teeth. *International Endodontic Journal* 55 Suppl 4. 1059–1084.

Mannocci, F., Bhuva, B., Roig, M. et al. (2021). European Society of Endodontology position statement: the restoration of root filled teeth. *International Endodontic Journal* 54: 1974–1981.

Mannocci, F., Cavalli, G., and Gagliani, M. (2008). The restorability of broken-down teeth. In: *Adhesive Restoration of Endodontically Treated Teeth* (ed. F. Mannocci, G. Cavalli, and M. Gagliani). Berlin: Quintessence, ch. 8.

Randow, K. and Glantz, P.O. (1986). On cantilever loading of vital and non-vital teeth-an experimental study. *Acta Odontologica Scandinavica* 44: 271–277.

Reeh, E.S., Messer, H.H., and Douglas, W.H. (1989). Reduction in tooth stiffness as a result of endodontic and restorative procedures. *Journal of Endodontics* 15: 512–516.

Thomas, R.M., Kelly, A., Tagiyeva, N., and Kanagasingam, S. (2020). Comparing endocrown restorations on permanent molars and premolars: a systematic review and meta-analysis. *British Dental Journal* https://doi.org/10.1038/s41415-020-2279-y.

6.3 *Internal Bleaching*

Neha Patel

Objectives

At the end of this case, the reader should understand the aetiology of discoloration and know how to manage a discoloured non-vital tooth.

Introduction

A 19-year-old female attended complaining of pain and discoloration of her upper left central incisor (UL1).

Complaint

The patient was suffering from an intermittent dull ache from tooth UL1 for the past year, which has progressively worsened along with a brown discoloration of the tooth (Figure 6.3.1).

Medical History

The patient was fit and healthy.

Dental History

Regular attender with no dental anxiety.

Social History

Non-smoker and non-drinker.

Pitt Ford's Problem-Based Learning in Endodontology, Second Edition. Edited by Elizabeth Shin Perry, Shanon Patel, Shalini Kanagasingam, and Samantha Hamer. © 2025 John Wiley & Sons Ltd. Published 2025 by John Wiley & Sons Ltd.

Examination

The patient presented with an unrestored dentition and discoloration of the UL1. The UL1 was tender to percussion and buccal palpation and was unresponsive to thermal test (Endo-Frost) and electric pulp test.

Radiographic Examination

- Normal bone levels.
- An apical radiolucency associated with the UL1.
- A wide pulp canal space (Figure 6.3.2).

Cone beam computed tomography

A small-volume cone beam computed tomography (CBCT) scan of tooth UL1 was taken to assess the location, size and spread of the periapical lesion. There was a large periapical radiolucency and associated thinning of the buccal alveolar plate (Figure 6.3.3).

Diagnosis

A diagnosis of pulpal necrosis with symptomatic apical periodontitis and immature apex was reached regarding the UL1.

What is extrinsic staining?

Extrinsic staining is staining of the outer enamel surface that can be removed and is the result of topical or extrinsic agents.

What are the factors predisposing to extrinsic staining?

- *Enamel defects*: Pits and defects can accumulate substances.
- *Salivary dysfunction*: Saliva helps remove food particles and plaque, which cause discoloration.
- *Poor oral hygiene*: Plaque and calculus build up results in black and brown staining.

What are the causes of extrinsic staining?

- *Food and beverages*: Coffee, tea and wines contain tannins, which result in brown staining. Foods containing polyphenols also can cause discoloration.
- *Tobacco*: Smoking cigarettes or cigars or chewing tobacco results in very dark brown and black stains, usually involving the cervical third to half of the tooth.
- *Chromogenic bacteria*: Bacterial species such as *Actinomyces* result in black staining due to poor oral hygiene. Fluorescent bacteria and fungi (*Penicillum* and *Aspergillum*) can result in green staining.

- *Topical medications*: Chlorhexidine/stannous fluoride can lead to brown staining.
- *Metallic compounds*: Exposure to iron, manganese and silver can result in black staining.

How are pigmentations classified?

Pigmentations are classified as follows:

- N1: Direct dental stain binding to tooth surface chromogenically. Chromogens are coloured particles that adhere to the enamel, e.g. coffee, tea, wine, metals and bacterial products.
- N2: Direct dental stain, whereby the chromogen changes colour after binding to the tooth.
- N3: Indirect dental stain, where a colourless pre-chromogen undergoes a chemical reaction after binding to the tooth, resulting in a stain.

What is intrinsic staining?

Intrinsic staining is discoloration incorporated into the structure of the tooth and cannot be removed physically. This can be in the enamel and/or the dentine and has varied distribution (regional, generalised, primary or secondary teeth).

What are the pre-eruptive causes of intrinsic staining?

- Tetracycline staining:
  - Susceptibility occurs in the second trimester in vitro → eight years post birth.
  - Severity/degree of staining is dependent on time and duration.
- Systemic conditions:
  - *Hyperbilirubinemia* results in bilirubin deposition in the enamel and dentine.
  - *Erthyropoietic porphyria* increases porphyrins, resulting in erythrodontia.
  - *Amelogenesis imperfecta*, caused by mutations of *AMELX*, *ENAM* or *MMP20* genes.
  - *Dentinogenesis imperfecta*, caused by changes in the *DSPP* gene.
  - *Enamel hypoplasia*, caused by vitamin A, C, D and calcium and phosphorous deficiency.
  - *Alkaptonuria*, an inherited metabolic disease.

What are the post-eruptive causes of intrinsic staining?

- Fluorosis:
  - Excess fluoride intake during the maturation stage of enamel formation, resulting in white streaks or patches.

- Trauma:
  - Ruptured blood vessels where product diffuses into tubules.
  - Haemoglobin degrades, resulting in a dark discoloration.
- Iatrogenic:
  - Failure to remove all pulpal remnants.
  - Amalgam/gold restorations cause dark grey/brown stains.
  - Silver in root canal sealers – Grossman/Kerr/silver points.
  - Mineral trioxide aggregate (MTA).

Treatment

What are the treatment options for this case?

- No treatment.
- Root canal treatment of the UL1 + internal/external bleaching.
- Root canal treatment of the UL1 + veneer/crown.
- Extraction.

Treatment plan

- Root canal treatment of tooth UL1.
- Internal/external bleaching of tooth UL1.

Access was gained and chemo-mechanical preparation was completed in the first visit. Minimal mechanical preparation was required and the canal was copiously irrigated with sodium hypochlorite and ethylenediaminetetraacetic acid (EDTA) solution.

Tooth UL1 was obturated using MTA followed by gutta percha. A 6–7 mm apical plug of MTA was packed into position incrementally using a Machtou plugger assisted by ultrasonics, then backfilled with gutta percha and pulp canal sealer, using a warm vertical condensation technique (Figure 6.3.4). The gutta percha was kept 3 mm below the cemento-enamel junction (CEJ) and a 2 mm glass ionomer cement plug was placed over the gutta percha. This allows for the tooth to be bleached from the gingival third upwards (Figure 6.3.5). The access cavity was cleaned with ultrasonic and water irrigation, removing any debris. The bleaching tray was tried in the patient's mouth to check it was well fitting and that minimal saliva would enter, ensuring no dilution of the gel.

A pre-operative shade was taken including photographs. The patient was given bleaching trays and instructions on how to load bleach into the tooth and how to keep the area clean. Tooth UL1 was successfully bleached and post-operative photographs were taken (Figure 6.3.6). The tooth was reviewed a year later and signs of healing were noted (Figure 6.3.7).

What needs to be considered prior to bleaching?

- Patient selection and compliance.
- Diagnosis/symptoms.
- Periapical status of tooth in question.
- Quality of the root filling.
- Pre-operative shade.

What instructions are given to the patient?

- Bleaching can be carried out over two-hourly sessions.
- You can bleach as many times as you like over the course of a day.
- Avoid coloured foods such as red wines, coffee and turmeric.
- Store bleach in the fridge and keep it away from sunlight.
- Brush your teeth prior to bleaching and swallow any excess saliva.
- Ensure the access cavity is clean and free from debris.
- Use a mirror and ensure your bleaching tray is ready.
- Place the tip of the bleaching syringe behind the tooth undergoing bleaching and move it forward until it drops into the hole.
- Push the syringe up and pump bleach in until some of the gel drops below the incisal edge.
- Any excess can be placed into the bleaching tray.
- Place the bleaching tray into your mouth.
- Once two hours have passed, remove the tray and clean it with cold water. Remove any excess gel from the access cavity.
- Once you feels that the tooth has sufficiently lightened, you can stop bleaching.

What Is in a Bleaching Kit?

- Two or three syringes of bleach.
- Syringe tips (check that they fit inside the access cavity).
- Teepees, monojet syringe and microbrushes to keep the access cavity clean.
- Instruction sheet.

A specialised tray can be made with cut-out windows on the teeth adjacent to that being bleached. This ensures that only the affected tooth will be whitened.

What is the mechanism of bleaching?

- Redox reaction (oxidation/reduction).
- Oxidising agent (bleach) has free radicals and impaired electrons that become reduced when they are given up.
- The reducing agent (substance being bleached) accepts the electrons and becomes oxidised.
- 10% carbamide peroxide is equivalent to 3.6% hydrogen peroxide.

What are the causes of failure to bleach?

- Lack of patient compliance.
- Prolonged treatment and open access.
- Existing restorations.
- Incomplete removal of access cavity restoration.
- Incomplete removal of gutta percha or sealer remnants.
- Extension of tray cervically.

Discussion and Conclusion

The use of internal bleaching can achieve the desired results without resorting to more aggressive or irreversible techniques, such as crowns or veneers. It also provides a less invasive and often more cost-effective approach. It is key, however, that the true nature and cause of the discolouration are identified, to understand whether internal bleaching will be successful or even possible. The internal/external bleaching technique is dependent on a compliant patient who has the dexterity to place the bleach into the tooth. It is important that it can be placed to below the level of the CEJ to allow for the entire crown of the tooth to be evenly bleached. The access cavity must therefore also be clean, free of any debris and the gutta percha reduced to the correct level. Any existing restorations will not bleach and must be replaced post bleaching for an ideal aesthetic result.

Alternative techniques include the walking bleach technique and the chairside power bleaching technique. The bleaching agents commonly used for these techniques include hydrogen peroxide (5–35%), carbamide peroxide (10–16%) or sodium perborate. The walking bleach technique involves replacement of the bleaching agent on a weekly basis until the desired colour change is achieved, usually after two to four visits.

When choosing the appropriate bleaching agent and effective concentration, clinicians will be guided by their local regulations. In the UK and the European Union (since 2010), whitening treatment can only be prescribed by a registered dental professional after a clinical examination, in concentrations of up to 6% hydrogen peroxide. Such products cannot be used on any person under the age of 18 unless it is for the prevention or treatment of disease. Sodium perborate is no longer used due to safety concerns, as the European Union has classified all 'borate substances' as carcinogenic, mutagenic or toxic for reproduction. By law, teeth whitening products can only be sold directly to the public if they contain a maximum of 0.1% hydrogen peroxide. All other products above this concentration and up to 6% must be provided by a dentist.

There is a risk of external cervical resorption associated with non-vital bleaching procedures. External cervical resorption can occur more frequently with the use of higher concentrations of bleach and thermo-catalytic techniques, especially in teeth with a history of trauma. Patients must be informed of the risk of root resorption as well as the possibility of reoccurrence of discoloration in the long term.

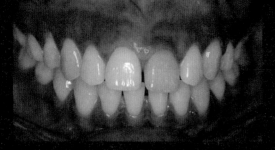

Figure 6.3.1 Clinical pre-operative labial photograph.

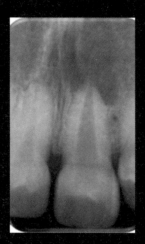

Figure 6.3.2 Pre-operative periapical radiograph of tooth UL1.

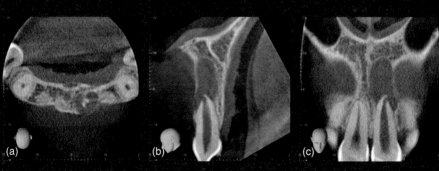

Figure 6.3.3 Pre-operative cone beam computed tomography of tooth UL1: (a) axial view, (b) sagittal view, (c) coronal view.

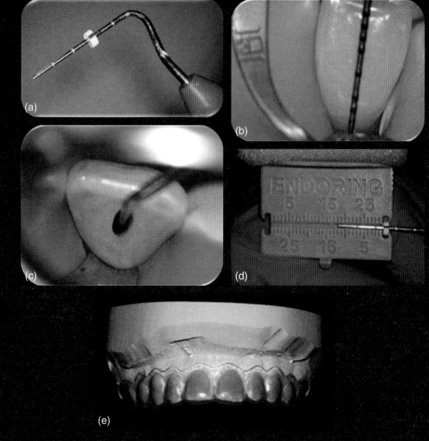

Figure 6.3.4 (a) Machtou plugger. (b) Cemento-enamel junction (CEJ) measured with plugger labially. (c) Level of CEJ recorded. (d) CEJ can now be measured internally through the access cavity. (e) Bleaching tray.

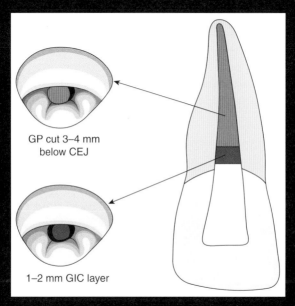

GP cut 3–4 mm below CEJ

1–2 mm GIC layer

Figure 6.3.5 Layers of filling material in relation to the cemento-enamel junction.

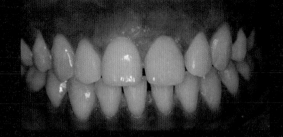

Figure 6.3.6 Clinical post-operative labial photograph.

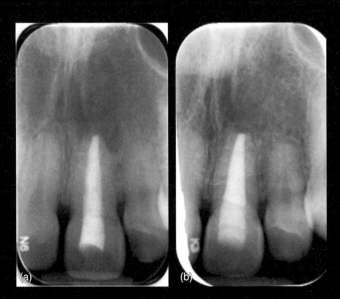

Figure 6.3.7 (a) Post-operative periapical radiograph. (b) One-year review periapical radiograph.

Further Reading

Abbott, P. and Heah, S.Y. (2009). Internal bleaching of teeth: an analysis of 255 teeth. *Australian Dental Journal* 54 (4): 326–333.

Coelho, A.S., Garrido, L., Mota, M. et al. (2020). Non-vital tooth bleaching techniques: a systematic review. *Coatings* 10 (1): 61.

Frank, A.C., Kanzow, P., Rödig, T., and Wiegand, A. (2022). Comparison of the bleaching efficacy of different agents used for internal bleaching: a systematic review and meta-analysis. *Journal of Endodontics* 48 (2): 171–178.

Kahler, B. (2022). Present status and future directions – Managing discoloured teeth. *International Endodontic Journal* 55 (Suppl. 4), 922–950.

Plotino, G., Buono, L., Grande, N.M. et al. (2008). Nonvital tooth bleaching: a review of the literature and clinical procedures. *Journal of Endodontics* 34 (4): 394–407.

Poyser, N.J., Kelleher, M.G., and Briggs, P.F. (2004). Managing discoloured non-vital teeth: the inside/outside bleaching technique. *Dental Update* 31 (4): 204–14.

VII Dental Trauma

7.1 *Complicated Crown Fracture*

Elizabeth Shin Perry

Objectives

At the end of this case the reader should understand the diagnosis and management of a complicated crown fracture. In addition, the reader should understand the treatment decisions involved in determining whether vital pulp therapy should be performed in such cases.

Introduction

A 13-year-old male patient presented with an enamel–dentine fracture and pulp exposure of the upper left central incisor (UL1) after an accident playing basketball two days previously. He was seen by his dentist, who recommended that he be seen by the endodontist for treatment.

Chief Complaint

The patient reported that the tooth was sensitive to hot and cold for less than 10 seconds. There was no lingering or spontaneous pain.

Medical History

Unremarkable.

Dental History

The patient was a regular attender and visited his dentist every six months.

Pitt Ford's Problem-Based Learning in Endodontology, Second Edition. Edited by Elizabeth Shin Perry, Shanon Patel, Shalini Kanagasingam, and Samantha Hamer. © 2025 John Wiley & Sons Ltd. Published 2025 by John Wiley & Sons Ltd.

Clinical Examination

Extraoral examination was unremarkable and intraoral examination revealed a mixed dentition with good oral hygiene. The incisal half of the crown of the UL1 had fractured off (Figure 7.1.1) and there was a 2 mm exposure of the pulp (Figure 7.1.2a). All four upper incisors were non-tender to percussion or palpation. The teeth had a positive response to thermal testing (cold). Tooth UL1 responded normally to pulp sensibility testing. The patient's mother had saved the fractured segment of tooth with the hope that it could be used in the repair of the tooth.

What did the radiograph reveal about tooth UL1?

- An angulated fracture across the mesial pulp horn with loss of half of the crown.
- A large root canal space with an open apex (Figure 7.1.3).
- Thin root walls.

Diagnosis and Treatment Planning

Diagnosis of tooth UL1 was reversible pulpitis associated with a complicated enamel–dentine fracture. The root apex appeared to be open and the tooth had an immature root anatomy with a large root canal space.

What are the treatment options for tooth UL1?

- Vital pulp therapy
  - Pulp cap
  - Partial pulpotomy
  - Deep pulpotomy
- Root canal treatment
- Extraction

In cases of complicated crown fracture and exposure of the pulp, vital pulp therapy is the preferred option when possible. By maintaining the vitality of the pulp in a tooth with immature root anatomy, the physiological development of the root continues. In mature teeth with complicated crown fracture, the vitality of the pulp may be maintained and is desirable in many cases over complete removal of the pulp. In these patients, removal of the pulp should only be performed if the pulp appears to be irreversibly inflamed, vital pulp therapy is not successful and the pulp becomes necrotic, or if the patient exhibits symptoms that are not resolving.

Conversations with the parents of the young patient should include the possibility that root canal treatment may become necessary in the future, but that vital pulp therapy gives the tooth the best chance for maturation of the root and long-term survival. In addition, due to the nature of traumatic dental injuries, the neighbouring teeth should be assessed regularly for clinical and radiographic changes.

What is the difference between an uncomplicated and a complicated crown fracture?

An uncomplicated crown fracture is a fracture of the enamel and dentine only, while a complicated crown fracture is a fracture of the enamel and dentine with exposure of the pulp (Figure 7.1.2b).

Treatment

Local anaesthetic was administered and dental dam isolation was performed. The external surface of the tooth was disinfected with sodium hypochlorite. The exposed pulp appeared to be inflamed and bled easily. The exposed pulp was removed stepwise using a sterile round diamond bur in a high-speed dental handpiece with water coolant until haemostasis could be achieved. Placement of a cotton pellet moistened with 2.5% sodium hypochlorite gently over the exposed pulp for several minutes controls the bleeding in healthy non-inflamed pulp tissue.

In this case the pulp tissue was removed to the level of the cemento-enamel junction before healthy non-bleeding tissue was observed (Figure 7.1.4). Subsequently, 3 mm of Biodentine was placed directly over the exposed pulp followed by glass ionomer (Figures 7.1.5 and 7.1.6). The fractured segment was carefully reattached. A groove was made in the fractured fragment to increase the bonding surface area. The exposed dentine on the fragment and tooth surface was acid etched and a dual-cure bonded composite resin was used to reattach the fragment. After the position was confirmed through the surgical microscope, the area was light cured on the buccal and palatal (Figures 7.1.7, 7.1.8 and Table 7.1.1).

What material should be used in vital pulp therapy?

Historically, calcium hydroxide has been used to seal pulpal exposures due to its antimicrobial activity and formation of mineralised hard tissue. However, its limitations are well documented, including high solubility, poor sealing ability and porous defects found in the resultant dentinal bridge.

Currently, the use of calcium silicate cements for vital pulp therapy procedures has consistently demonstrated excellent results. The calcium silicate cements are biocompatible, osteogenic and bioactive and have been shown to yield a consistently superior dentine layer over the affected pulp

Table 7.1.1 Clinical decisions following crown fracture with pulp exposure.

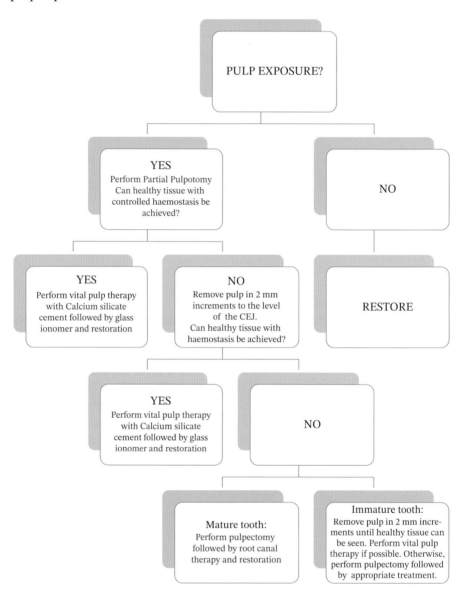

compared to calcium hydroxide. The dentine layer formed in prior cases treated by calcium hydroxide has been shown to have tunnelling defects that are prone to microleakage. Early calcium silicate cements have had difficult handling properties and setting times, and mineral trioxide aggregate (MTA) in particular has been linked to tooth discoloration. The latest generation of calcium silicate cements has overcome these issues and the material of choice should depend on evidence-based studies and patient-centred outcomes (Table 7.1.2).

Table 7.1.2 Calcium silicate cements.

Biodentine	Endosequence Root Repair Material	MTA	Bioaggregate
• Powder: Tricalcium silicate, dicalcium silicate, calcium carbonate, calcium oxide, and zirconium oxide as radiopacifier • Liquid: Water, calcium chloride, hydrosoluble polymer (plasticizing agent)	• Pre-mixed paste or putty: calcium silicates, monobasic calcium phosphate, zirconium oxide, tantalum oxide, proprietary fillers and thickening agents	• Powder: Dicalcium silicate, tricalcium silicate, tricalcium aluminate, calcium sulfate, tricalcium aluminoferrite, bismuth oxide as radiopacifier • Liquid: Distilled water	• Powder: Tricalcium silicate, dicalcium silicate, hydroxyapatite, calcium silicate oxide, tantalum oxide, calcium phosphate silicate • Liquid: Distilled water

What are the options for restoration of a complicated crown fracture?

- Reattach fractured fragment if available.
- Bonded composite restoration.
- Partial-coverage porcelain restoration (veneer).
- Full-coverage crown restoration.
- Post and core, full-coverage crown (in cases with significant loss of tooth structure).

When assessing options for restoration of a tooth with a complicated crown fracture, the age of the patient and the anticipated longevity of the restoration should be considered. In the very young patient a conservative restoration is preferable, especially if the growth and development of the tooth and bony structures are incomplete. In this case, reattachment of the fractured segment allowed for maximal preservation of tooth structure. The patient will be able to proceed with further restoration of the tooth as he matures.

What follow-up is needed for a complicated crown fracture?

Regular follow-up is recommended to evaluate the resolution of the symptoms as well as to evaluate the other teeth that may have been affected by the trauma. Because a traumatic dental injury is rarely limited to one tooth, the surrounding teeth can often experience concussion or luxation injuries that manifest endodontic disease at a later date. Thus, follow-up visits should include assessment of symptoms and vitality of the pulp if it was maintained in the fractured tooth as well as the surrounding teeth.

The patient was followed at regular intervals and the symptoms of achiness and thermal sensitivity resolved immediately. An eight-month review revealed formation of a calcific bridge adjacent to the Biodentine (Figure 7.1.9). The tooth responded to sensibility testing and the adjacent teeth also responded within normal limits to endodontic testing. At the

Table 7.1.3 Parameters of successful vital pulp therapy.

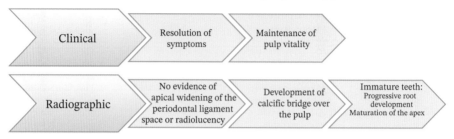

| Clinical | Resolution of symptoms | Maintenance of pulp vitality | |
| Radiographic | No evidence of apical widening of the periodontal ligament space or radiolucency | Development of calcific bridge over the pulp | Immature teeth: Progressive root development Maturation of the apex |

20- and 26-month reviews, continued calcific bridge formation as well as apical closure and root maturation were noted (Figures 7.1.10, 7.1.11 and Table 7.1.3).

Discussion

Appropriate management of the complicated crown fracture is essential for the long-term health of the tooth. With the exposure of the pulp, the situation must be assessed carefully to administer the best treatment option for each patient. In the young patient with immature root anatomy, it is preferable to maintain the vitality of the pulp for the continued growth and development of the root. For the mature patient, maintenance of the vitality of the pulp tissue, when possible, is an excellent option for conservative treatment of the tooth. After removal of the inflamed coronal pulp tissue, if haemostasis can be achieved and healthy pulp tissue is observed, vital pulp therapy should be considered as the first line of treatment. With all teeth, a quality well-sealed restoration is important for the protection of the tooth as well as for the patient's confidence and well-being.

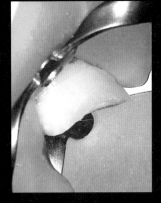

Figure 7.1.1 Clinical photograph showing fractured incisal edge.

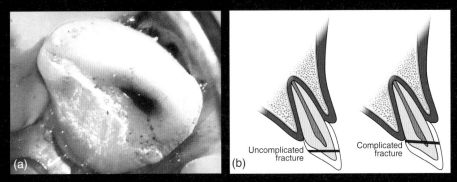

Figure 7.1.2 (a) Clinical photograph showing exposed pulp. (b) Diagram of uncomplicated and complicated crown fractures.

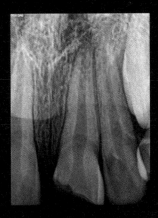

Figure 7.1.3 Pre-operative radiograph showing an immature root with an open apex.

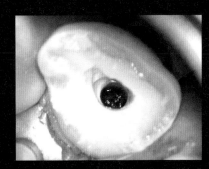

Figure 7.1.4 Pulpotomy was performed and inflamed pulp tissue was removed until healthy non-bleeding tissue was observed.

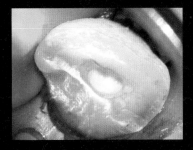

Figure 7.1.5 Biodentine was placed directly over the pulp.

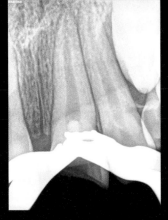

Figure 7.1.6 Radiograph showing Biodentine placed directly over the pulp tissue.

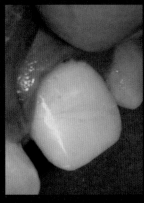

Figure 7.1.7 The access opening was sealed with glass ionomer and the fractured segment was reattached with dual-cure bonded composite.

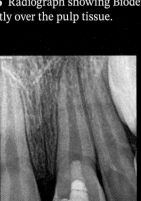

Figure 7.1.8 Immediate post-operative radiograph.

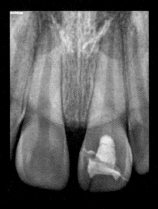

Figure 7.1.9 Eight-month follow-up radiograph showing a small calcific bridge forming below the Biodentine.

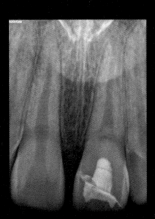

Figure 7.1.10 20-month follow-up radiograph showing continued calcific bridge formation and apical closure and root maturation.

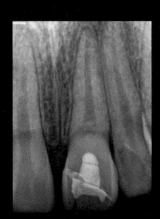

Figure 7.1.11 26-month follow-up radiograph showing a significant calcific bridge, increased root width and apical closure indicating continued root maturation.

Further Reading

American Association of Endodontists (2021). AAE position statement on vital pulp therapy. Chicago, IL: AAE. https://www.aae.org/wp-content/uploads/2021/05/VitalPulpTherapyPositionStatement_v2.pdf.

Bogen, G., Dammaschke, T., and Chandler, N. (2021). Vital pulp therapy. In: *Pathways of the Pulp*, 12e (ed. L. Berman and K.M. Hargreaves), 849–876. St. Louis, MO: Elsevier.

Bourguignon, C., Cohenca, N., Lauridsen, E. et al. (2020). et al, International Association of Dental Traumatology guidelines for the management of traumatic dental injuries: 1. Fractures and luxations. *Dental Traumatology.* 36 (4): 314–330.

Cvek (1993). Partial pulpotomy in crown-fractured incisors-results 3–15 years after treatment. *Acta Stomatologica Croatica* 27: 167–173.

Duncan, H.F., El-Karim, I., Dummer, P.M.H., Whitworth, J., and Nagendrababu, V. (2023). Factors that influence the outcome of pulpotomy in permanent teeth. *International Endodontic Journal 56*, suppl 2: 62.81.

Parirokh, M., Torabinejad, M., and Dummer, P.M.H. (2018). Mineral trioxide aggregate and other bioactive endodontic cements: an updated overview – Part 1: Vital pulp therapy. *International Endodontic Journal* 51 (2): 177–205.

Smith, A.J. (2012). Dentin formation and repair. In: *Dental Pulp* (ed. K.M. Hargreaves, H.E. Goodis, F.R. Tay, et al.). Chicago, IL: Quintessence, ch. 3.

7.2 *Horizontal Root Fracture*
Peng-Hui Teng

Objectives

At the end of this case, the reader should be able to diagnose and manage root fracture cases and be able to formulate a follow-up protocol for such injuries.

Introduction

A 45-year-old male presented with mild intermittent throbbing pain associated with his upper left central incisor (UL1). He had also noticed that the tooth had discoloured.

Chief Complaint

The patient was asymptomatic when he presented to the clinic. There had been previous episodes of spontaneous pain; each episode lingered for a few minutes before the pain resolved by itself. He recalled a history of trauma to the UL1 tooth more than 10 years ago after being accidentally elbowed while playing football.

Medical History

Unremarkable.

Dental History

The patient was a regular dental attender, with a minimally restored dentition.

Pitt Ford's Problem-Based Learning in Endodontology, Second Edition. Edited by Elizabeth Shin Perry, Shanon Patel, Shalini Kanagasingam, and Samantha Hamer.
© 2025 John Wiley & Sons Ltd. Published 2025 by John Wiley & Sons Ltd.

Clinical Examination

The crown of the UL1 had greyish discolouration. The tooth was unrestored. It was not tender to percussion and responded negatively to pulp sensibility testing. There was no swelling or sinus tract associated with the UL1. The adjacent maxillary teeth were asymptomatic and responded normally to sensibility testing. The periodontal probing depths and mobility of UL1 and the adjacent maxillary teeth were within the normal range. Clinical findings associated with root fracture were listed in Table 7.2.1.

Radiographic evaluation (Figure 7.2.1) revealed an oblique fracture line at the middle third of the root of the UL1. The radiolucent line was more evident in the mesial aspect crossing the root canal centrally and was less discernible at the distal half of the root. The root canal of UL1 was patent and clearly visible from the radiograph. There was no displacement of the coronal and apical segment. The periodontal ligament (PDL) space was intact and no periapical radiolucency was associated with the UL1. There was no abnormality detected for the adjacent teeth (UL2 and UL3). No sign of alveolar fracture was seen in the radiograph. A periapical radiograph of UR1 and UR2 was also taken to rule out any traumatic dental injuries (TDI) and periapical radiolucency (Figure 7.2.1). A list of radiographic findings associated with root fracture can be found in Table 7.2.2.

A small field-of-view (FOV) cone beam computed tomography (CBCT) scan was taken to assess the true nature of the injury (Figure 7.2.2). The CBCT scan confirmed the presence of an oblique root fracture in the mid-root level. The root fracture was incomplete and only involved the labial aspect of the root canal.

Table 7.2.1 Clinical features of a horizontal root fracture.

- Coronal segment of the affected tooth may be mobile and may be displaced
- The affected tooth may be tender to percussion
- Bleeding from the gingival sulcus of the affected tooth may be seen
- There may be a negative response to pulp sensibility testing initially, indicating transient or permanent nerve damage
- Transient discolouration of the crown of the affected tooth may occur

Table 7.2.2 Radiographic features of a horizontal root fracture.

- Complete/incomplete radiolucent line of varying diameter between the coronal and apical root segment
- Pulp obliteration of coronal segment as a complication of healing
- Periradicular radiolucency adjacent to the necrotic coronal segment if the coronal segment has turned necrotic and developed periradicular periodontitis

Diagnosis and Treatment Planning

What is the diagnosis?

A diagnosis of horizontal root fracture with necrotic coronal segment was reached for the UL1.

Why was a cone beam computed tomography scan taken?

The latest International Association of Dental Traumatology (IADT) guidelines recommend taking a parallel periapical radiograph, two additional periapical radiographs at different horizontal and/or vertical angulations and a standard occlusal radiograph for the assessment of root fracture (Bourguignon et al. 2020). Conventional radiographs such as standard occlusal radiographs are subjected to various limitations and errors, such as image elongation or foreshortening, cone cutting, overlapping and anatomical noise. Moreover, conventional radiographs could only assess the proximal aspect of the tooth, which is not always the case in complex TDI such as root fracture. For instance, an oblique root fracture in the sagittal plane could easily be missed by a conventional radiograph, even with the help of a parallax technique. A root fracture will only be detected if the x-ray beam passes directly through the fracture line.

IADT guidelines and the European Society of Endodontology (ESE) position statement recommend that a CBCT scan should be taken as an adjunct for complex TDI that could be under-appreciated in conventional radiographs. CBCT, although with a lower resolution than a periapical radiograph, produces diagnostically sufficient three-dimensional images that can accurately illustrate the location, extent and true nature of a root fracture. As a CBCT scanner was available in this case, it was considered appropriate to opt for CBCT to allow us to assess the UL1 and adjacent teeth in three dimensions with one scan. In cases where CBCT is not available, the recommendations in the IADT guidelines should be followed.

How does the radiation dose of a cone beam computed tomography scan compare to conventional radiographs?

It is widely accepted that a CBCT scan has a higher radiation dose compared to a conventional radiograph. An intraoral radiograph has an effective dose of 2–9 μSv, whereas a small FOV CBCT has an effective dose of 19–44 μSv. The cumulative radiation dose of a series of intraoral radiographs (periapical radiographs at different angles and standard occlusal radiograph) used in root fracture assessment is comparable to a CBCT scan, which allows detailed assessment of the affected tooth and the associated root fracture in any view. The radiation dose of CBCT is similar to the cosmic radiation dose of two to three long-haul flights from London to New York.

What is the treatment plan for this patient?

The treatment plan was to perform root canal treatment (RCT) for the UL1 followed by non-vital bleaching of the tooth.

Treatment

RCT for the UL1 was initiated under dental dam isolation. The RCT was done to the coronal segment up to the fracture line only. The working length was estimated using a pre-operative CBCT scan (Figure 7.2.3). The root canal was chemo-mechanically prepared and obturated with mineral trioxide aggregate (MTA) (Figure 7.2.4). The access cavity was then restored with a composite resin restoration. The post-operative radiograph revealed good root canal filling up to the fracture line (Figures 7.2.5 and 7.2.6). The patient was referred back to the referring dentist for internal bleaching.

Why was root canal treatment done only to the coronal segment?

Pulpal healing in a root fracture is normally favourable, therefore RCT is usually not required unless the tooth becomes necrotic. Pulp necrosis typically involves only the coronal segment. The apical root segment usually remains vital and requires no further treatment, as the blood supply for the apical root segment is unaffected. Hence RCT is only indicated for the necrotic coronal root segment.

What challenges might the clinician face during root canal treatment?

RCT in the coronal segment can pose various technical challenges to the clinician. As RCT is only performed to the level of the fracture line, the coronal segment is similar to an immature root with a wide apical foramen. Caution is required to prevent inadvertent over-instrumentation and extrusion of root filling material. Apexification using calcium silicate cement maybe beneficial over conventional gutta percha root filling due to its biocompatibility and ability to promote hard tissue repair.

The clinician may also face difficulty in achieving a consistent working length in a wide apical foramen of the coronal root segment. Measurement of working length from a pre-operative CBCT scan provides a feasible solution for this problem. In this case, CBCT was used to measure the working length for instrumentation (Figure 7.2.3). The post-operative radiograph confirmed the accuracy of CBCT in measuring the working length of tooth UL1.

What type of healing is expected with a horizontal root fracture?

The healing of root fracture can be divided into four types of healing pattern (Table 7.2.3).

Table 7.2.3 The four types of healing patterns of horizontal root fractures.

Types of healing in root fracture	Details
Healing with hard tissue	• Most favourable healing • Usually seen in root fracture with intact pulp and minimal/no displacement of coronal segment
Healing with connective tissue	• Often seen in root fracture with displacement of coronal segment such as extrusion or lateral luxation • Dominated by periodontal ligament (PDL) cells
Healing with bone and connective tissue	• Similar to healing with connective tissue, but only observed in growing patient • Bone tissue is formed between coronal and apical segments, with intact PDL surrounding both segments
Non-healing with granulation tissue	• Seen in root fracture with necrotic and infected coronal segment • Formation of granulation tissue between coronal and apical segment • Granulation tissue resembles granulation tissue formed in apical periodontitis

In this case, as the root fracture is incomplete and RCT has been performed to the necrotic coronal segment, we expect favourable healing by hard tissue in the UL1.

What is the follow-up protocol for horizontal root fracture cases?

In fresh root fracture cases, IADT guidelines recommend clinical and radiographic evaluations after four weeks, after six to eight weeks, after six months, after one year and then yearly review for at least five years. If splinting is required, the splint should be removed after four weeks in mid-root or apical root fracture cases. However, if the root fracture is located cervically, splinting of the mobile coronal segment for up to four months may be needed. In this case, tooth UL1 was not displaced and had normal physiological mobility, therefore no splinting was required.

Maintaining pulp vitality is essential in promoting hard tissue repair by dentine. It is recommended to monitor the pulp status of fresh root fracture cases for at least one year, as pulp necrosis and infection of the coronal root segment may occur later. In the current case, RCT was done to the coronal segment due to pulp necrosis, therefore the UL1 should be reviewed at yearly intervals like other root canal–treated teeth.

Discussion

This case is an example of a late diagnosis of horizontal root fracture. If the root fracture is not associated with the displacement and increased mobility of the coronal segment, the symptoms are usually mild and patients often choose not to seek dental treatment. Hence, the root fracture may remain undetected. Most cases of horizontal root fracture may heal without intervention.

If the patient presented with a luxated or mobile coronal fragment, the coronal segment should be repositioned as soon as possible and stabilised with a passive and flexible splint for four weeks. If the root fracture is located at the cervical third of the root, splinting for up to four months may be needed.

In cases where the root fracture extends supracrestally and the coronal segment is very mobile, removal of the coronal segment may be recommended. Root canal treatment of the apical segment followed by restoration with a post-retained crown, orthodontic or surgical extrusion of the apical segment, crown-lengthening procedure or even extraction and replacement may be considered in the treatment planning of such cases.

Most horizontal root fracture cases will have favourable pulpal healing. Therefore, no RCT should be initiated in the first visit for fresh root fracture cases. However, the pulp status should be monitored regularly as pulp necrosis may develop later. Pulp necrosis usually involves the coronal segment only. Hence, RCT is indicated solely for the coronal segment.

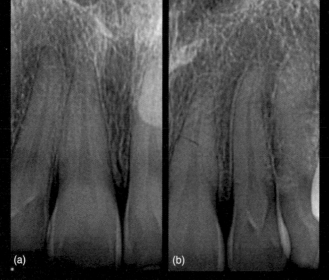

Figure 7.2.1 (a) Pre-operative periapical radiograph of UR1 and UR2 shows unaffected adjacent teeth. (b) Periapical radiograph of UL1 and UL2 shows an oblique radiolucent line in the mid-root of UL1 and unaffected UL2.

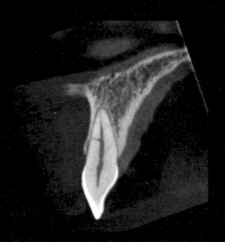

Figure 7.2.2 Sagittal view of cone beam computed tomography of the UL1.

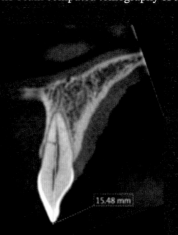

Figure 7.2.3 Estimation of working length using a pre-operative cone beam computed tomography scan (sagittal view).

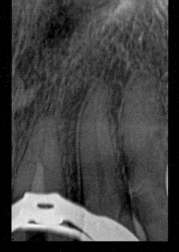

Figure 7.2.4 Mineral trioxide aggregate obturation of the UL1.

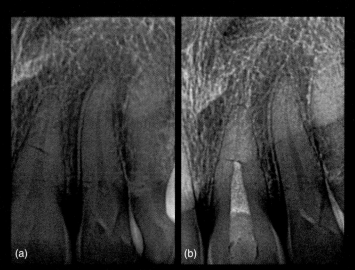

Figure 7.2.5 (a) Pre-operative and (b) post-operative periapical radiographs of the UL1

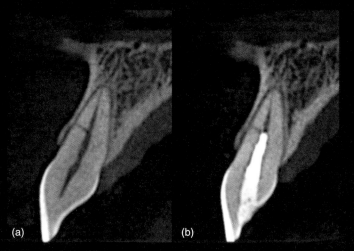

Figure 7.2.6 (a) Pre-operative and (b) post-operative cone beam computed tomography

Further Reading

Andreasen, J.O., Andreasen, F.M., and Andersson, L. (2019). *Textbook and Color Atlas of Traumatic Injuries to the Teeth*, 5e. Oxford: Blackwell.

Andreasen, J.O., Bakland, L.K., Flores, M.T. et al. (2011). *Traumatic Dental Injuries: A Manual*, 3e. Oxford: Blackwell.

Bourguignon, C., Cohenca, N., Lauridsen, E. et al. (2020). International Association of Dental Traumatology guidelines for the management of traumatic dental injuries: 1. Fractures and luxations. *Dental Traumatology* 36: 314–330.

Krastl, G., Weiger, R., Filippi, A. et al. (2021). European Society of Endodontology position statement: Endodontic management of traumatized permanent teeth. *International Endodontic Journal* 54:1473–1481.

Patel, S., Brown, J., Semper, M. et al. (2019). European Society of Endodontology position statement: use of cone beam computed tomography in endodontics: European Society of Endodontology (ESE) developed by. *International Endodontic Journal*. 52 (12): 1675–1678.

7.3 *Traumatic Dental Injuries*

Elizabeth Shin Perry

Objectives

At the end of this case, the reader should appreciate the significance of traumatic dental injuries and understand the immediate management, long-term treatment and follow-up involved.

Introduction

A 14-year-old boy presented two days after a traumatic dental injury to his anterior teeth.

Chief Complaint

The patient was helping his father to build a fence on a hot summer day when he felt dizzy and fainted. When he regained consciousness, he saw that his face was bruised and bloody and his upper right central incisor (UR1) was missing, and his upper left central incisor (UL1) was out of the socket, hanging on his orthodontic wire by the bracket (Figure 7.3.1). The UR1 was found on the kitchen floor one hour after the accident and was then stored in milk. Three hours after the accident, the teeth were replanted and splinted in the local hospital emergency clinic (Figure 7.3.2). The patient reported to his general dentist, who referred him to the endodontic specialist for follow-up treatment.

Pitt Ford's Problem-Based Learning in Endodontology, Second Edition. Edited by Elizabeth Shin Perry, Shanon Patel, Shalini Kanagasingam, and Samantha Hamer.
© 2025 John Wiley & Sons Ltd. Published 2025 by John Wiley & Sons Ltd.

Medical History

Unremarkable.

Dental History

The patient was a regular dental attender and visited his dentist every six months for hygiene visits. He was undergoing orthodontic treatment.

Clinical Examination

The patient saw an endodontist two days after the traumatic injury. Clinical examination revealed a titanium splint previously placed apically to the orthodontic brackets extending from the upper right lateral incisor (UR2) to the upper left canine (UL3). The orthodontic bracket on the UR1 was missing and the orthodontic wire from the UR1 to the entire left side was previously removed. All maxillary and mandibular anterior teeth were examined for signs of injury. The UR1, UL1, UL2 and LL1 were tender to percussion and palpation, with no response to thermal (cold) or electric pulp sensibility testing, whereas the remaining anterior teeth were responsive within normal limits.

What did the periapical radiographs and limited-view cone beam computed tomography images reveal?

The periapical radiographs of the upper and lower anterior teeth revealed widening of the periodontal ligament space at the apex of the UR1 and periapical radiolucencies associated with the UL1 and UL2 (Figure 7.3.3). Further imaging with a cone beam computed tomography (CBCT) scan confirmed the exact nature of the traumatic dental injury and also confirmed the position of the replanted teeth. The CBCT scan revealed:

- UR1: widening of the periodontal ligament at the apex. The tooth had been well approximated in the bony socket on replantation (Figure 7.3.4).
- UR2: periapical radiolucency and widening of the periodontal ligament on the buccal aspect of the root (Figure 7.3.5).
- UL1: periapical radiolucency with expansion of the cortical plate buccal to the root apex and widening of the periodontal ligament space on the palatal root surface, suggestive of the tooth being palatally displaced during the avulsion injury (Figure 7.3.6).

Diagnosis and Treatment Planning

What was the diagnosis?

The diagnosis for the UR1 and UL1 was pulpal necrosis and symptomatic apical periodontitis associated with prior avulsion and replantation. The diagnosis for the UL2 was subluxation with symptomatic apical periodontitis and for the LL1 was concussion with symptomatic apical periodontitis.

What was the treatment plan?

The initial treatment of replantation, repositioning and splinting of the avulsed teeth had already been performed by the emergency clinic on the day of the trauma two days previously. After assessment of the already managed traumatic dental injury, the treatment plan recommended for the UR1 and UL1 was to initiate root canal therapy within two weeks. Although the present splint that had been placed in the hospital emergency clinic was sufficient for temporary stabilisation of the replanted teeth, it was positioned apical to the orthodontic brackets and was not ideal for soft tissue management, thus removal and replacement of the splint were recommended.

The treatment recommended was:

- Remove the existing titanium splint and orthodontic brackets.
- Initiate endodontic treatment followed by intracanal medication of the root canal with calcium hydroxide.
- Place a new flexible splint, utilising orthodontic brackets and arch wire to splint/stabilise the traumatised teeth.
- Complete root canal treatment of the UR1 and UL1 in four weeks.
- Monitor the UL2 and LL1 on a periodic basis to evaluate pulp vitality and the onset of possible endodontic complications.

What is the role of calcium hydroxide in the treatment of traumatic dental injuries?

Calcium hydroxide is the intracanal medicament of choice for most traumatic dental injuries due to its ability to disinfect the canal space and dentine. It is antibacterial to most species within the root canal system, although some anaerobic bacteria such as *Enterococcus faecalis* may exhibit resistance. Calcium hydroxide has the ability to diffuse into the dentine and aids in the disinfection of infected dentinal tubules. The high pH of calcium hydroxide (between 12.5 and 12.8) permeates through the dentine to increase the pH of the outer root surface after several weeks, thereby preventing migration of the bacteria to the outer root surface, and may decrease the risk of root resorption.

Treatment

The titanium trauma splint was removed, and bracket and root canal treatment of the UR1 and UL1 was initiated. Root canal treatment was commenced under local anaesthetic and dental dam, the canals were instrumented and irrigated with sodium hypochlorite, and the canals were dressed with calcium hydroxide paste and sealed (Figure 7.3.7). The patient was seen that same day by his orthodontist to replace the missing bracket on the UR1 and maxillary arch wire (Figure 7.3.8). At the next visit, four weeks later, the calcium hydroxide was removed thoroughly with passive ultrasonic irrigation and the root canals were obturated with gutta percha and BC Sealer (Brasseler USA, Savannah, GA, USA). The access cavities were permanently sealed with a bonded composite restoration (Figure 7.3.9).

What about the continued negative response to pulp sensibility testing of the other teeth?

On completion of the root canal treatment of the UR1 and UL1 and at subsequent follow-up four weeks later, the vitality of the UL2 and LL1 was reevaluated. In luxation traumatic dental injuries, pulp sensibility testing may initially exhibit no response due to transient pulpal damage. Thus, endodontic treatment should not be started solely on the basis of no response to pulp sensibility testing.

In these types of injuries, teeth will often initially exhibit percussion tenderness, which is expected after the trauma. In these cases, the pulp vitality should be monitored for at least three months before initiation of endodontic treatment unless pulpal necrosis with definitive signs and symptoms can be confirmed. A thorough discussion with the patient should include the possibility of root canal treatment in the future (Table 7.3.1).

The UL2 exhibited signs of radiographic periapical pathology and symptoms of percussion tenderness six months after the initial trauma and was diagnosed with pulpal necrosis and symptomatic periapical periodontitis. Root canal treatment was completed (Figure 7.3.10). One year after the initial trauma, the LL1 exhibited calcification of the root canal and tenderness to percussion and was non-responsive to pulp sensibility tests (Figure 7.3.11). A diagnosis of pulpal necrosis with symptomatic periapical periodontitis was made and root canal treatment was completed (Figure 7.3.12).

Five years post trauma, periapical radiographs and CBCT revealed no signs of periapical pathology or root resorption. The teeth maintained their aesthetic appearance and remained asymptomatic (Figures 7.3.13 and 7.3.14). The patient is attending university and is very pleased that he was able to save his smile.

Table 7.3.1 Clinical findings and management of concussion and luxation dental injuries.

Injury	Clinical findings	Treatment	Follow-up
Concussion	Normal mobility + percussion ± pulp vitality	• No treatment • Monitor pulp vitality[a]	4 weeks 1 year
Subluxation	+ percussion + mobility ± pulp vitality	• No treatment • Splint with passive flexible splint for 2 weeks if excessive mobility of tenderness • Monitor pulp vitality[a]	2 weeks 3, 6 months 1 year
Extrusive luxation	Tooth appears elongated + mobility − pulp vitality likely	• Reposition tooth • Splint with passive flexible splint for 2–4 weeks • Monitor pulp vitality	2 weeks 1, 2, 3, 6 months 1 year Yearly for 5 years
Lateral luxation	Tooth displaced to palatal, lingual or labial immobile due to apex locked in bone − Pulp vitality likely	• Reposition tooth by disengaging from the locked position splint with passive flexible splint for 4 weeks • Monitor pulp vitality[a] • 2 weeks after injury evaluate for signs of pulpal necrosis and external resorption, if present, initiate endodontic procedures appropriate for immature vs mature teeth	2 weeks 1, 2, 3, 6 months 1 year Yearly for 5 years
Intrusive luxation	Tooth is displayed apically − Mobility − Pulp vitality likely	Immature tooth: • Allow eruption without intervention • If no eruption after 4 weeks, initiate orthodontic repositioning • Monitor pulp vitality[a] Mature tooth: • Allow re-eruption, if no re-eruption within 8 weeks, reposition surgically or orthodontically before ankylosis develops • Initiate root canal therapy at 2 weeks or as position allows	2 weeks 1, 2, 3, 6 months 1 year Yearly for 5 years

[a] If pulpal necrosis becomes evident, initiate appropriate endodontic treatment for stage of root development.

Table 7.3.2 Complications and treatment of traumatic dental injuries.

```
┌─────────────────┐              ┌─────────────────┐
│     Pulpal      │              │   Pulp canal    │
│    necrosis     │              │  obliteration   │
└─────────────────┘              └─────────────────┘

┌──────────┐   ┌──────────┐      ┌─────────────────┐
│  Mature  │   │ Immature │      │ Pulpal necrosis │
│   tooth  │   │   tooth  │      │     evident?    │
└──────────┘   └──────────┘      └─────────────────┘

┌──────────┐   ┌──────────────┐  ┌─────────────────┐
│ Root canal│   │ Apexification │  │  Initiate root  │
│  therapy  │   │ or regenerative│ │  canal therapy  │
└──────────┘   │  endodontic   │  └─────────────────┘
               │   procedure   │
               └──────────────┘
```

```
                    ┌─────────────┐
                    │  Resorption │
                    └─────────────┘

┌──────────────┐ ┌──────────┐ ┌─────────────────┐ ┌─────────────────┐
│   External   │ │ Internal │ │ Cervical invasive│ │  Replacement    │
│ inflammatory │ │          │ │                 │ │  (ankylosis)    │
└──────────────┘ └──────────┘ └─────────────────┘ └─────────────────┘

┌──────────────┐ ┌──────────┐ ┌─────────────────┐ ┌──────────────────┐
│ Initiate root│ │ Initiate │ │Initiate appropriate│ │If >1 mm infraposition│
│ canal therapy│ │root canal│ │  non-surgical   │ │ in growing patient,│
│ with long-term│ │ therapy  │ │ and/or surgical │ │ initiate decoronation│
│ calcium      │ │          │ │   treatment     │ └──────────────────┘
│ hydroxide    │ └──────────┘ └─────────────────┘
└──────────────┘
```

What are the complications of traumatic dental injuries?

The severity of the complications of traumatic dental injuries are directly related to the extent of the injury and the stage of development of the tooth. The main complications following traumatic dental injuries are pulpal necrosis followed by infection, pulp canal obliteration (PCO) and root resorption (Table 7.3.2).

Damage to the pulp resulting in pulpal necrosis is one of the most common complications of all traumatic dental injuries. In teeth with immature root formation and open apices, revascularisation is more likely to occur. When pulpal necrosis does occur, the stage of development of the tooth should be considered before commencing endodontic treatment. Regenerative endodontic procedures or apexification would be performed for immature teeth, while root canal therapy would be performed for mature teeth.

Table 7.3.3 Factors influencing the prognosis of a replanted tooth after avulsion.

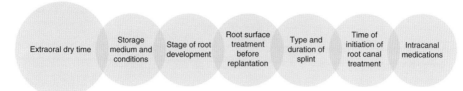

| Extraoral dry time | Storage medium and conditions | Stage of root development | Root surface treatment before replantation | Type and duration of splint | Time of initiation of root canal treatment | Intracanal medications |

Another sequela of traumatic dental injuries, especially severe luxation injuries, is PCO or narrowing of the root canal space. PCO alone is not an indication for intervention as many of these teeth contain vital tissue within the root canal, and endodontic treatment is not recommended in the absence of pulpal necrosis or other symptoms of symptomatic apical periodontitis.

Perhaps the most concerning complication of traumatic dental injuries is root resorption. External inflammatory resorption, replacement resorption (ankylosis), internal resorption and invasive cervical resorption have all been reported to be associated with traumatised teeth. Early detection and management of root resorption are essential to improve the long-term prognosis of these teeth.

In cases where the tooth is completely avulsed, there are additional factors that influence the prognosis after replantation (Table 7.3.3). It is essential to manage avulsed teeth in a timely and appropriate manner to ensure the best outcome (retention). Important prognostic factors include stage of root development, extra-oral time and storage medium (see Chapter 7.4, Table 7.4.1). The patient must be made aware of the importance of regular review appointments to assess for possible complications such as root resorption, pulp canal obliteration, discolouration as well as apical periodontitis.

Discussion

Knowledge of the appropriate management of traumatic dental injuries is essential to achieving successful outcomes for the patient. Timely, often immediate, treatment determines the patient's ability to retain the involved teeth for their lifetime. More often than not, an endodontist is not the first dental practitioner to see a patient after a traumatic dental injury has occurred. In complex cases, it is recommended that an early referral to an endodontist is made for advice and/or management. Regular follow-up appointments are essential.

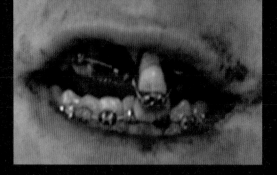

Figure 7.3.1 Immediate post trauma, avulsed UR1 and UR2.

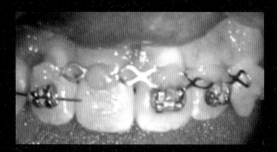

Figure 7.3.2 The hospital emergency clinic replanted, repositioned and splinted teeth three hours post trauma.

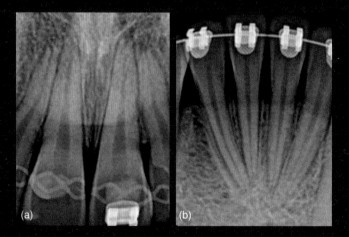

Figure 7.3.3 (a) Pre-operative radiograph shows widening of the periodontal ligament space at the apex of UR1 and apical radiolucency associated with UL1 and UL2. (b) Pre-operative radiograph shows normal appearance of lower anterior teeth.

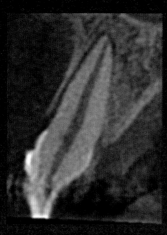

Figure 7.3.4 Cone beam computed tomography of UR1: widening of the periodontal ligament at the apex. The tooth had been well approximated in the bony socket on reimplantation.

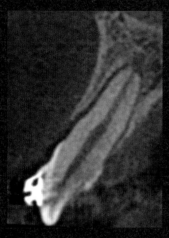

Figure 7.3.5 Cone beam computed tomography of UL2: apical radiolucency and widening of the periodontal ligament on the buccal root surface.

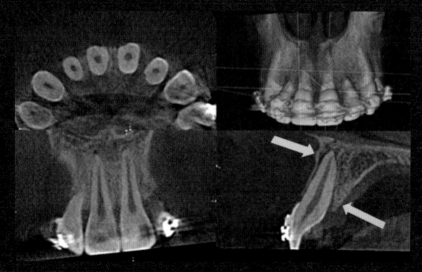

Figure 7.3.6 Cone beam computed tomography of UL1: apical radiolucency with expansion of the cortical plate buccal to the root apex and widening of the periodontal ligament space on the palatal root surface, suggestive of the tooth being palatally displaced during the avulsion injury.

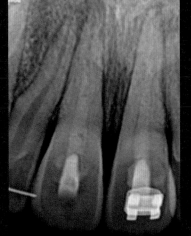

Figure 7.3.7 Root canal therapy was initiated and the canals were dressed with calcium hydroxide.

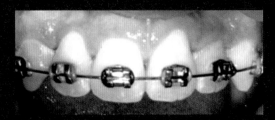

Figure 7.3.8 Titanium trauma splint was removed, and bracket and arch wire were replaced.

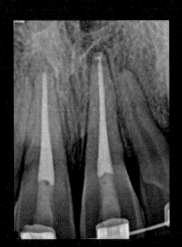

Figure 7.3.9 Four weeks later, the canals were obturated and the access openings

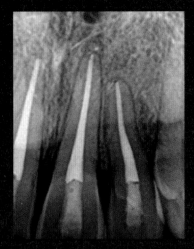

Figure 7.3.10 Six months post trauma, UL2 was treated for pulpal necrosis and symptomatic apical periodontitis.

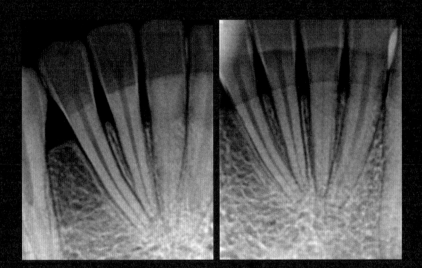

Figure 7.3.11 One year after the initial trauma, the LL1 exhibited pulp canal obliteration, widening of the periodontal ligament space at the apex and symptoms of tenderness to percussion.

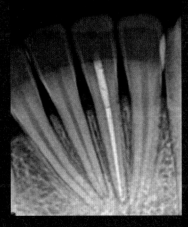

Figure 7.3.12 Root canal therapy of LL1 was completed.

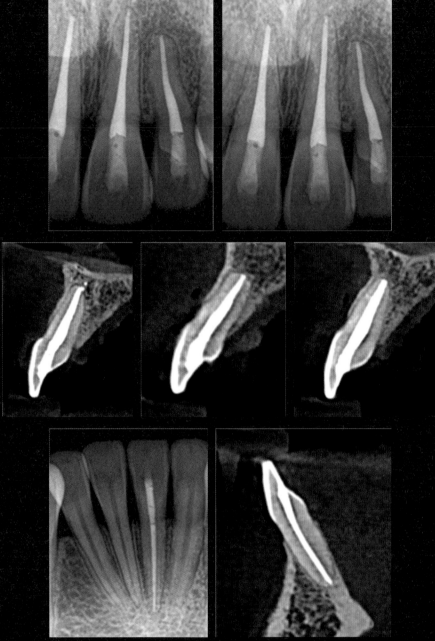

Figure 7.3.13 Five-year post trauma, follow-up with periapical radiographs and cone beam computed tomography shows no signs of resorption or endodontic pathology.

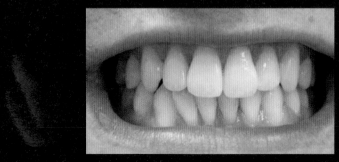

Figure 7.3.14 Five year follow-up shows an excellent aesthetic result.

Further Reading

Andreasen, J.O., Andreasen, F.M., and Andersson, L. (2019). *Textbook and Color Atlas of Traumatic Injuries to the Teeth*. Oxford: Wiley Blackwell.

Bakland, L. (ed.) (2006). Update on traumatic dental injuries. *Endodontic Topics* 14: 20–40.

Bourguignon, C., Cohenca, N., Lauridsen, E. et al. (2020). International Association of Dental Traumatology guidelines for the management of traumatic dental injuries: 1. Fractures and luxations. *Dental Traumatology*. 36 (4): 314–330.

Flores, M.T., Andersson, L., Andreasen, J.O. et al. (2007). Guidelines for the management of traumatic dental injuries. II. Avulsion of permanent teeth. *Dental Traumatology* 23: 130–136.

Fouad, A., Abbott, P., Tsillngaridis, G. et al. (2020). International Association of Dental Traumatology guidelines for the management of traumatic dental injuries: 2. Avulsion of permanent teeth. *Dental Traumatology* 36: 331–342.

International Association of Dental Traumatology (2020). Guidelines for the management of traumatic dental injuries. Redmond, WA: IADT. https://www.iadt-dentaltrauma.org/for-professionals.html.

7.4 *Avulsion*

Nestor Cohenca

Objectives

At the end of this case, the reader should appreciate the significance of avulsion injuries and understand the immediate management and long-term treatment involved with avulsed teeth.

Introduction

A 16-year-old boy presented one day after a traumatic injury in which the upper left central incisor was avulsed.

Chief Complaint

The patient reported that he was hit in the mouth with a baseball while playing catch. The patient never lost consciousness and remembers the details of the event. The upper left central incisor (UL1) was avulsed and remained dry for 30 minutes wrapped in a paper towel (Figure 7.4.1). The tooth was then placed back into the socket by his father (Figure 7.4.2), on the advice of their paediatric dentist. The patient went straight to his dentist, who confirmed the position (Figure 7.4.3) and splinted the tooth with a rigid composite resin splint (Figure 7.4.4). The patient was prescribed amoxicillin and chlorhexidine rinses and was referred to the endodontist for further management.

Medical History

The patient was fit and well.

Dental History

The patient is under regular dental care with his paediatric dentist. He completed orthodontic treatment two years ago.

Pitt Ford's Problem-Based Learning in Endodontology, Second Edition. Edited by Elizabeth Shin Perry, Shanon Patel, Shalini Kanagasingam, and Samantha Hamer.
© 2025 John Wiley & Sons Ltd. Published 2025 by John Wiley & Sons Ltd.

Clinical Examination

Clinical examination revealed a rigid composite splint extending from the upper right lateral incisor (UR2) to the upper left canine (UL3). All maxillary and mandibular anterior teeth were examined for signs of injury. The UR1, UL1 and UL2 were tender to percussion. Only the UL1 was sensitive to palpation. All anterior maxillary teeth responded positively and within normal limits to sensibility tests (cold and electric pulp testing), except for tooth UL1 (avulsed).

What did the periapical radiographs and limited field-of-view cone beam computed tomography images reveal?

Two periapical radiographs and a limited field-of-view (FOV) cone beam computed tomography (CBCT) scan were taken and reviewed. The periapical radiographs revealed a normal periodontal ligament (PDL) space around the UL1 and UL2 (Figures 7.4.3 and 7.4.5). Further analysis of the 3D CBCT scan confirmed the correct repositioning of the replanted tooth and ruled out an alveolar bone fracture. (Figures 7.4.6 and 7.4.7). Widening of the PDL on the buccal root surface of the UL1 was noted (Figure 7.4.7). The avulsed tooth appeared to be well repositioned.

What imaging is recommended in the assessment of dental trauma?

Current guidelines advise multiple parallax, two-dimensional periapical radiographs. The clinician should evaluate each case and determine which radiographs are appropriate, depending on the nature of the traumatic dental injuries. Diagnostic radiographs also provide a baseline for future comparisons at follow-up examinations. The use of film holders is highly recommended to allow standardisation and reproducible radiographs.

CBCT provides enhanced visualisation of traumatic dental injuries, particularly root fractures, crown/root fractures and lateral luxations. In cases of crown/root fractures, the scan provides critical information such as the location, extent and direction of a fracture. In these specific injuries, three-dimensional imaging is important for diagnosis and treatment planning, and should be considered, where available. A guiding principle when considering exposing a patient to ionising radiation is whether the image is likely to change the management of the injury.

Radiographic examination of avulsions should include two periapical radiographs (mesial and distal) and a CBCT scan should be considered if available. The CBCT scan may be used before and after tooth replantation to rule out alveolar bone fractures and to confirm satisfactory tooth repositioning.

Diagnosis and Treatment Planning

Diagnosis of the UL1 was prior avulsion with pulpal necrosis and symptomatic apical periodontitis.

The immediate treatment of replantation and splinting of the avulsed tooth was performed by the paediatric dentist within an hour of the trauma. Treatment recommended for the UL1 included:

- Replacement of the current rigid splint with a flexible splint (Figure 7.4.8).
- Endodontic access for pulp debridement, root canal disinfection and intracanal medication with calcium hydroxide (Figure 7.4.9).
- Splint removal at two weeks post trauma. Clinical evaluation of all anterior maxillary teeth.
- Completion of endodontic therapy three to four weeks post trauma (Figure 7.4.10).
- Follow-up at 3 and 6 weeks followed by 3, 6, 12 and 24 months.

What type of splint should be used in traumatic dental injuries and how long should the splint remain in place?

Current protocols supports the use of a flexible splint to stabilise avulsed teeth, allowing physiological movement for better healing of the periodontium. A passive stainless steel wire of a diameter up to 0.0016 inches or 0.4 mm, or a nylon fishing line (0.13–0.25 mm) can be used and bonded to the teeth with composite resin. Splinting time varies based on the presence of alveolar fracture and the type or severity of the injury. Excessive and/or inappropriate splinting increases the likelihood of root resorption.

Treatment

Root canal treatment of the UL1 was initiated within 24 hours after the replantation and the rigid composite splint was replaced by a flexible splint. The initial endodontic therapy included pulp debridement, root canal disinfection and intracanal medication with calcium hydroxide. Three weeks later, endodontic treatment was completed using gutta percha and calcium silicate cement sealer. The coronal access was sealed with a composite restoration. The patient was followed-up at 3, 6 and 12 months for clinical and radiographic examination (Figure 7.4.11). The UL1 remained asymptomatic and fully functional. The adjacent teeth were found to be asymptomatic and responsive to sensibility testing. No replacement resorption was diagnosed clinically or radiographically at the review appointments.

Discussion

Avulsion is a complex traumatic injury characterised by the complete dislodgement of the tooth from its socket. Among all types of injuries, avulsions are the most challenging with regard to management. Avulsion results in the tooth's blood supply, innervation and PDL being severely damaged. At present, dental replantation is considered the therapy of choice for traumatic tooth avulsion. Inflammatory and replacement root resorption are common complications after an avulsion. Complete repair of the periodontium is only possible if the tooth is replanted immediately following current treatment protocols.

The way the avulsed tooth was handled, the extraoral time and storage medium are key factors that have an impact on the healing potential and complications expected. Ideally, tooth replantation should enable regeneration of the histologically normal and functional PDL, due to the progenitor and stem cells localised in this tissue. However, a decrease in the quantity of viable remnant tissue, cells and collagen fibres will result in a decrease in the chances for repair. Replacement root resorption (ankylosis-related resorption) is considered the most serious type of root resorption after tooth avulsion and replantation. This process leads to dentoalveolar ankylosis, due to lack of a viable periodontal ligament leading into fusion of bone and dental tissues as part of the bone remodeling process.

Recently, the International Association of Dental Traumatology (IADT) published new and revised guidelines for the treatment of avulsed teeth. From a clinical point of view, it is important for the clinician to assess the condition of the PDL cells by classifying the avulsed tooth into one of the following three groups before commencing treatment (Table 7.4.1):

- *The PDL cells are most likely viable.* The tooth has been replanted immediately or within a very short time (about 15 minutes) at the place of the accident.
- *The PDL cells may be viable but compromised.* The tooth has been kept in a storage medium such as milk, Hank's balanced salt solution (e.g. Save-a-Tooth or a similar product), saliva or saline, and the total extraoral dry time has been less than 60 minutes.
- *The PDL cells are likely to be non-viable.* The total extraoral dry time has been more than 60 minutes, regardless of whether the tooth has been stored in an additional medium or not.

Table 7.4.1 Summary of protocols for the management of avulsed permanent teeth.

The tooth was replanted immediately (or not more than 15 minutes extraoral time)	The tooth has been kept in a storage medium (milk, HBSS, saliva or saline) and the total extraoral dry time has been less than 60 minutes	The tooth has had a total extraoral dry time of more than 60 minutes
<ul><li>Clean the affected area (saline or chlorhexidine)</li><li>Verify the position (clinically/radiographically)</li><li>Local anaesthesia (without vasoconstrictor)</li><li>If needed, reposition the tooth correctly (up to 48 hours post implantation)</li></ul>	<ul><li>Rinse root with saline or HBSS</li><li>Local anaesthesia (without vaso-constrictor)</li><li>Rinse socket and replant the tooth (slight digital pressure)</li><li>Verify the position (clinically/radio-graphically)</li></ul>	<ul><li>Agitate the tooth in a physiological storage medium, or with gauze soaked in saline, to remove visible contaminants or loose debris</li><li>While the patient is being examined, the tooth may be left in the storage medium</li><li>Local anaesthesia (without vasoconstrictor)</li><li>Rinse and examine the socket</li><li>Remove coagulum if necessary</li><li>Reposition any fractured alveolar fragment</li><li>Replant the tooth gently</li><li>Verify the position (clinically/radiographically)</li></ul>

Flexible splint for 2 weeks (flexible wire diameter of 0.016 in. or 0.4 mm)[a]

Suture lacerations as needed

Endodontic therapy within 2 weeks (calcium hydroxide intracanal medicament)[b]

Systemic antibiotics (amoxicillin or doxycycline for 1 week)

Chlorhexidine rinses (for 1 week)

Check tetanus vaccination

Post-operative instructions (soft diet, no contact sports, oral hygiene maintenance)

Endodontic therapy must be initiated within 2 weeks of the traumatic injury

Review (at 2 weeks, 4 weeks, 3 months, 6 months, 1 year, and yearly for 5 years)

HBSS, Hank's balanced salt solution.
[a] In cases with alveolar fracture, a more rigid splint may be used for about 4 weeks.
[b] Revascularisation should be considered when replanting immature teeth in children.

What root canal medicaments are recommended in the treatment of traumatic dental injuries?

Endodontic therapy needs to be initiated within 2 weeks. Calcium hydroxide remains the recommended intracanal medicament followed by root canal filling. Current strategies also include the use of corticosteroids, which have the potential to facilitate fibroblastic regeneration as an anti-inflammatory and anticlastic intracanal medicament. Timing is significantly different as it needs to be placed immediately or shortly following replantation and left in situ for at least six weeks. Recommended topical steroids include 0.5% triamcinolone, 0.05% clobetasol and 0.05% fluocinonide.

What is the recommended follow-up for replanted avulsed teeth?

Replanted teeth should be monitored clinically and radiographically at one to two weeks (when the splint is removed and endodontic therapy initiated), four weeks, three months, six months, one year and yearly thereafter for at least five years. Clinical and radiographic examination at the follow-up examinations will provide information to determine the outcome.

- *Favourable outcome*: Asymptomatic, functional, normal mobility, no sensitivity to percussion, normal percussion sound. No radiolucencies and no radiographic evidence of root resorption. The lamina dura should appear normal.
- *Unfavourable outcome*: Patient may or may not have symptoms; presence of swelling or sinus tract; the tooth may have excessive mobility or no mobility (ankylosis) with high-pitched (metallic) percussion tone. Presence of radiolucencies. Radiographic evidence of resorption: infection-related (inflammatory) resorption, or ankylosis-related (replacement) resorption. When ankylosis occurs in a growing patient, infra-position of the tooth is highly likely, leading to disturbances in alveolar and facial growth over the short, medium and long term.

What factors influence the prognosis of a replanted tooth?

Several factors influence the prognosis of a replanted tooth, including extraoral dry time, storage medium and storage conditions, stage of root development, root surface treatment before replantation, preparation of the dental socket, type and duration of the splint, time of initiation of root canal treatment, intracanal medications and systemic antibiotic therapy. Yet, above all, extraoral time remains the most important factor to favour a successful outcome. In the case presented, the immediate action taken by the father, who repositioned the avulsed tooth within 30 minutes at the site of injury, provided favourable conditions for periodontal healing.

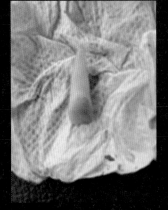

Figure 7.4.1 Photograph of avulsed UL1, dry for 30 minutes.

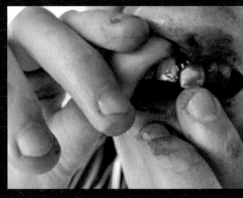

Figure 7.4.2 Photograph of UL1 reimplanted by patient's father.

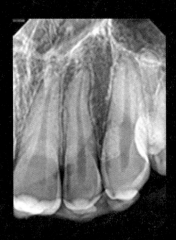

Figure 7.4.3 Periapical radiograph of UL1 and UL2.

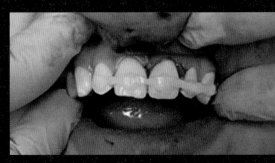

Figure 7.4.4 Photograph of a rigid composite splint.

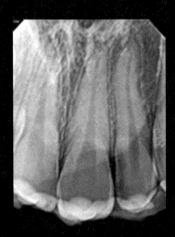

Figure 7.4.5 Periapical radiograph of UL1 and UL2.

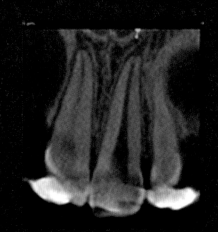

Figure 7.4.6 Cone beam computed tomography scan showing coronal view of UL1.

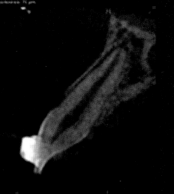

Figure 7.4.7 Cone beam computed tomography scan showing sagittal views of UL1.

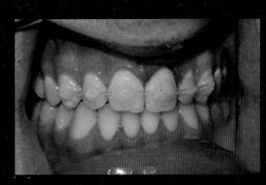

Figure 7.4.8 Photograph of a flexible splint.

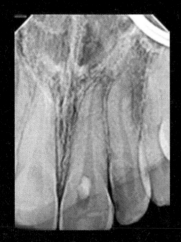

Figure 7.4.9 Periapical radiograph of UL1 with intracanal dressing.

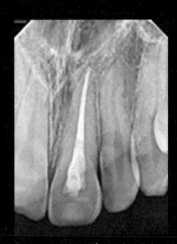

Figure 7.4.10 Post-operative periapical radiograph of UL1

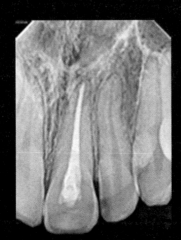

Figure 7.4.11 One-year follow-up periapical radiograph of UL1.

Further Reading

Andreasen, J.O., Andreasen, F.M., and Andersson, L. (2007). *Textbook and Color Atlas of Traumatic Injuries to the Teeth*, 4e. Oxford: Blackwell Munksgaard.

Andersson, L. (2007). Tooth avulsion and replantation. *Dental Traumatology* 23: 129.

Bourguignon, C., Cohenca, N., Lauridsen, E. et al. (2020). International Association of Dental Traumatology guidelines for the management of traumatic dental injuries: 1. Fractures and luxations. *Dental Traumatology* 36: 314–330.

Cohenca, N. and Silberman, A. (2017). Contemporary imaging for the diagnosis and treatment of traumatic dental injuries: a review. *Dental Traumatology* 33: 321–328.

Day, P.F., Gregg, T.A., Ashley, P. et al. (2012). Periodontal healing following avulsion and replantation of teeth: a multi-centre randomized controlled trial to compare two root canal medicaments. *Dental Traumatology* 28: 55–64.

Fouad, A.F., Abbott, P.V., Tsilingaridis, G. et al. (2020). International Association of Dental Traumatology guidelines for the management of traumatic dental injuries: 2. Avulsion of permanent teeth. *Dental Traumatology* 00: 1–12.

Isaksson, H., Koch, G., Bakland, L.K., and Andreasen, J.O. (2021). Effect of splinting times on the healing of intra-alveolar root fractures in 512 permanent teeth in humans: a Scandinavian multicenter study. *Dental Traumatology* 37: 672–676.

Kinirons, M.J., Boyd, D.H., and Gregg, T.A. (1999). Inflammatory and replacement resorption in reimplanted permanent incisor teeth: a study of the characteristics of 84 teeth. *Endodontics & Dental Traumatology* 15 (6): 269–272.

Krastl, G., Weiger, R., Filippi, A. et al. (2021). European Society of Endodontology position statement: Endodontic management of traumatized permanent teeth. *International Endodontic Journal* 54:1473–1481.

VIII Root Resorption

8.1 *External Cervical Resorption*

Shanon Patel

Objectives

At the end of this case the reader should appreciate the pathogenesis, diagnosis and management of external cervical resorption (ECR).

Introduction

A 22-year-old male medical student presented with persistent bleeding on brushing teeth and spontaneous pain localised to the lower left canine (LL3).

Chief Complaint

Hot/cold foods and liquids resulted in a localised throbbing pain lasting approximately 20 minutes. The symptoms had been present for three weeks and had been getting progressively worse.

Medical History

Unremarkable.

Dental History

Attended annually for dental check-up appointments and twice a year for hygienist maintenance. The patient recalled having the tooth restored with a direct plastic restoration two to three years ago after his dentist detected a buccal caries. The patient had Invisalign orthodontic treatment 10 years ago for 18 months.

Pitt Ford's Problem-Based Learning in Endodontology, Second Edition. Edited by Elizabeth Shin Perry, Shanon Patel, Shalini Kanagasingam, and Samantha Hamer.
© 2025 John Wiley & Sons Ltd. Published 2025 by John Wiley & Sons Ltd.

Clinical Examination

The extraoral examination was unremarkable. The patient had a minimally restored dentition and his oral hygiene status was satisfactory.

The LL3 was restored with a buccal composite restoration that extended subgingivally. Periodontal probing resulted in significant bleeding; the base of the restoration did not feel like it was very well adapted to the base of the cavity. Sensibility testing with EndoFrost reproduced the patient's symptoms. The adjacent teeth were healthy and responded normally to sensibility testing (Table 8.1.1).

A periapical radiograph of the tooth revealed a radiopaque restoration in the cervical region of the LL3, the inferior border of which appeared to be poorly adapted (Figure 8.1.1a). Beneath the restoration was a radiolucency extending across the width of the tooth; the root canal borders can be traced through the radiolucency. There were no other signs of endodontic or periodontal disease detected on the radiograph. Small field-of-view cone beam computed tomography (CBCT) confirmed a poorly adapted restoration and ECR in close proximity to or even perforating the root canal (Figure 8.1.1b–d).

There are no 'classic' symptoms or signs for ECR. The radiographic symptoms are also highly variable (Table 8.1.2).

Table 8.1.1 Clinical signs of external cervical resorption.

- Located in the cervical region of tooth
- 'Pink spot' may be noticed by patient or dentist
- Tooth usually responds positively to vitality testing unless there is pulpal involvement (in very advanced cases)
- Probing elicits spontaneous and profuse bleeding
- Sharp, thinned edges around the resorptive cavity

Table 8.1.2 Radiological signs of external cervical resorption.

- Detected as chance radiological finding, as tooth is usually asymptomatic
- Varies from asymmetrically located radiolucency with irregular margins in cervical/proximal region of tooth to uniformly round radiolucency centred over the root
- Early lesions are usually radiolucent in appearance
- Advanced lesions may have mottled appearance due to fibro-osseous nature of the lesion
- Root canal often visible and intact (indicating lesion is external)

Would a parallax radiograph have been beneficial?

Parallax radiographs may be indicated if a CBCT is not possible. With ECR, a second (parallax) radiograph will result in a change in position of radio-lucency, while with internal inflammatory resorption the radiolucency will stay centred. Parallax radiographs can also be used to locate the position of ECR using the 'SLOB' (**S**ame **L**ingual **O**pposite **B**uccal) rule (Figure 8.1.2).

In this case, the clinical examination confirmed the position (buccal) of the ECR defect. The CBCT scan revealed that the lesion was confirmed to the buccal aspect of the tooth. There is good evidence that CBCT overcomes the limitations of periapical radiographs, thus improving the diagnosis and/ or management of ECR, by giving the clinician a precise appreciation of the nature and extent of the lesion; that is, three-dimensional (3D) morphology, degree of circumferential spread and proximity to the root canal.

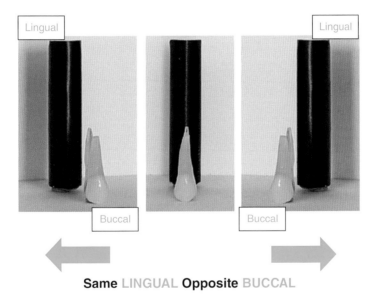

Same LINGUAL **Opposite** BUCCAL

Figure 8.1.2 'SLOB' rule. As the tubehead moves mesially, the root that appears more mesial will be the lingual/palatal, and if the tubehead moves distally, the root that appears more distal will be the lingual/palatal (moves in the same direction as the tubehead).

What are the limitations of periapical radiographs when diagnosing resorptive lesions?

The two-dimensional (2D) nature of radiographs compresses the complex anatomy into a 2D shadowgraph. Therefore, it is often not possible to accurately appreciate the exact location, nature (i.e. size and shape) and extent (whether or not the canal has been perforated) of the root resorption. In addition, the overlying anatomy (anatomical noise) may obscure the area of interest, resulting in a challenging radiographic interpretation.

Are There Any Classifications for External Cervical Resorption?

The Heithersay classification describes the extent of ECR based on (2D) radiographs, thus resulting in under-estimation and/or inadequate appreciation of the true nature of ECR. The Patel classification is 3D, based on periapical radiographs and CBCT (Table 8.1.3). The aim of this descriptive classification is to ensure an accurate diagnosis and aid communication of ECR between clinicians. It has been shown to be more accurate than the Heithersay classification. In this case the ECR is a Patel 2Ap.

Table 8.1.3 Patel classification of external cervical resorption lesions.

Height	Circumferential spread	Proximity to the root canal
1. At cemento-enamel junction level or coronal to the bone crest (supracrestal)	A: ≤90°	d: Lesion confined to dentine
2. Extends into coronal third of the root and apical to the bone crest (subcrestal)	B: >90° to ≤180°	p: Probable pulpal involement
3. Extends into mid-third of the root	C: >180° to ≤270°	
4. Extends into apical third of the root	D: >270°	

Diagnosis and Treatment Planning

What was the diagnosis?

The diagnosis of the LL3 was ECR associated with irreversible pulpitis.

What are the stages of external cervical resorption?

There are three stages: resorptive (initiation), resorptive (propagation) and reparative (remodelling). Resorption and repair may occur simultaneously in different regions of the resorptive defect.

What is the aetiology of external cervical resorption?

The aetiology is poorly understood; however, it is accepted that cementum provides a protective barrier against resorption of the underlying dentine. Damage to or deficiency of this protective layer, below the epithelial attachment, is believed to predispose the dentine to resorption by osteoclasts. Several potential aetiological factors have been suggested, although there is no cause-and-effect evidence for any of these factors (Table 8.1.4). The literature is polarised as to whether the resorptive process is sustained by stimulation of the osteoclasts by bacteria emanating from the gingival sulcus.

Table 8.1.4 Factors predisposing the patient to external cervical resorption.

- Trauma
- Intracoronal bleaching
- Orthodontics
- Periodontal therapy
- Surgical procedures
- Other factors: bruxism, developmental defects, intracoronal restorations, systemic diseases

What are the aims of treatment with external cervical resorption?

- Arrest the resorptive process.
- Restore the damaged root surface.
- Improve the aesthetics of the tooth (e.g. 'pink spot').
- Prevent further resorption.

What are the treatment options for external cervical resorption?

See Table 8.1.5.

Table 8.1.5 Treatment options for external cervical resorption.

- External repair of the resorptive defect ± root canal treatment
- Internal repair + root canal treatment
- Intentional replantation
- Periodic review (untreatable teeth)
- Extraction (untreatable teeth)

- *External repair of the resorptive defect ± root canal treatment.* Excavation and restoration of the ECR defect with a direct restoration (e.g. Patel class 1Ad, 2Ad, 2Bd). Root canal treatment is indicated in cases where there is (probable) pulp involvement or necrosis (e.g. Patel class 1Ap, 2Ap, 2Bp).
- *Internal repair and root canal treatment.* Root canal treatment, excavation and restoration of the resorptive defect with a Bioceramic or direct plastic restoration (e.g. Patel class 2Cp, 2Dp, 3Cp, 3Dp).
- *Intentional replantation.* (Elective) endodontic treatment and extraction to allow access to the otherwise inaccessible ECR for restoration and/or recontouring (e.g. Patel class 3Ad, 3Bd).
- *Periodic review.* Untreatable teeth (e.g. Patel class 2-4Dd, 2-4Dp, or cases with significant reparative tissue within the ECR lesion).
- *Extraction.* Symptomatic untreatable teeth – as above.

Treatment options depend on the severity, nature and accessibility of the resorptive process; in some cases, a mucoperiosteal flap may have to be raised to gain adequate access to the ECR defect.

The objectives of treatment are elimination of the resorptive tissue, sealing of the resultant defect and portal of entry, and prevention of recurrence.

The decision to leave the tooth alone is one that should be made by the patient only when they are made aware that the condition will deteriorate without intervention. However, this may be the most appropriate option if the tooth has a hopeless prognosis, and is to be left for as long as possible in situ in order to maintain alveolar bone levels prior to implant placement.

Extraction of the tooth is indicated if the tooth is extensively damaged resulting in it being unrestorable, or if ECR is inaccessible to treatment (for example, when it has progressed too subgingivally and/or interproximally).

What treatment would you carry out in this case?

Endodontic treatment is indicated as the tooth is irreversibly inflamed. The root canal should be located and then temporarily occluded with a gutta percha point, which will prevent the canal being inadvertently blocked when the resorptive defect is restored (Figure 8.1.1e, f). A mucogingival flap is then reflected to allow the resorptive defect to be excavated (Figure 8.1.1g). The undermined enamel is then removed with a diamond bur in a high-speed, reverse turbine handpiece. The resorptive cavity is restored with a composite resin restoration (Figure 8.1.1h), after which root canal treatment is completed (Figure 8.1.1i,j). A periapical radiograph is taken prior to repositioning and suturing of the mucogingival flap (Figure 8.1.1k). The sutures are then removed three to four days later. The patient should be reviewed one year later (Figure 8.1.1l).

Discussion

The clinical and radiographic presentation of ECR is highly variable, with no classic presentation, which often can result in misdiagnosis and/or inappropriate management. Due to the limitations of radiographs in diagnosis as well as in precisely determining the nature of ECR lesions, CBCT is recommended when considering treatment of treatable ECR lesions.

Early ECR lesions are usually resorptive in nature, and providing they are accessible to treatment have a good prognosis. As the resorptive lesions and tooth destruction progress, the prognosis decreases as the tooth is weakened. In addition, with advanced ECR lesions, the entire lesion may not be accessible, resulting in incomplete removal of ECR and ultimately recurrence of the lesion.

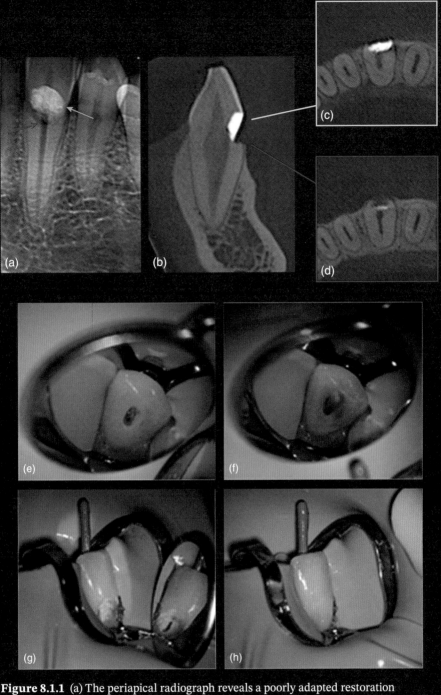

Figure 8.1.1 (a) The periapical radiograph reveals a poorly adapted restoration (green arrow); note that the canal is visible through the radiolucency (purple arrow). (b) Sagittal and (c, d) coronal cone beam computed tomography images reveal the close proximity of the external cervical resorption to the root canal as well as a poorly adapted restoration. (e, f) The root canal would be accessed in the normal manner for non-surgical endodontic treatment. (g) With the dental dam still in situ, a mucogingival flap is reflected to expose the resorption lesion. The granulomatous tissue occupying the defect is excavated and the margins of the defects are refined to remove any grossly undermined enamel or dentine, and (h) restored with a composite resin restoration. The flap is then sutured in position, the dental dam is replaced and root canal treatment is completed as normal. Radiographs

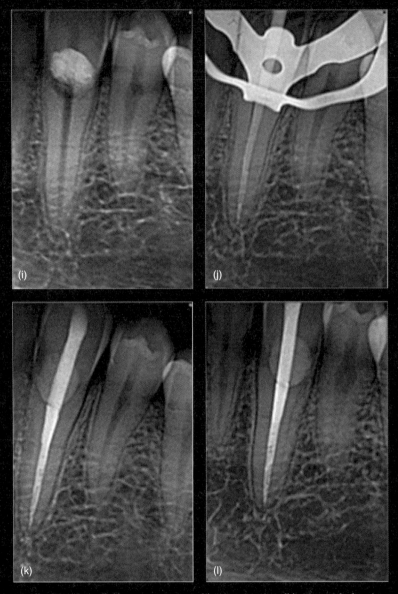

Figure 8.1.1 (Continued) (i) pre-treatment, (j) master point, (k) post-endodontic (note how well adapted the restoration is) and (l) at one-year review.

Further Reading

ESE (2014). European Society of Endodontology position statement: the use of CBCT in endodontics. *International Endodontic Journal* 47: 502–504.

Heithersay, G.S. (1999). Clinical, radiologic, and histopathologic features of invasive cervical resorption. *Quintessence International* 30: 27–37.

Mavridou, A.M., Bergmans, L., Barendregt, D., and Lambrechts, P. (2017). Descriptive analysis of factors associated with external cervical resorption. *Journal of Endodontics* 43: 1602–1610.

Mavridou, A.M., Pyka, G., Kerckhofs, G. et al. (2016). A novel multimodular methodology to investigate external cervical tooth resorption. *International Endodontic Journal* 49: 287–300.

Patel, K., Mannocci, F., and Patel, S. (2016). The assessment and management of external cervical resorption with periapical radiographs and cone-beam computed tomography: a clinical study. *Journal of Endodontics* 42: 1435–1440.

Patel, S., Abella, F., Patel, K. et al. (2023). Clinical and radiographic features of external cervical resorption – An observational study. *International Endodontic Journal* 56: 1475–1487.

Patel S, Foschi F, Condon R, Pimentel T, Bhuva B (2018) External cervical resorption: part 2 - management. International Endodontic Journal 51(11): 1224–1238.

Patel, S., Foschi, F., Mannocci, F., and Patel, K. (2018). External cervical resorption: a three-dimensional classification. *International Endodontic Journal* 51: 206–214.

Patel S, Mavridou AM, Lambrechts P, Saberi N (2018) External cervical resorption-part 1: histopathology, distribution and presentation. International Endodontic Journal 51(11): 1205–1223.

Rodriguez, G., Abella, F., Durán-Sindreu, F. et al. (2017a). Influence of cone-beam computed tomography in clinical decision making among specialists. *Journal of Endodontics* 43: 194–199.

Vaz de Souza, D., Schirru, E., Mannocci, F. et al. (2017). External cervical resorption: a comparison of the diagnostic efficacy using 2 different cone-beam computed tomographic units and periapical radiographs. *Journal of Endodontics* 43: 121–125.

8.2 *Internal Inflammatory Resorption*

Shanon Patel

Objectives

At the end of this case the reader should have an appreciation of the diagnosis and management of internal inflammatory root resorption.

Introduction

A 43-year-old female presented as a new patient. She was asymptomatic; however, she gave a history of intermittent discomfort localised to her upper right central incisor (UR1) for several months, which she managed with over-the-counter analgesics.

Chief Complaint

The UR1 was tender to chewing for three to four months and the patient also complained of an occasional spontaneous throbbing ache from the upper right incisor region. These symptoms resolved approximately four months ago.

Medical History

Asthmatic.

Dental History

The patient's upper anterior teeth were traumatically injured in a car accident 19 years ago; these teeth were subsequently restored with crowns. Approximately one year ago the patient had these crowns replaced to improve the appearance of her smile.

Pitt Ford's Problem-Based Learning in Endodontology, Second Edition. Edited by Elizabeth Shin Perry, Shanon Patel, Shalini Kanagasingam, and Samantha Hamer. © 2025 John Wiley & Sons Ltd. Published 2025 by John Wiley & Sons Ltd.

Clinical Examination

Extraoral examination was unremarkable. Intraoral examination revealed a moderately restored dentition, with good oral hygiene with periodontal probing depths of 1–3 mm.

The upper incisor teeth were restored with well-adapted and contoured crowns. The UR1 was tender to percussion and palpation and did not respond to thermal (cold) or electric pulp testing. There were no other signs of endodontic or periodontal disease associated with the upper anterior teeth.

What did the radiographs reveal?

- Alveolar bone height within normal limits (Figure 8.2.1a).
- UR2 was root filled and there appeared to be a small amount of sealer extrusion apically. The tooth was restored with a well-adapted crown that was retained in placed with a fibre post.
- UR1 was restored with a well-adapted crown, there was a well-demarcated, symmetrical radiolucency in the coronal third of the canal and the periphery was slightly more radiopaque. The periodontal ligament space appeared to be a normal width and the canal apical to the radiolucency was sclerosed. The cone beam computed tomography (CBCT) scan confirmed that the root was not perforated, meaning that root canal treatment was potentially viable (Figure 8.2.1b, c).

Radiographically, internal inflammatory resorption lesions may be round or oval, with a circumscribed border and radiolucent. The resorptive defect is always a continuity (or ballooning out) of the root canal (Table 8.2.1).

Table 8.2.1 Features of internal inflammatory resorption.

Clinical features

- Discoloured tooth
- Pink spot
- Periapical periodontitis signs (e.g. sinus, tenderness to percussion, etc.)

Sensitivity testing

- + or – depending on stage

Radiographic features

- Symmetrical 'ballooning' out of the root canal
- Resorption cavity stays centred with parallax radiographs
- Cone beam computed tomography scan may reveal a perforation

Is a cone beam computed tomography scan indicated?

A CBCT scan is essential when a provisional diagnosis of internal inflammatory resorption (IIR) is reached that appears to be amenable to treatment. The three-dimensional (3D) views will provide essential information on the nature of the resorptive lesion, whether there is perforation of the external root wall and also the restorability of the tooth; these factors will have an impact on treatment planning. Differentiating IIR and external cervical resorption (ECR) from each can often be challenging with radiographs. There is good evidence that CBCT improves not only the accuracy of diagnosis of resorptive lesions, but also the confidence of diagnosis, and improves selection of the most appropriate treatment plan.

Is there any benefit of taking a parallax radiograph?

A parallax radiograph is indicated when CBCT is not available. A second angled radiograph at a different angle will often confirm the nature of the resorption lesion. ECR will move in the same direction as the x-ray tube shift if they are lingually/palatally positioned. They will move in the opposite direction to the tube shift if they are buccally positioned (refer to Case 8.1 for a diagram on the SLOB rule). However, the position of IIR will not change position relative to the canal on both radiographs.

While the canal walls will be visible with horizontal parallax radiographs, the ECR lesion will appear to move with the change of horizontal angle of the x-ray tube.

Diagnosis and Treatment Planning

What was the diagnosis for the UR1?

Asymptomatic periapical periodontitis associated with an infected necrotic root canal system and internal inflammatory resorption.

What are the treatment options that should be discussed with the patient?

- Endodontic treatment
- Leave alone
- Extraction

What does the internal root resorption lesion contain?

These lesions consist of granulomatous tissue, bacteria and odontoclasts adjacent to the resorbing dentine.

What causes internal root resorption?

Osteoclasts are responsible for IIR. They are formed by the fusion of mononuclear precursor cells of the monocyte–macrophage lineage derived from the spleen or bone marrow. They are recruited to the site of injury or irritation by the release of proinflammatory cytokines.

For internal resorption to occur, the pulp tissue apical to the resorptive lesion must be vital, thus providing the blood supply to provide clastic cells and their nutrients; the infected coronal necrotic pulp tissue provides stimulation for those clastic cells. Bacteria typically enter the root canal through dentinal tubules, carious cavities or cracks or fractures (Table 8.2.2). The interface between the necrotic and vital pulp tissue drives the lesions, therefore, subject to restorability, endodontic treatment is indicated to eliminate IIR.

Treatment

Endodontic treatment was carried out over one visit under local anaesthetic and dental dam. The crown was removed, the sclerosed apical third identified (Figure 8.2.1d), prepared and disinfected with NaOCl and obturated with gutta percha. The resorptive cavity was irrigated with NaOCl using ultrasonic activation to enhance its penetrability into the resorptive defect. However, due to the inaccessible nature of the resorptive defect, predictably debriding the resorptive cavity was challenging.

The resorptive defect was obturated with a bioactive endodontic cement (Biodentine). This bioactive material group not only has excellent sealing ability, its high pH will impair the osteoclastic action of any residual IIR remnants within the large resorptive cavity, thus arresting the resorptive process (Figure 8.2.1e).

Would a two-visit treatment be more appropriate?

After the tooth had been prepared, it could have been medicated with calcium hydroxide for a few weeks to predictably disinfect the root canal, especially the instrumented root canal. At the second visit, the combination of the calcium hydroxide dressing and sodium hypochlorite irrigant would have a synergistic effect on dissolving any remaining necrotic tissue remnants within the root canal. However, the editors believe that with its high pH, a similar if not better outcome may be achieved with bioactive cements.

Table 8.2.2 Aetiological factors for internal resorption.

- Idiopathic
- Trauma
- Chronic inflammation (pulpitis)
- Restorative treatment
- Previous pulpotomy treatment
- Orthodontic treatment
- Autotransplantation

Alternatively, a thermoplastic root filling technique may be used to ensure obturation of the entire root canal space.

What is the prognosis for this tooth?

There is minimal remaining root volume in the coronal third of the tooth; however, this may have been the situation for several months or years. The prognosis for the tooth is fair to good, especially as the tooth is not in occlusion in lateral excursions, and only has a light contact in the intercuspal position. The patient is aware that the tooth is more 'light use only'. The patient should be advised that as the tooth is extensively restored it may not last a lifetime, especially as she is relatively young, and that an implant-retained crown may be indicated if the tooth becomes symptomatic. At the one-year review, the patient was asymptomatic and the radiograph showed no apical pathology (Figure 8.2.1f).

What other special considerations are there when carrying out endodontic treatment on teeth with internal resorption?

Because of its shape, the resorptive cavity cannot be instrumented, therefore copious amounts of sodium hypochlorite must be used to dissolve and wash out any pulpal (necrotic) tissue within this cavity. The irrigant can also be 'energised' using an ultrasonic file. This will allow the irrigant to penetrate the otherwise inaccessible part of the resorptive cavity and help break up necrotic pulp tissue.

How does internal replacement resorption differ from internal inflammatory resorption?

There are metaplastic hard tissue deposits within the internal replacement resorptive defect, which is reflected radiographically as a hazy, mottled radiopacity with an irregular and often poorly defined border. Clinically, internal replacement resorption will present in the same way as IIR.

Discussion

IIR is often detected in later stages; that is, when the patient presents with symptoms of pulpitis and/or periapical periodontitis. Vitality testing may give positive results in early lesions when vital tissue is still present; however, a negative response to vitality testing is likely with advanced lesions. Bleeding during preparation may indicate either an active resorptive process and/or a perforation of the resorptive lesion through the root wall.

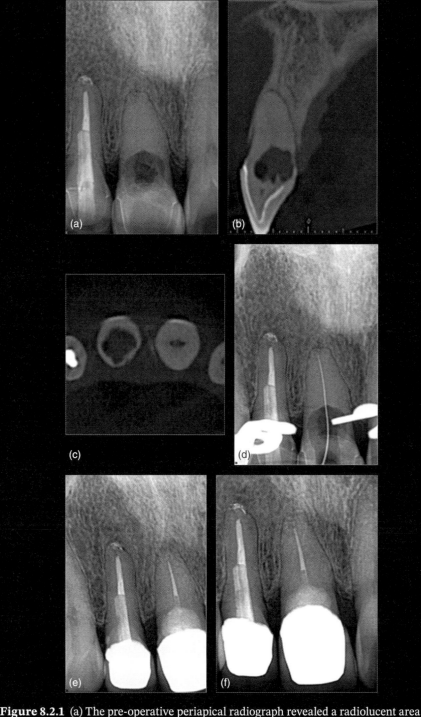

Figure 8.2.1 (a) The pre-operative periapical radiograph revealed a radiolucent area over the coronal third region of the UR1; note the different radiolucencies due to the overlap of the palatal wall. (b, c) Sagittal and axial CBCT reconstructed images reveal the nature of the internal inflammatory resorptive lesion. (d) Working length, (e) post endodontic treatment, (f) one-year review.

Further Reading

Çalişkan, M.K. and Türkün, M. (1997). Prognosis of permanent teeth with internal resorption: a clinical review. *Endodontics and Dental Traumatology* 13: 75–81.

Haapasalo, M. and Endal, U. (2206). Internal inflammatory root resorption. *Endodontic Topics* 14: 60–79.

Wedenberg, C. and Lindskog, S. (1985). Experimental internal resorption in monkey teeth. *Endodontics and Dental Traumatology* 1: 221–227.

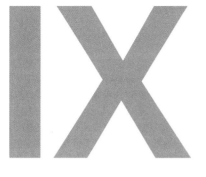

IX Additional Considerations for Patient Management

9.1 Apical Periodontitis and Systemic Disease

Shalini Kanagasingam,
Abdulaziz A. Bakhsh, and Philip Mitchell

Objectives

At the end of this case, the reader should be able to recognise the potential associations between apical periodontitis and systemic diseases. This includes the effects of diabetes mellitus and cardiovascular disease on endodontic outcomes.

Introduction

A 51-year-old male presented for a routine one-year review after having had root canal treatment of his upper right second molar (UR7).

Chief Complaint

The patient was asymptomatic since the root canal treatment was carried out by an endodontist, followed by restoration with a gold crown by a prosthodontist.

Medical History

The patient has a history of diabetes mellitus (DM), hypertension, high cholesterol levels and a history of myocardial infarction about five years ago. He had been taking multiple medications including metformin, metoprolol succinate, atorvastatin, aspirin and clopidogrel.

Dental History

The patient was a regular attender. The UR6 and UR7 had been restored with gold crowns 11 months previously. He had also recently had implant treatment to replace the missing UR5, with no complications.

Pitt Ford's Problem-Based Learning in Endodontology, Second Edition. Edited by Elizabeth Shin Perry, Shanon Patel, Shalini Kanagasingam, and Samantha Hamer.
© 2025 John Wiley & Sons Ltd. Published 2025 by John Wiley & Sons Ltd.

Clinical Examination

The patient had a moderately restored dentition and the soft tissues were healthy. Tooth UR7 was not tender to percussion and not painful on biting. Probing depths were within normal limits.

A radiograph of the UR7 revealed the presence of a periapical radiolucency that appeared larger and more distinct when compared to the immediate post-treatment radiograph taken a year ago (Figure 9.1.1a, b).

A cone beam computed tomography (CBCT) scan was taken to assess the extent of the periapical lesion and any untreated (missed) canals (Figure 9.1.1c–f). The scan revealed that all the root canals had been filled and a periapical radiolucency associated with mesio-buccal 1, mesio-buccal 2, disto-buccal and palatal canals. No missed canals were detected.

Diagnosis and Treatment Planning

A diagnosis of asymptomatic apical periodontitis associated with the previously treated UR7 was made.

The treatment options for the UR7 were:

- No treatment (continue to monitor)
- Non-surgical root canal retreatment
- Surgical treatment (apicectomy)
- Extraction

The patient was very concerned that the periapical lesion had not healed and, in fact, appeared to have radiographically worsened over the past year. He shared that he was particularly anxious about this due to his medical history, as he had come across information on social media regarding root canal treatment being linked to poor general health.

What are the potential pathways by which apical periodontitis can impact the development of systemic diseases?

Apical periodontitis can act as a reservoir for microbes and/or microbial by-product dissemination via the periapical vasculature into the patient's systemic circulation. Raised levels of inflammatory biomarkers can induce a systemic inflammatory response, eventually leading to an increased frequency of cardiovascular events. Endodontic pathogens may directly seed into the arterial wall via bacteraemia. This initiates a local inflammatory reaction including adaptive immune responses, inducing cellular changes, eventually forming atherosclerotic plaques.

Apical periodontitis may go undiagnosed for years, which can potentially lead to increased systemic inflammation. Repeated or chronic infections may be

Table 9.1.1 Potential pathways linking endodontic disease to systemic disorders.

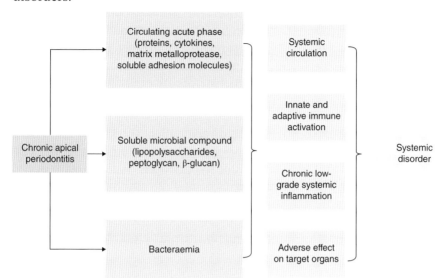

another additional causal element for DM. Inflammatory mediators, especially cytokines, can decrease insulin sensitivity, incur changes to adipocyte function and damping of endothelial nitric oxide production, leading to the development of DM. These mechanisms warrant further investigations (Table 9.1.1).

What is the association between apical periodontitis and cardiovascular disease?

Recent advances in the understanding of disease processes have led to a significant interest in the role of apical periodontitis in cardiovascular disease (CVD), and in particular atherosclerosis. Atherosclerosis is associated with a multitude of risk factors, including smoking, DM, high blood pressure and a sedentary lifestyle. Creating causation from association can be very difficult in the presence of so many confounding factors, but recent research in the field of biochemical mediators of inflammation has shed light on this relationship. Cytokines (interleukins [IL] 2 and 6) immunoglobulins, (IgM, IgG, IgA), C-reactive protein (CRP), asymmetric dimethylarginine (ADMA) and fibroblast growth factor-23 (FGF-23) have been shown to have a positive correlation with the severity of apical periodontitis.

The levels of CRP, a non-specific systemic inflammatory biomarker, can be elevated in infectious and inflammatory conditions. CRP serum levels can be a predictor of vascular events and have been implicated directly in atherosclerosis by causing endothelial cell dysfunction, oxidative stress and coagulation. Increased IL-6 levels in apical periodontitis enhance CRP synthesis, which can sustain a low-level systemic inflammatory response, thus increasing the risk for atherosclerotic CVD.

ADMA is a chemical that is naturally found in blood plasma. It is an analogue of L-arginine and acts to inhibit the production of nitric oxide, which plays a key role in normal endothelial function and cardiovascular health. Recent clinical studies have found that patients with apical periodontitis had significantly elevated levels of ADMA compared to the controls. This may escalate the risk of atherosclerosis. The increased ADMA levels at baseline have also been shown to reduce the proportion of successful endodontic outcomes.

FGF-23 is a bone-derived hormone that regulates phosphate levels and vitamin D. High levels of FGF-23 can directly affect the kidney and heart, thereby increasing the risk of hypertension, subclinical atherosclerosis, cardiovascular events and left ventricular hypertrophy. Patients with apical periodontitis had higher baseline levels of FGF-23 and this was positively correlated with the size of the periapical radiolucency. Interestingly, this biomarker continued to decline at every review appointment, with a significant reduction at one year after surgical and non-surgical root canal retreatment had been carried out.

Apical periodontitis contributes to the increased levels of systemic inflammatory markers, thus contributing to the risk of chronic systemic inflammatory conditions such as atherosclerosis and CVD. In susceptible patients, even a short-term increase of inflammatory marker levels immediately after root canal retreatment and apical surgery could potentially heighten the risk of vascular events. Having said this, the evidence suggests that successful endodontic treatment may provide long-term benefits on vascular and systemic health, which outweighs the transient adverse effect.

What is the effect of diabetes mellitus on the levels of inflammatory markers and how is it linked to apical periodontitis?

DM is a complex multisystem metabolic syndrome that can affect the immune system by upregulation of proinflammatory cytokines along with downregulation of growth factors, resulting in a predisposition to chronic inflammation, degradation of tissues and reduced capacity for wound healing. Proinflammatory biomarkers such as tumour necrosis factor (TNF)-α, IL-1α, IL-1β, IL-6 and CRP are elevated in patients with DM, which can be detrimental to periapical healing. Patients with DM have been shown to have a higher prevalence of apical periodontitis, larger periapical lesion size and increased incidence of periapical infections compared to non-diabetic patients. Studies have reported higher prevalence of untreated periapical lesions, flare-ups and failed endodontic treatment in patients with DM.

Conversely, apical periodontitis correlates with higher glycated haemoglobin (HbA1C) levels and contributes to poor diabetic metabolic control. Diabetic patients experience heightened inflammatory periapical response, resulting in worsening hyperglycaemia and poorly controlled DM, thus compromising therapeutic management while increasing the likelihood of further systemic complications.

What is the role of statin intake in the outcome of non-surgical root canal treatment?

Statins are a group of medicines that can help lower the levels of low-density lipoprotein (LDL) cholesterol in the blood and are administered to patients with hypercholesterolaemia with associated increased risk of atherosclerosis and heart diseases, including coronary heart disease and risk of cardiac infarction.

In animals, statins were found to reduce bone resorption in an induced periapical lesion. This is due to its anti-inflammatory and immunomodulatory effect. Furthermore, on investigating the long-term intake of statins in humans, studies have shown that there was a significant association between statins and healing of apical periodontitis.

How should clinicians incorporate the evidence linking systemic diseases and outcomes of endodontic treatment when obtaining informed consent?

Diabetic patients, particularly those with poor glycaemic control, should be informed about the evidence of poor outcome of endodontic treatment, with increased risk of failure due to delayed or arrested periapical repair. Apical periodontitis has been reported to raise the serum levels of multiple inflammatory biomarkers that could increase the risk of vascular events. In line with shared decision making, this information should be incorporated into the informed consent process when discussing treatment options with vulnerable patients. Dentists should consider liaising with the patient's physician.

Treatment

The patient was aware that tooth UR7 appeared to be well root treated by the previous endodontist; however, the presence of a larger and more distinct periapical lesion at the one-year review denotes treatment failure. It was explained that there could be multiple reasons for failed primary root canal treatment, including microbial and non-microbial factors. The impact of the patient's medical condition was also discussed. He then shared that he had poor diabetic control and he was concerned that this would reduce the chances of success of non-surgical retreatment of UR7.

The risks and benefits of each treatment option were discussed with the patient. He was not keen to undergo further complex treatment and after further consideration over the next few days, he returned to request an extraction of UR7. The tooth was subsequently extracted with no complications.

Discussion

The link between dental and systemic disease has long been a matter of interest for clinicians. The idea of dental infections causing or exacerbating systemic disease is not new. In 1925, Weston Price published methodologically flawed animal-based research suggesting that infected teeth were to blame for diseases such as rheumatoid arthritis and psychiatric disorders. In the early days of focal infection theory, it was believed that microbes had the ability to migrate from sites of disease to cause inflammation at distant sites. More recently, there has been much research on the role of inflammatory mediators in the aetiology of systemic disease.

There has been much recent research on the association between systemic disease and the prevalence and healing of apical periodontitis. The problem with cohort studies is that they report association rather than causation. It is likely that uncontrolled DM does impair the healing response. The cellular effect of hyperglycaemic conditions has been well documented. It would make sense to treat the poorly controlled diabetic patient with caution.

The causal relationship for apical periodontitis, raised levels of inflammatory mediators and their role in CVD is compelling. This evidence comes from interventive cohort studies that demonstrate a reduction in the level of some inflammatory mediators following successful treatment. Apical periodontitis should be managed proactively in patients with a high CVD risk. This may include root canal treatment, retreatment or, indeed, if it is in the patient's best interest, an extraction.

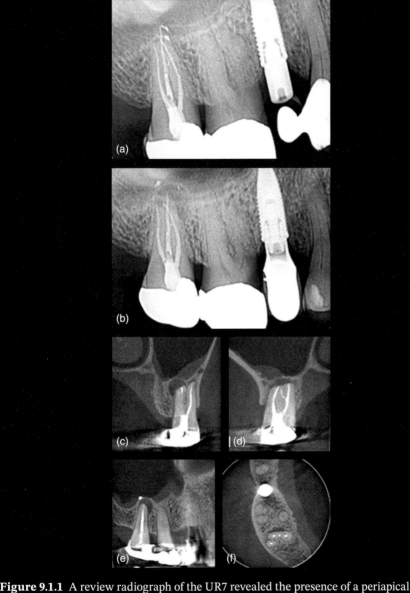

Figure 9.1.1 A review radiograph of the UR7 revealed the presence of a periapical lesion which appeared larger and more distinct as compared to the post-treatment radiograph taken a year ago (a, b). Tooth UR6 and the implant which replaced UR5 were asymptomatic. A CBCT scan was taken to assess the extent of the periapical lesion and the presence of missed canals. The coronal (c, d), sagittal (e) and axial (f) sections showed a periapical lesion associated with well filled mesiobuccal 1, mesiobuccal 2, distobuccal and palatal canals. The mesiobuccal root appears to be merged with the palatal root. No missed canals were detected.

Further Reading

Allihaibi, M., Niazi, S.A., Farzadi, S., Austin, R., Ideo, F., Cotti, E., and Mannocci, F. (2023). Prevalence of apical periodontitis in patients with autoimmune diseases: A case-control study. *International Endodontic Journal* 56: 573–83.

Bakhsh, A., Moyes, D., Proctor, G. et al. (2022). The impact of apical periodontitis, non-surgical root canal retreatment and periapical surgery on serum inflammatory biomarkers. *International Endodontic Journal* 55 (9): 923–937.

Cotti, E., Cairo, F., Bassareo, P.P. et al. (2019). Perioperative dental screening and treatment in patients undergoing cardio-thoracic surgery and interventional cardiovascular procedures. A consensus report based on RAND/UCLA methodology. *International Journal of Cardiology* 1 (292): 78–86.

Gomes, M.S., Blattner, T.C., Sant'Ana Filho, M. et al. (2013). Can apical periodontitis modify systemic levels of inflammatory markers? A systematic review and meta-analysis. *Journal of Endodontics* 39 (10): 1205–1217.

Segura-Egea, J.J., Martín-González, J., and Castellanos-Cosano, L. (2015). Endodontic medicine: connections between apical periodontitis and systemic diseases. *International Endodontic Journal* 48 (10): 933–951.

Vidal, F., Fontes, T.V., Marques, T.V., and Gonçalves, L.S. (2016). Association between apical periodontitis lesions and plasmatic levels of C-reactive protein, interleukin 6 and fibrinogen in hypertensive patients. *International Endodontic Journal* 49 (12): 1107–1115.

Zhang, J., Huang, X., Lu, B. et al. (2016). Can apical periodontitis affect serum levels of CRP, IL-2, and IL-6 as well as induce pathological changes in remote organs? *Clinical Oral Investigations* 20 (7): 1617–1624.

9.2 Medicolegal Issues in Endodontics

Garry L. Myers

Objectives

At the end of this case, the reader should understand (i) the difference between adverse clinical events and dental negligence, (ii) what defines the 'Standard of Care', (iii) some basic risk management principles and (iv) the importance of dental ethics.

Introduction

A 72-year-old female was referred by her general dentist for a consultation to evaluate pain symptoms that had developed two months following the completion of root canal treatment on the lower left first molar (LL6).

Chief Complaint

The patient's chief complaint was expressed as 'I am having pain when I chew on my left side'. These symptoms had been present for six weeks (although they had briefly subsided after she had been prescribed a course of antibiotics by her dentist before the symptoms returned). She reported no spontaneous or thermal pain when she first presented to the office for the consultation.

Medical History

The patient reported that she had mild hypertension and mild kidney problems (reduced function of the kidneys). She was currently taking the medication enalapril and reported that she was allergic to sulfa drugs.

Dental History

She presented to her dentist with a toothache. After the tooth had been assessed, root canal treatment had been initiated on tooth LL6. She returned to the office three weeks later and reported that her symptoms had resolved,

Pitt Ford's Problem-Based Learning in Endodontology, Second Edition. Edited by Elizabeth Shin Perry, Shanon Patel, Shalini Kanagasingam, and Samantha Hamer.

and therefore root canal was completed. Two months later she developed pain localised to the lower left quadrant and after a discussion she was referred to an endodontist for a specialist consultation.

Clinical and Radiographic Examination

The extraoral examination was unremarkable. The intraoral exam confirmed that the soft tissues were healthy. The LL6 was tender to percussion; there were no other signs of endodontic or periodontal disease in the lower left quadrant. The LL6 was restored with a porcelain fused to metal crown that had an access cavity restored with a composite resin restoration. Periodontal probing depths were all 2–3 mm. Teeth LL5 and LL7 responded normally to all sensibility testing.

A periapical radiograph showed that endodontic treatment had been carried out on LL6. However, the following were noted: (i) a furcation perforation was evident with obturation materials and a separated instrument in the bony furcation area down to the root apex, (ii) the mesial canals were untreated and (iii) the distal canal had been accessed, but the obturation was well short of the canal terminus (Figure 9.2.1a).

On further discussion with the patient, it was evident that she was unaware of the separated instrument that had been left behind from the prior treatment. She also expressed that she was very unhappy with her dentist and that he had refunded her fees incurred for treatment provided on LL6. On review of the referral paperwork, no mention was made regarding the separated instrument from the general dentist's endodontic treatment.

Diagnosis and Treatment Planning

What was the diagnosis?

Previously treated LL6 associated with symptomatic apical periodontitis.

The patient was informed about the separated instrument along with the furcation perforation and untreated canals. A questionable prognosis was given.

What were the treatment options?

- Non-surgical retreatment, with the understanding that it would be unlikely that the separated instrument could be retrieved with this option.
- Surgical treatment of tooth LL6, which would include removal of the separated instrument.
- A combination of the previous two choices.
- Extraction of tooth LL6.
- No further treatment at this time, although it was mentioned that symptoms would probably not resolve on their own.

After discussing the various treatment options with the patient, non-surgical retreatment was planned as she did not want to have the tooth extracted if at all possible.

It is clear from the radiograph that a few inadvertent mishaps had occurred during the initial root canal treatment provided on LL6, the two most obvious being the separated instrument and a perforation out of the tooth into the furcation area of the tooth. In many situations, separation of an instrument or a perforation of the tooth during routine endodontic treatment is not usually considered dental negligence except in the following circumstances: (i) this risk was not covered in the informed consent discussion, (ii) the patient was not informed of this incident at the time of the appointment, (iii) a proper referral to a specialist was not made when indicated and (iv) the patient was not followed up once treatment had been completed.

In this case, it was apparent that this patient was not informed of the separated instrument, nor was the error likely recognised at the time of treatment and a referral to a specialist was not made until three months after the treatment when symptoms developed with the tooth. There are several areas of negligence in this case.

It is important to appreciate that mistakes or untoward events do occur during dental treatment and when they occur, it is essential that the patient be informed of these incidents. While these situations can be embarrassing, disclosing such untoward events will not generally erode the patient's confidence in the clinician, but rather will often increase the trust the patient has in the clinician through truthful disclosures and sincere apologies.

After completing a thorough evaluation and discussing the findings in this case, the decision was made to provide non-surgical retreatment on tooth LL6. The treatment was completed in two visits with the use of calcium hydroxide intracanal medicament between visits. While the separated instrument was not retrieved, the perforation was repaired, the untreated canals were located and the retreatment was completed to more optimal lengths (Figure 9.2.1b). The patient was followed up annually for three years, during which time she remained asymptomatic and functional on the LL6 (Figure 9.2.1c).

Discussion

It is apparent that some adverse events occurred during the initial root canal treatment provided to this patient. As clinicians, we will all make mistakes during treatment. There are many risks associated with endodontic care, which include separated instruments, perforations, missed canals, treatment of the wrong tooth, overfills and nerve paraesthesias.

Risk management is a concept that has become very prominent in today's clinical world and simply defined is 'reducing the likelihood that an adverse event will occur during treatment'. It comprises three primary aspects:

- The clinician should be able to identify potential risks of treatment pre-operatively. Each case will present with different risks and these need to be discussed with the patient. The clinician should also determine if their skill set is sufficient to manage these risks should they arise.
- Obtaining informed consent from the patient prior to any treatment is essential. Proper informed consent involves a joint decisional process between provider and patient on whether to proceed with treatment or not. Informed consent states that the patient has been made aware of the benefits of the proposed treatment, the potential risks/complications of treatment, reasonable treatment alternatives to the proposed treatment and finally the consequences of non-treatment.
- Good record keeping (documentation) of the evaluation and treatment is the third aspect of good risk management. Documentation should be contemporaneous and include the informed consent along with justifying the treatment that is ultimately provided. Accuracy matters! If something is not documented, then the implication is that it never happened.

Standard of Care has evolved over time as a result of 'expert witness testimony' in the courts of law along with new emerging technologies and improved clinical procedures that have developed over time. Standard of Care has been defined as 'that reasonable care and diligence ordinarily exercised by similar members of the profession in similar cases under like conditions'. It needs to be understood that Standard of Care does *not* require perfect results or ideal endodontic care. It is a minimal standard of reasonably acceptable practice rather than the ideal result. Standard of Care does require that the clinician avoid unreasonable risks that may harm the patient receiving the care. A similar concept that has been introduced is a Standard of Practice. An example of this has been outlined and described by the American Association of Endodontists (AAE). It was delineated to serve as a guideline for endodontic care that clinicians are expected to adhere to during their course of treatment. The guideline, however, *does not* legally set the standard of care; it simply provides a template for care as published by the AAE.

Negligence is in essence a violation of Standard of Care. While negligent errors are often unintentional acts, of either omission or commission, they are generally associated with either carelessness or inattentiveness during the provided treatment. Four elements need to be met to prove dental negligence in a court of law: (i) the creation of a duty (acceptance of a patient for care), (ii) breach of duty, (iii) causation (departure from the Standard of Care) and

(iv) damages incurred. One example that has proven to be a common illustration of dental negligence involves those cases where a foreign material has been inadvertently extruded into the mandibular canal during root canal therapy on mandibular molars. In each of these types of situations it can be straightforward to meet the four elements that are needed to prove dental negligence. Other examples that can lead to negligence include (i) failure to inform the patient when an inadvertent mishap has occurred, (ii) failure to use a dental dam during treatment if a foreign object is swallowed or aspirated during treatment, (iii) failure to refer a patient to a specialist for management of complex cases or complications arising during treatment and (iv) failure to obtain the patient's 'informed consent' prior to treatment.

Conclusion

Endodontic procedures have become a prominent part of the daily practice of dentistry today. As newer technologies (e.g. heat-treated nickel-titanium rotary instruments, microscopes and cone beam computed tomography) have become incorporated into endodontic treatment procedures, the perception has grown that providing root canal treatment has become much easier to achieve than in the past. The reality remains, however, that endodontic procedural errors (Table 9.2.1) can, and will, still occur, with the potential for significant consequences. A thorough examination resulting in a proper diagnosis remains essential and as a part of this process the clinician should be able to identify cases where risks may be high for mishaps to

Table 9.2.1 Endodontic procedural errors that can occur.

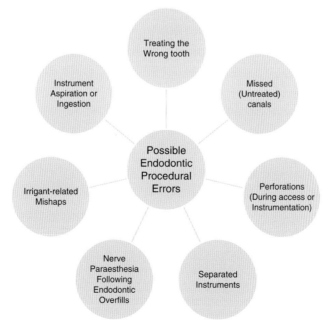

Table 9.2.2 Mismanagement of procedural errors.

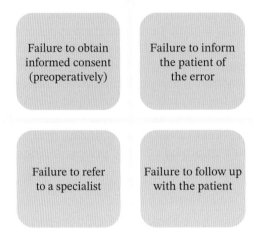

occur. When procedural errors do occur, these teeth can often be managed in an ethical and successful manner, but proper steps need to be taken to minimise the medico-legal consequences (Table 9.2.2).

Maintaining a careful and thoughtful approach to endodontic care will lead to great results and a professionally satisfying practice experience. The American Dental Association Code of Ethics and the General Dental Council's Standards for the Dental Team emphasise that patients' interests should be placed above all else when providing dental care. Healthcare professionals have a duty to be honest and trustworthy in their dealings with people. *Primum non nocere* – this Latin phrase comes from the Hippocratic Oath, an oath of ethics in medical and dental care. Its meaning? 'First, do no harm.'

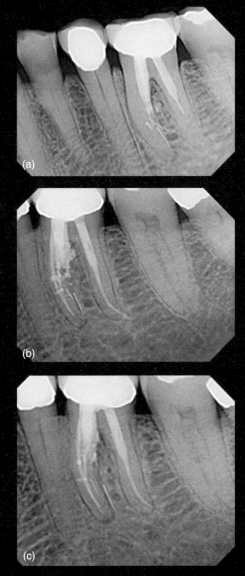

Figure 9.2.1 (a) Previous endodontic treatment with a furcation perforation and a separated instrument in the bony furcation area extending to the root apex. The mesial canals were untreated and the distal canal had been accessed, but obturation was well short of the canal terminus. (b) Post-operative radiograph following root canal retreatment and perforation repair. The untreated canals were located and the retreatment was completed to more optimal lengths. (c) The patient was followed up annually for three years, during which time she remained asymptomatic and functional on the LL6.

Further Reading

Alrahabi, M., Zafar, M.S., and Adanir, N. (2019). Aspects of Clinical Malpractice in Endodontics. *European Journal of Dentistry* 13: 450–8.

American Association of Endodontists (2017). Endodontic competency. White paper. Chicago, IL: AAE. https://www.aae.org/specialty/wp-content/uploads/sites/2/2017/10/endo-competency-whitepaper.pdf.

American Association of Endodontists (2020). Treatment standards. White paper. Chicago, IL: AAE. https://www.aae.org/specialty/wp-content/uploads/sites/2/2018/04/TreatmentStandards_Whitepaper.pdf.

American Association of Endodontists (2014). Endodontics: Colleagues for excellence. The standard of practice in contemporary endodontics. Chicago, IL: AAE. https://www.aae.org/specialty/wp-content/uploads/sites/2/2017/06/ecfefall-2014standardofpractice.pdf.

Cohen, S. and Schwartz, S. (1987). Endodontic complications and the law. *Journal of Endodontics* 13: 191.

Gluskin, A.H., Lai, G., Peters, C.I., and Peters, O.A. (2020). The double-edged sword of calcium hydroxide in endodontics. *Journal of the American Dental Association* 151: 317–326.

Siedberg, B.H. (2008). The law and endodontics. In: *Ingle's Endodontics*, 6e (ed. J.I. Ingle, L.K. Bakland, and C. Baumgartner), 86–104. Ontario, Canada: B.C. Decker.

Zinman, E.J. (2016). Endodontic records and legal responsibilities. In: *Cohen's Pathways of the Pulp (Online Content)*, 11e (ed. K.M. Hargreaves and L.H. Berman), 124–190. St. Louis: Elsevier.

Prognosis and Outcome Assessment of Endodontically Treated Teeth

Nadia Chugal and Elizabeth Shin Perry

Objectives

At the end of this case, the reader should be able to appreciate pre-operative diagnosis and its relationship to the outcome of endodontic treatment. In addition, the reader should understand the rationale for debridement of the root canal system, be aware of protocols to disinfect and obturate the root canal system and be able to assess endodontic outcome over time.

Introduction

A 72-year-old female presents with sensitivity associated with the maxillary left second premolar (UL5) following buccal cusp fracture. The tooth was very painful at the time of fracture; however, the pain had subsided.

Chief Complaint

Patient complained of mild sensitivity that is present all the time.

Medical History

Unremarkable.

Dental History

The patient receives regular dental and hygiene care. She has a full complement of teeth except for third molars and a moderately restored dentition. The patient reports that she sustained fracture of the UL5 that extended subgingivally. The tooth was very painful at the time of fracture, but only mildly sensitive at the time of examination. The tooth was subsequently crown lengthened and restored with a direct composite restoration.

Pitt Ford's Problem-Based Learning in Endodontology, Second Edition. Edited by Elizabeth Shin Perry, Shanon Patel, Shalini Kanagasingam, and Samantha Hamer.
© 2025 John Wiley & Sons Ltd. Published 2025 by John Wiley & Sons Ltd.

Clinical Examination

Extraoral examination was unremarkable. Intraoral examination revealed a moderately restored dentition and good level of oral hygiene. The soft tissues were healthy. The periodontal probing depths were all <4mm and mobility was physiological. The tooth was in occlusion with the mandibular second premolar. The UL5 was non-responsive to cold and electric pulp testing and was tender to percussion [++] and palpation [+] but not to biting [−]. Control teeth UL3 and UL7 responded within normal limits to cold test, electric pulp test, percussion, palpation and biting.

What did the radiographs reveal?

Preoperative diagnostic periapical radiographs of tooth UL5 reveal the following:

- The bucco-lingual view shows apical and distal-lateral radiolucency, suggestive of the presence of a lateral canal and/or resorption (Figure 9.3.1a).
- The angled radiograph shows more distinctly the location and extent of bone destruction. The ascending radiolucency on the apical portion of the distal aspect of the tooth may suggest vertical root fracture (Figure 9.3.1b).

Diagnosis and Treatment Planning

Diagnosis of the UL5 was pulpal necrosis with symptomatic apical periodontitis.

Treatment options discussed with the patient were:

- No treatment (not a recommendation).
- Root canal treatment (recommendation).
- Extraction (not a recommendation, always an option)

The patient wished to retain her tooth and root canal treatment followed by a cuspal coverage restoration were planned. The pre-treatment prognosis was favourable as the tooth was restorable and had a good crown-to-root ratio and no periodontal disease or issues.

What should be discussed with the patient prior to treatment?

- Findings and prognosis of the root canal treatment versus alternative treatment options (e.g. dental implant).
- Pros/cons of different treatment options.
- Possible outcomes.

- Additional treatment needed after endodontic treatment.
- Any patient concerns.
- Obtaining of informed consent.

Before commencing endodontic treatment, it is important to perform a thorough examination and arrive at a correct diagnosis. It is essential to assess all risk factors that may influence the outcome of endodontic treatment. This is part of informed consent.

What is the cause of apical periodontitis?

It is an established fact in endodontics that necrotic teeth with apical periodontitis are infected by microorganisms, primarily bacteria. The cause of pulpal necrosis is always the result of microbial invasion of the root canal space. The predisposing events, conditions or portals of entry of microorganisms leading to this infection may be dental caries, traumatic injuries, dentinal cracks and/or periodontal disease.

What is the goal of endodontic treatment?

The ultimate goal of endodontic treatment is to preserve the tooth in a healthy and functional state. In cases of pulp necrosis and apical periodontitis, this is achieved by means of root canal treatment and quality coronal restoration. Treating necrotic teeth with apical periodontitis rests on understanding the aetiology of the presenting condition and measures needed to achieve successful clinical outcome.

Treatment

Root canal treatment was carried out under local anaesthesia and dental dam isolation. The operating field was disinfected with sodium hypochlorite. The access was observed under a surgical operating microscope and no second canal was observed. Working length was determined with the aid of an electronic apex locator and confirmed radiographically (Figure 9.3.2a). Biomechanical preparation was completed with a combination of stainless steel hand files and nickel titanium rotary files and the canal was irrigated with sodium hypochlorite and ethylenediaminetetraacetic acid (EDTA). The canal was dressed with an aqueous paste of calcium hydroxide between treatment visits. The tooth was restored with a provisional restoration.

A non-routine post-treatment radiograph was taken to evaluate placement of calcium hydroxide relative to the resorption site on the apical-distal area (Figure 9.3.2b). The radiograph revealed calcium hydroxide at the site of a likely lateral canal and infection-induced resorption at the portal of exit. At the second appointment, the patient was asymptomatic. Root canal treatment was completed with gutta percha and sealer using warm vertical condensation obturation (Figure 9.3.2c). The tooth was temporised with intermediate restorative material (IRM). The occlusion was checked and post-operative instructions were given. The patient was advised to proceed with the restorative phase of treatment as soon as possible.

The post-treatment prognosis was favourable, endodontic treatment was executed to a high standard and there were no untoward events.

Follow-Up and Outcome Assessment

The first follow-up visit was conducted six months post treatment. The patient was asymptomatic. The tooth was restored with a well-adapted cuspal coverage restoration, and clinical examination of the upper left quadrant was unremarkable. Radiographic evaluation revealed significant healing of the periapical lesion (Figure 9.3.3a). At the next follow-up visit 12 months after root canal treatment completion, the patient remained asymptomatic. Clinical exam was non-remarkable and radiographic exam demonstrated further bony fill of the periapical lesion (Figure 9.3.3b). A long-term follow-up radiograph at seven years confirmed complete healing of the periapical lesion and restoration of normal width of the periodontal ligament and lamina dura (Figure 9.3.3c).

Prognostic Factors Influencing the Outcome of Endodontic Treatment

Risk assessment before endodontic treatment

The multifactorial nature of endodontic outcomes has been demonstrated in numerous studies that have addressed a wide range of factors with a potential impact on endodontic treatment outcome. An understanding of these high-impact factors may guide the practitioner's decision-making process about the appropriate treatment procedures and prognosis of the proposed treatment. It may confirm or deter a practitioner's decision to treat or to refer a tooth for treatment by a specialist. It also has practical implications related to treatment execution and preparation of armamentariums necessary to treat various endodontic conditions. For example, protocols may be different for immature and mature teeth, or teeth with or without a periapical lesion, and for non-surgical or surgical management.

It is paramount that both the patient and dentist have a full understanding of the prognostic factors and the risks to subsequent outcomes before commencing root canal treatment. For clarity of analysis and comprehension, the factors that have impact on the outcome of endodontic treatment can be grouped into three major categories: pre-operative, intra-operative and post-operative.

Pre-operative factors

Some prognostic factors, such as the presence and extent of the periapical lesion, the complexity of the root canal system, obliterated canal(s) due to hyper-mineralisation, pathological or idiopathic root resorption and infection-induced apical root resorption are the presenting conditions that are not under the control of treatment providers. Often, a complex presenting condition of the tooth has multiple risk factors. The presence of apical periodontitis is an important prognostic factor that may result in a less favourable outcome compared to teeth without apical periodontitis. Therefore, when apical periodontitis is diagnosed, the dentist should recommend root canal treatment at the earliest sign. This will in turn improve prognosis and expected outcome. Pre-operative medical conditions such as diabetes can negatively affect the success of endodontic treatment of teeth with apical periodontitis.

Intra-operative factors

Dental practitioners, through systematic and thorough pre-operative evaluation and well-executed clinical protocol, can manage most intra-operative factors, such as level of instrumentation, quality of root canal obturation and procedural mishaps. Over-instrumentation could introduce necrotic tissue and bacteria in the root canal into the periapical tissues. Under-instrumentation could leave bacteria in the apical few millimetres of the root canal. The level of instrumentation of root canals is especially important for elimination of infection in teeth with apical periodontitis. Studies have shown that a 1 mm loss of working length is associated with a 12–14% decrease in favourable outcome. Inadequate root canal obturation with voids may allow coronal leakage of oral bacteria to reach the periapical tissues. A separated instrument or root perforation may prevent complete chemo-mechanical debridement of the canal system apical to the separated instrument or perforation, thus preventing effective elimination of bacteria in the root canal system and compromising the treatment outcome.

Post-operative factors

Post-operative factors include timely placement of a quality coronal restoration following endodontic treatment. The restorative phase of treatment is under the control of the dentist and the patient. The importance of an adequate coronal restoration of endodontically treated teeth in relation to the success of root canal treatment has been demonstrated in many studies. A permanent coronal restoration is critical for the prevention of reinfection and further damage to the structural integrity of the tooth.

Discussion

Endodontic treatment outcome is the consequence or the result of the treatment of a disease that is profoundly influenced by a multitude of pre-operative, intra-operative and post-operative prognostic factors (Table 9.3.1). Through each phase of treatment, the prognosis of endodontically treated teeth relies on the proper disinfection and prevention of reinfection of the root canals. Following completion of endodontic treatment, it is important to follow the patient and monitor the resolution of apical periodontitis for at least one year after treatment.

Methods used to evaluate the outcome of endodontic therapy include clinical examination for resolution of clinical signs and symptoms, radiographic evaluation of periapical osseous status and histopathological findings of biopsy specimens.

Symptoms associated with endodontically involved teeth include the presence of swelling, draining sinus tract, spontaneous pain and pain to percussion, palpation or biting. Clinical examination following endodontic treatment is conducted to evaluate the presence or absence of signs and symptoms as well as any improvement of any preexisting symptoms. Persistent pain may be due to non-odontogenic causes or persistent infection.

Table 9.3.1 Multifactorial nature of endodontic outcome. Possible relationships between prognostic factors and endodontic treatment outcome.

Radiographic examination is conducted to detect the presence or absence of a periapical lesion. In cases where a periapical lesion is present pre-operatively, a decrease in the size of the lesion is an indicator that healing is progressing. Both conventional periapical radiography and cone beam computed tomography have been employed for radiographic examination in endodontics.

A landmark study on endodontic outcome assessment by Strindberg laid the foundation for conduct of future endodontic outcome studies. The terminology and definitions for outcome assessment are summarised in Table 9.3.2. Strindberg's criteria include clinical and radiographic assessment. Some of the criteria are particularly strict, for instance that lamina dura is intact, a criterion that may not always be achieved despite a clinically successful outcome.

Table 9.3.2 Strindberg's criteria for endodontic outcomes.

	Clinical	Radiographic
Success	No symptoms	<ul><li>Contours and width of periodontal ligament (PDL) are normal</li><li>PDL contours are widened, mainly around excess root filling</li><li>Lamina dura is intact</li></ul>
Failure	Symptoms present	<ul><li>Unchanged periradicular rarefaction</li><li>Decrease in periradicular rarefaction, but no resolution</li><li>Appearance of new rarefaction or an increase in the size of initial rarefaction</li></ul>
Uncertain		<ul><li>Ambiguous or technically unsatisfactory radiograph that could not be interpreted with certainty</li><li>Periradicular rarefaction less than 1 mm and disrupted lamina dura</li><li>Tooth was extracted prior to recall due to reasons not related to endodontic outcome</li></ul>

These criteria differentiate between the clinical and radiographic status of a treated tooth.

Outcome assessment of endodontic therapy has evolved from Strindberg's stringent criteria to patient-centred criteria that emphasise the function and survivability of the endodontically treated tooth. Although the absence of clinical signs and symptoms and radiographic restoration of normal structures of the periapical tissues is the ultimate goal, a tooth may be functional for many years despite minimal symptoms or the persistence of small and stable periapical lesions (Table 9.3.3).

Ultimately, the patient should be fully informed of the difference between disease, survival and function of a tooth. As periapical pathosis (apical periodontitis) is considered a disease, then a tooth with a persistent inflammatory periapical lesion after treatment, regardless of its size, should be considered as incomplete elimination of the disease. Therefore, complete elimination of disease remains the ultimate goal of root canal treatment.

Table 9.3.3 The American Association of Endodontists approved definitions of endodontic outcomes.

Healed	Functional[a], asymptomatic teeth with no or minimal radiographic periradicular pathosis
Nonhealed	Non-functional, symptomatic teeth with or without radiographic periradicular pathosis
Healing	Teeth with periradicular pathosis, which are asymptomatic and functional, or Teeth with or without radiographic periradicular pathosis, which are symptomatic but whose intended function is not altered
Functional[a]	A treated tooth or root that is serving its intended purpose in the dentition

[a] These definitions integrate the clinical, radiographic and functional status of a treated tooth.

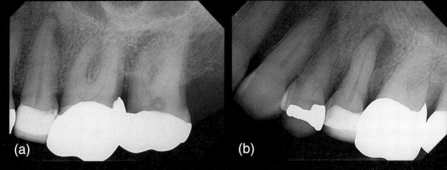

Figure 9.3.1 Diagnostic periapical radiographs of upper left maxillary premolar, UL5. (a) Bucco-lingual view demonstrates radiolucent area associated with a root of the tooth. This is suggestive of the presence of a lateral canal and infection-induced resorption. (b) Angled radiograph demonstrates more distinctly the location and the extent of bone destruction. The ascending radiolucency on the apical portion of the distal aspect of the tooth may suggest vertical root fracture.

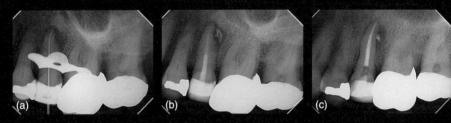

Figure 9.3.2 Treatment periapical radiographs of upper left maxillary premolar, UL5. (a) Working length radiograph. (b) Radiograph taken to evaluate placement of calcium hydroxide relative to the resorption site on the apical-distal area. (c) Post-treatment final radiograph at the completion of root canal treatment.

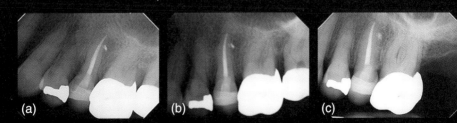

Figure 9.3.3 Follow-up radiographs of upper left maxillary premolar, UL5. (a) Six-month follow-up radiograph shows healing periapical lesion. (b) One-year follow-up shows progressive resolution of periapical radiolucency with bone filling the area of initial apical periodontitis. (c) Long-term follow-up radiograph, seven years and eight months post treatment, shows complete resolution of periapical lesion and restoration of normal width of periodontal ligament and lamina dura.

Further Reading

Burns, L.E., Kim, J., Wu, Y., Alzwaideh, R., McGowan, R., and Sigurdsson, A. (2022). Outcomes of primary root canal therapy: An updated systematic review of longitudinal clinical studies published between 2003 and 2020. *International Endodontic Journal* 55, 714–731.

Chugal, N.M., Clive, J.M., and Spångberg, L.S. (2003). Endodontic infection: some biologic and treatment factors associated with outcome. *Oral Surgery, Oral Medicine, Oral Pathology, Oral Radiology, and Endodontics* 96 (1): 81–90.

Chugal, N., Mallya, S.M., Kahler, B., and Lin, L.M. (2017). Endodontic treatment outcomes. *Dental Clinics of North America* 61 (1): 59–80.

Friedman, S. and Mor, C. (2004). The success of endodontic therapy—healing and functionality. *Journal of the California Dental Association* 32: 493–503.

Ng, Y.L., Mann, V., and Gulabivala, K. (2011). A prospective study of the factors affecting outcomes of nonsurgical root canal treatment: Part 1: Periapical health. *International Endodontic Journal* 44 (7): 583–609.

Pak, J.G. and White, S.N. (2011). Pain prevalence and severity before, during, and after root canal treatment: a systematic review. *Journal of Endodontics* 37: 429–438.

Sjogren, U., Hagglund, B., Sundqvist, G., and Wing, K. (1990). Factors affecting the long-term results of endodontic treatment. *Journal of Endodontics* 16 (10): 498–504.

Index

Note: Page numbers with *f* and *t* refer to figures and tables, respectively.

Pitt Ford's Problem-Based Learning in Endodontology, Second Edition. Edited by
Elizabeth Shin Perry, Shanon Patel, Shalini Kanagasingam, and Samantha Hamer.
© 2025 John Wiley & Sons Ltd. Published 2025 by John Wiley & Sons Ltd.